PROMOTING HEALTH
A Practical Guide

To all those working to reduce inequalities in health

For Baillière Tindall

Commissioning Editor: Susan Young
Project Development Manager: Katrina Mather
Project Manager: Joannah Duncan
Design: Judith Wright
Cartoonist: Chris Flook

PROMOTING HEALTH
A Practical Guide

Linda Ewles BSc MSc MA
Bristol, UK

Ina Simnett MA(Oxon) DPhil CertEd
Bristol, UK

FIFTH EDITION

⚜ Baillière Tindall

Edinburgh   London   New York   Oxford   Philadelphia   St Louis   Sydney   Toronto   2003

BAILLIÈRE TINDALL
An imprint of Elsevier Science Limited

First edition 1985
Second edition 1992
Third edition 1995
Fourth edition 1999
Fifth edition 2003
 Reprinted 2003

ISBN 0 7020 2663 8

British Library Cataloguing in Publication Data
A catalogue record for this book is available from the British Library

Library of Congress Cataloging in Publication Data
A catalog record for this book is available from the Library of Congress

Note
Medical knowledge is constantly changing. Standard safety precautions must be followed, but as new research and clinical experience broaden our knowledge, changes in treatment and drug therapy may become necessary or appropriate. Readers are advised to check the most current product information provided by the manufacturer of each drug to be administered to verify the recommended dose, the method and duration of administration, and contraindications. It is the responsibility of the practitioner, relying on experience and knowledge of the patient, to determine dosages and the best treatment for each individual patient. Neither the Publisher nor the authors assume any liability for any injury and/or damage to persons or property arising from this publication.

The Publisher

Printed in China

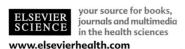

**ELSEVIER
SCIENCE** your source for books,
journals and multimedia
in the health sciences
www.elsevierhealth.com

The
publisher's
policy is to use
**paper manufactured
from sustainable forests**

Linda Ewles BSc MSc MA

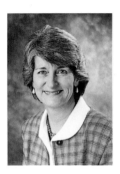

Following over 30 years' work in the NHS and local authority public health, Linda Ewles is now a freelance public health writer, editor, and trainer.

She started her career as a hospital dietitian but soon moved into health education and community dietetics in the UK and overseas. After that, she held various posts in health promotion and public health, including 5 years at Bristol Polytechnic teaching health education, nutrition, and communication. When working for the NHS her responsibilities included managing health promotion departments in East Sussex and Bristol. In the 1990s at Avon Health Authority she worked at a more strategic level, developing health promotion in collaboration with local authorities and other agencies; and commissioning public health services and programmes from NHS trusts and other organisations.

She is a member of the UK Public Health Association, and has published numerous papers and contributions to health promotion textbooks.

Ina Simnett MA(Oxon) DPhil CertEd

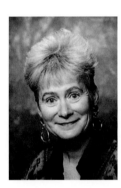

Dr Ina Simnett is a freelance researcher, trainer and health promotion consultant and has worked in the UK and Australia. Current activities include external examination and consultancy work with universities in England and Ireland.

She started her career as a research physiologist, and then worked in health promotion for 12 years, including managing the Northumberland Health Education Department. She later became a training consultant with the NHS Training Authority and ran management training programmes for health service managers. She has extensive experience of planning and teaching health promotion to health professionals, teachers and social services staff in the UK.

She has published numerous papers and contributed to a number of open learning materials in health promotion, is the author of *Managing Health Promotion – a practical guide to the management of health promotion*, and contributed to *Evidence-based Health Promotion,* edited by ER Perkins, I Simnett and L Wright.

Contents

Acknowledgements

We are indebted to the following people who so willingly and knowledgeably updated text and contributed new material for this fifth edition.

Natalie Field BSc SRD PGDip   is a project manager (HIMP Performance Scheme) in the Public Health Department at Avon Health Authority. Previously, she worked for Health Promotion Service Avon for 6 years on a variety of initiatives using different approaches and in different settings. In addition, she has practised as a dietitian for 10 years, working in hospital, primary care, and the community.

Mary Hart SRN MSc   spent 20 years working as a community nurse in rural India and Bangladesh, where she developed particular interests in child health issues and leprosy control. On returning to the UK, she began a new career in health promotion and has held a variety of posts during the last 12 years. She is currently the Health Promotion Manager for North Somerset Primary Care Trust.

Linda Lawton BSc PGCE MSc MBA   worked within the NHS for 19 years, during which time she held posts in health promotion, commissioning and public health, latterly as Assistant Director of Public Health and Head of Health Development. She now works freelance in the areas of management and organisational development as well as in health promotion and public health, undertaking a variety of projects including research, evaluation, facilitation, and training.

Hazel Millar BA MSc   has over 20 years' experience in health promotion, in the voluntary and statutory sectors. Her work in adult basic education and community health development focused predominantly on women's health issues. Since 1990 she has worked for Health Promotion Gloucestershire and as manager of Health Promotion Service Avon. She is currently Director of Health and Community Development for South Gloucestershire Primary Care Trust.

Judy Orme BSc MSc   has worked in the field of public health for more than 20 years. She is Principal Lecturer and Programme Leader for the MSc Public Health in the Faculty of Health and Social Care at the University of the West of England, Bristol. She is also the Director of the Centre for Research in Public Health and Primary Care Development. Her research interests include drugs, alcohol and young people, and the sociology of public health.

Angela Scriven BA MEd CertEd FRSH   is the Course Leader for the MSc in Health Promotion at Brunel University. She has been teaching and researching in the field of health promotion for over 20 years and has published widely, including the two edited books *Health promotion alliances: theory and practice* and *Health promotion:*

professional perspectives. Her research is centred on the relationship between health promotion policy and practice within specific contexts.

We would also like to acknowledge and thank the numerous people who have influenced the development of our own learning and ideas throughout the years of our health promotion experience and writing. Many others have also helped in practical ways with editions of this book; they include colleagues in the health promotion departments and other organisations we have worked in, and tutors and students who have tried out the exercises.

For the various ways in which they helped, we especially thank Peter Allen, Ian Baker, Alan Beattie, Donna Brandes, Stella Carpenter, Peter England, Martin Evans, Ian Fairfax, Stewart Greenwell, Sue Habeshaw, Trevor Habeshaw, Iain Harkess, Keith Hazeltine, John Heron, Hazel Johns, Penny Mares, Kieran Morgan, Jane Randell, Liz Rolls, Dali Sidebottom, Roger Silver, Jan Smithies, Sue Steel, Bob Ticktum, Sylvia Tilford, Jane Villa, Kathy Weare, Elizabeth Williams and Linda Wright.

Finally, we thank Chris Flook for ideas and skill in livening up the text with cartoons; our husbands, Jim Pimpernell and Jack Humphreys, for practical and moral support; and our editors and publishing staff – Patrick West and Jim McCarthy for the first three editions, and Jacqueline Curthoys, Karen Gilmour and Katrina Mather for the fourth and fifth editions – for their unfailing help and skill in turning our words into a lively book.

Linda Ewles and Ina Simnett
2003

Note on Terminology

We have tried to practise non-sexist writing throughout this book, using the principles and ideas we discuss in the paragraphs on non-sexist writing in Chapter 11. We have not always succeeded, and there are times when, for the sake of clarity, we have needed to refer to a health promoter or a client as 'he' or 'she'. In these instances, we have chosen to refer to the health promoter as 'she' and to the recipient of health promotion as 'he'. This is not, of course, intended to imply that all health promoters are female, or that those people receiving or using health promotion are always male. It is simply to avoid confusion and clumsy repetition of 'he/she' and 'himself/herself'.

Also, we have often referred to the people health promoters are working with as 'patients', 'consumers', 'users' or 'clients'. This does not imply, for example, that where we have referred to patients the text is irrelevant to healthy clients or vice-versa. It is solely to avoid the use of awkward terms such as 'patient or client'.

A Reflection

This poem was pinned above the desk of one of us (LE) for many years. It was first published in 1953 in the *Journal of Soil Association* 7 (4), 24. It came to light again in 1980, in the *Proceedings of the British Student Health Association*, where it was quoted in an article by Walter Yellowlees, a general practitioner from Aberfeldy. It seems to have been part of health promotion folklore for decades.

We are encouraged by the emphasis on improving public health, preventing ill health and tackling health inequalities in recent years. But we feel that the message of this poem is still highly relevant 50 years after it was written.

The Ambulance in the Valley

*by **Maline***

T'was a dangerous cliff, as they freely confessed
Though to walk near its crest was so pleasant;
But over its terrible edge there had slipped
A duke and full many a peasant.

The people said something would have to be done
But their projects did not at all tally
Some said 'put a fence around the edge of the cliff'
Some 'an ambulance down in the valley.'

The lament of the crowd was profound and was loud
As their hearts overflowed with their pity,
But the cry for the ambulance carried the day
As it spread through the neighbouring city.

A collection was made to accumulate aid
And dwellers in high-rise and alley
Gave pounds or pence, not to furnish a fence,
But an ambulance down in the valley.

For the cliff is quite safe, if you're careful they said,
'And if people should slip and are dropping –
It isn't the slipping that hurts them so much
As the shock down below when they're stopping.'

So for years we have heard as these mishaps occurred,
Quick forth would the rescuers sally.

To pick up the victims who fell from the cliff
With the ambulance down in the valley.

Said one as his plea 'It's amazing to me
That you'd give so much greater attention
To repairing the results than to curing the cause,
You had much better aim at prevention.

'For the mischief of course, should be stopped at its source –
Come, neighbours and friends, let us rally.
It is far better sense to rely on a fence
Than an ambulance down in the valley.'

'He's daft in the head' the majority said.
'He would end all our earnest endeavour.
He's a man who would shirk this responsible work
But we will support it forever.'

'Aren't we picking up all, just as fast as they fall.
And giving them care liberally?
A superfluous fence is of no consequence
If the ambulance works in the valley.'

We are grateful to Jean Hall and Pam Cooper, readers from Teesside, who told us about the author and origin of the poem.

Introduction to the Fifth Edition

The aim of this book is to provide an easy-to-read, practical guide for all those who practise health promotion in their everyday work. It was first published in 1985, and in response to demand we have produced a new updated edition every few years. Earlier editions have also been published in Italian, Finnish, Swedish, Hungarian and Indonesian.

The book is addressed to all health promoters, including health professionals such as health promotion specialists and public health specialists, hospital and community nurses, health visitors and midwives, hospital doctors and general practitioners, dentists and dental hygienists, pharmacists, health service managers, and the professions allied to medicine, for example dietitians and chiropodists. It is also for a wide range of workers in statutory and non-statutory organisations, for example local authority staff such as environmental health officers and social workers, voluntary organisations, community groups and self-help groups, youth and community workers, teachers in schools, colleges and institutions of higher education, probation officers, prison officers, and police officers.

Health promotion in the UK today encompasses a wide variety of activities, with the common purpose of improving the health of individuals and communities. This book is concerned with the what, why, who and how of health promotion. It aims to help you explore important questions such as:

- What is health?
- What affects health?
- What is health promotion? How is it part of a wider public health movement?
- Who are the agents and agencies of health promotion?
- Who needs health promotion and what are these needs? How can priorities be set?
- How can health promotion be planned, managed, and evaluated?
- How can health promoters best carry out health promotion? What are the competencies they require? How do you actually *do* it?
- What are the key issues currently facing health promotion?

We focus on the theories, principles and competencies you need to consider, whatever your background and wherever you work. The range of health issues (such as mental health, sexual health or physical fitness) and settings for health promotion (such as people's homes, schools, GP surgeries or hospitals) is clearly enormous, and we do not aim to cover all these in depth. Different lines of work will all have their own areas of expert knowledge and specialist skills to be employed alongside the specific expertise in promoting health addressed in this book.

As in previous editions, we have organised the book into three parts. *Part 1 Thinking About Health and Health Promotion* deals with basic ideas of what health, health promotion and health education are about, and the different approaches and ethical issues that need to be considered, and identifies the agencies and people who have a part to play in health promotion and public health.

Part 2 Planning and Managing for Effective Practice looks at planning and evaluation at the level of a health promoter's daily work and starts by introducing a basic planning and evaluation framework. It continues with a discussion of how to identify and assess needs and priorities, and develop skills to manage yourself and your work effectively.

Part 3 Developing Competence in Health Promotion looks at how you can develop your competence in carrying out a range of activities, including helping people to learn in one-to-one and group settings, helping people towards healthier living, working with communities, and changing policies and practices. The fundamentals of communication and of using communication tools are also addressed.

This fifth edition is fully revised and updated to take account of developments in the new millennium, such as revised national strategies for health, efforts to modernise the National Health Service, and the advent of national programmes to tackle the root causes of inequalities in health. New issues we especially highlight are:

- changes to the structure and organisation of the National Health Service in the UK
- the developing public health system in the UK
- national standards for work in public health and the emergence of a multi-disciplinary public health workforce
- new research on the comparative effectiveness of different approaches to health promotion
- the impact of new technology, such as the Internet, on our work.

We have retained the 'user-friendly' approach adopted in the previous editions and introduced two innovations:

- a glossary explaining jargon commonly used in public health and health promotion
- many website addresses for further information.

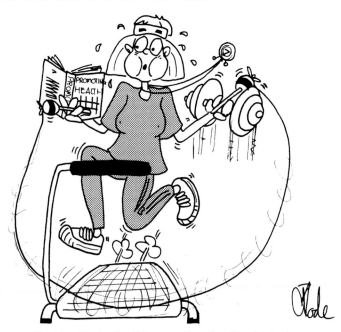

Studying this book will be an active educational experience

We aim to keep you involved, so that studying this book will be an active educational experience. We have included exercises to do as an individual or in a group, and examples and case studies to help you to apply ideas to your own situation. Often the exercises are designed to stimulate thought and discussion and, as there may be no 'right' answers, we do not provide them. Some readers may find this frustrating or uncomfortable. If so, we ask you to think it through, talk it over and work it out for yourself. In this way the 'answers' will have personal meaning and application. This is an example of how education can play a part in personal empowerment, and models the sort of approach we advocate in health promotion.

Linda Ewles and Ina Simnett
2003

1 THINKING ABOUT HEALTH AND HEALTH PROMOTION

Part 1 has three purposes:

- It sets the context for the whole book, by introducing key concepts, principles and ideas and by providing you with a shared language in which to communicate about health promotion.
- It provides an introduction to the dimensions and scope of health and health promotion, which enables you to focus on the wide range of activities and approaches and on the current movement towards multi-disciplinary public health.
- It highlights important philosophical and ethical issues, which are explored in a practical context later in the book.

Health is an extremely difficult word to define but it is clearly important that you know what you mean by it. We discuss this in Chapter 1, along with a description of the major influences on health and inequalities in health. We provide a historical overview of international and national movements towards better health.

In Chapter 2 we define health gain and health promotion and demonstrate that they encompass a wide range of activities. We offer frameworks for classifying the major areas of health gain and health promotion activity. We outline the national occupational standards for public health and provide an exercise to help you to explore the scope of your health promotion work.

In Chapter 3 we analyse the aims and values associated with different approaches to health promotion, explore a number of ethical dilemmas, and provide guidance on how to make ethical decisions.

In Chapter 4 we outline the developing public health system in the United Kingdom and identify the agents and agencies of health promotion. We provide you with help in clarifying your own health promotion role.

1   What is Health?

S U M M A R Y

We start with an exercise about what 'being healthy' means to you, and review the wide variation in people's concepts of health. We identify dimensions of health (physical, mental, emotional, social, spiritual and societal) and discuss a holistic concept. We then look at factors that affect health, and include discussions on the role of medicine and inequalities in health. Case studies illustrate the factors that shape the health of people in widely differing circumstances. In the final section we provide a historical overview of the contribution of international and national movements towards better health.

What Does 'Being Healthy' Mean to You?

'Being healthy' means different things to different people and much has been researched and written about people's varying concepts of health.[1] It is fundamental that you, as a health promoter, explore and define for yourself what being healthy means to you and may mean to your clients. This is the aim of Exercise 1.1.

Exercise 1.1 generally shows that different people identify different aspects of 'being healthy' as important. What you choose is often a reflection of your particular circumstances at the time. For example, if you are feeling stressed at work you are likely to identify 'enjoying my work without too much stress' as important, but if you have just given up smoking you are likely to identify 'never smoking'. As your circumstances change, your idea of what 'being healthy' means to you is likely to change too.

Lay and Professional Concepts of Health

To the general public, being healthy may just mean 'not being ill'. Health is taken for granted, only considered when illness or health problems are interfering with people's everyday lives. This may be summed up as 'you don't think about your health until you've lost it'.

There are perhaps some more positive ways in which the general public thinks of health. One way is reflected in phrases like 'building up strength' and having 'resistance' to infection. This implies that health means strength and robustness, and having reserves that can be called on to fight illness and cope with stress and fatigue.

Secondly, people may talk about being 'off-colour', 'run down', 'out of sorts' or, conversely, being 'in good form'. In this way, health may be closely associated with moods and feelings, and a sense of balance and equilibrium.[3]

Health may also be popularly portrayed, for example in magazines, as closely linked with youth, beauty and vitality.[4]

Exercise 1.1   What Does 'Being Healthy' Mean to You?[2]

In Column 1, tick any of the statements that seem to you to be important aspects of your health. Tick as many as you like.

For me, being healthy involves:	Column 1	Column 2	Column 3
1. Enjoying being with my family and friends	☐	☐	☐
2. Living to a ripe old age	☐	☐	☐
3. Feeling happy most of the time	☐	☐	☐
4. Having a job	☐	☐	☐
5. Hardly ever taking tablets or medicines	☐	☐	☐
6. Being the ideal weight for my height	☐	☐	☐
7. Taking regular exercise	☐	☐	☐
8. Feeling at peace with myself	☐	☐	☐
9. Never smoking	☐	☐	☐
10. Never suffering from anything more serious than a mild cold, flu or stomach upset	☐	☐	☐
11. Not getting things confused or out of proportion – assessing situations realistically	☐	☐	☐
12. Being able to adapt easily to big changes in my life such as moving house or a new job	☐	☐	☐
13. Drinking only moderate amounts of alcohol or none at all	☐	☐	☐
14. Enjoying my work without too much stress	☐	☐	☐
15. Having all the parts of my body in good working condition	☐	☐	☐
16. Getting on well with other people most of the time	☐	☐	☐
17. Eating the 'right' foods	☐	☐	☐
18. Enjoying some form of relaxation or recreation	☐	☐	☐

In Column 2, tick the six statements which are the *most important* aspects of 'being healthy' to you.

Then in Column 3, rank these six in the order of importance – put 1 by the most important, 2 by the next most important and so on down to 6.

If you are working in a group, compare your list with other people's. Look at the similarities and differences, and discuss the reasons for your choices.

Researchers in different settings have found a wealth of complex notions about health. For example:

- Mothers of small children in Wales said that having the capacity to cope and function as expected was an important aspect of 'health' for them; they also associated positive health with being cheerful and enthusiastic.[5]
- People may see health and illness as moral categories: some socially disadvantaged women in a Scottish study thought of illness in terms of spiritual or moral malaise.[6]
- Elderly Scottish people saw three major dimensions of health: the absence of illness and disease, a dimension of strength–weakness, and being fit to do the jobs expected.[7]
- Australian men responded to the question 'what does it mean to be a healthy person?' in terms of functional capacity, psychological well-being, absence of illness, and physical fitness.[8]
- Some South Asians in Britain have been found to hold a theory of health as a consequence of the bodily balance between 'hot' and 'cold'.[9]

Exploration of children's concepts of health is another area of study. Studies have shown that British children's ideas of being healthy and what makes them healthy are strongly tied up with being physically active and eating 'healthy' foods such as fruit and vegetables.[10] Children link smoking, the environment and 'unhealthy' food and drinks (such as sweets, crisps and fizzy drinks) with being unhealthy.[11]

Concepts of health are linked with people's social and cultural situations. Thus, to the mothers of small children in the Welsh study, coping with the family was their key concern. Middle-class women are more likely to identify aspects of emotional or mental well-being as part of their idea of health than working-class women, who more frequently concentrate on being physically fit.[12] 'Folk knowledge' of illness, prevention and treatment can also be powerful in shaping people's concept of health. Such knowledge may be part of a cultural heritage, passed on through generations.[13]

Standards of what may be considered 'healthy' also vary. An elderly woman may say she is in good health on a day when her chronic bronchitis and arthritis have eased up enough to enable her to hobble down to the shops. A man who smokes may not report his early morning cough as a symptom of ill health, because to him it is normal. People assess their own health subjectively, according to their own norms and expectations.

People may also 'trade-off' different aspects of health.[14] A common example is that people may accept the physical health damage from smoking as the price they pay for the emotional benefit: 'I know smoking is bad for me but it calms me down and I'd be in a worse state if I didn't'.

Because of this variety and complexity of the ways in which people think about health, it is difficult to measure health (as distinct from measuring illness).[15]

For more about measuring health, see Chapter 6, section on Finding and Using Information.

To summarise, then, people's ideas of 'health' and 'being healthy' vary widely. They are shaped by their experiences, knowledge, values and expectations, as well as their view of what they are expected to do in their everyday lives, and the fitness they need to fulfil that role.

To professionals in the field, 'health' may be viewed more objectively as freedom from medically defined disease and disability. But there may be a world of difference between a lay and a professional person's perception of what 'counts' as illness or disability, what causes it and what to do about it.[16] There will also be differences between health workers themselves, who may have widely varied concepts of health. For example, practitioners of complementary medicine hold to a range of beliefs about what health is, with different concepts of how health can be restored or improved.[17]

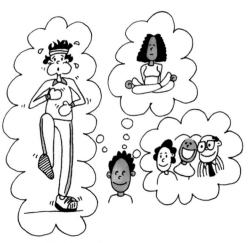

People's ideas of being healthy vary widely

Towards a Holistic Concept of Health

Over half a century ago the World Health Organization (WHO) defined health as 'a state of complete physical, mental and social well-being, and not merely the absence of disease and infirmity.'[18] In its time this was quite an innovatory statement, since it encompassed the three aspects of physical, mental and social well-being. Before that, in the 19th and earlier 20th century, as medical discoveries were made and medical practice developed, there had been a preoccupation with a mechanistic view of the body and consequently with physical health. Earlier still, of course, there had been centuries of many philosophies of health across the world in different civilisations, such as Greek and Chinese.

The 1948 WHO statement is still sometimes quoted, although the WHO has developed its view considerably since that time.[19] This historic definition has been heavily criticised, mainly on two grounds: it is totally unrealistic and idealistic (how often does anyone truly feel in a state of 'complete . . . well-being'?), and it implies a static position, whereas life and living are anything but static. The idea that health means having the ability to adapt continually to constantly changing demands, expectations and stimuli can be seen to be preferable.

Another criticism of the WHO definition is that it appears to assume that someone, somewhere, has the ability and right to define a state of health, whereas we have seen that people define their own state of health in many different ways. On the other hand, the definition can be defended on the grounds that it embraces the notion of positive health and acknowledges the central place of social and mental well-being.

Exercise 1.1 involved you in identifying different dimensions in the concept of health. These may be classified as follows.

Physical health This is, perhaps, the most obvious dimension of health, and is concerned with the mechanistic functioning of the body.

Mental health By mental health we mean the ability to think clearly and coherently. We distinguish this from emotional and social health, although there is a close association between the three.[20]

Emotional health This means the ability to recognise emotions such as fear, joy, grief and anger and to express such emotions appropriately. Emotional health (sometimes called 'affective' health) also means coping with stress, tension, depression and anxiety.

Social health Social health means the ability to make and maintain relationships with other people.

Spiritual health For some people, spiritual health is connected with religious beliefs and practices; for other people it is do with personal creeds, principles of behaviour and ways of achieving peace of mind and being at peace with oneself.

Societal health So far, we have considered health at the level of the individual, but a person's health is inextricably related to everything surrounding that person. It is impossible to be healthy in a 'sick' society that does not provide the resources for basic physical and emotional needs. For example, people obviously cannot be healthy if they cannot afford necessities for food, clothing and shelter, but neither can they be healthy in countries of extreme political oppression where basic human rights are denied. Women cannot be healthy when their contribution to society is undervalued, and neither black nor white can be healthy in a racist society where racism undermines human worth, self-esteem and social relationships. Unemployed people cannot be healthy in a society that values only people in paid employment, and it is very unlikely that anyone can be healthy if they live in an area that lacks basic services and facilities such as health care, transport and recreation.

The Holistic View

The identification of these different aspects of health is a useful exercise in raising awareness of the complexity of the concept of health. But in practice it is obvious that dividing people's lives into categories such as 'physical' and 'mental' often imposes artificial divisions and unhelpful distortions of a situation. Sexual health, for example, crosses all these boundaries.[21] All aspects of health are interrelated and interdependent, and we subscribe to the view that a holistic view of health is of greater value to you and the people you work with.

Other writers have provided useful analyses of what 'health' means from the viewpoint of a philosopher and a sociologist, and these are recommended for further study.[22]

The first of these (Seedhouse) proposes the idea of health as the foundation for achieving a person's realistic potential: enabling people to fulfil their own potential. It is about empowering people: enabling them to become all that they are capable of becoming.[23] Working for health is thus linked closely with improving people's quality of life.

This notion of health as the foundation for achieving human potential has much to offer the health worker. It recognises that health is a dynamic state, that each person's potential is different, and that each person's health needs are different. Working for health is both an individual and a societal responsibility, and involves empowering people to improve their quality of life.

The WHO also identify key aspects of 'health' which encompass these notions. They propose:

a conception of health as the extent to which an individual or group is able, on the one hand, to realize aspirations and satisfy needs; and, on the other hand, to change or cope with the environment. Health is, therefore, seen as a resource

Exercise 1.2　Dimensions of Health

1. Go back to your answers in Exercise 1.1 'What does being healthy mean to you?' Tick if any of the following dimensions of health are reflected in the statements you ticked in Column 1:

    Physical　　　　☐　　　　Emotional　☐
    Mental　　　　　☐　　　　Spiritual　☐
    Social　　　　　☐　　　　Societal　☐

    Is any one of these dimensions more important to you than the others? How do they relate to each other?

2. Has your idea of 'health' changed since childhood? If so, how and why? How do you think your idea of health may change as you grow older?

3. If you have had professional training in health or a related area of work, what difference has this made to your idea of health?

4. What do you think 'being healthy' may mean to someone who:

    ■ has learning difficulties?
    ■ has a permanent physical disability such as deafness or paralysis?
    ■ has an illness or infection for which there is currently no known cure such as diabetes, arthritis, HIV, schizophrenia?
    ■ lives in poverty?

5. Identify three or four key points you have learnt from this exercise about your own ideas of 'being healthy'.

for everyday life, not the objective of living; it is a positive concept emphasizing social and personal resources, as well as physical capacities.[24]

This is a rich definition, worth considering carefully. It encompasses ideas of:

■ personal growth and development ('realise aspirations')
■ meeting personal basic needs ('satisfy needs')
■ ability to adapt to environmental changes ('change or cope with the environment')
■ a means to an end, not an end in itself ('a resource for everyday life, not the objective of living')
■ not just 'absence of disease' (a 'positive concept')
■ a holistic concept ('social and personal resources ... physical capacities').

This discussion of 'what is health' leads on to thinking about what affects people's health.

What Affects Health?

Being healthy is rarely, if ever, the result of chance or luck. A state of health or ill health, however defined, is the result of a combination of factors having a particular effect on a particular individual at any one time. In order to work towards better health, we need to identify these influential factors. We suggest that you begin by identifying factors that influence your own health, using Exercise 1.3.

Exercise 1.3   What Affects Your Health?[25]

The aim of this radiating circle exercise is to identify factors that affect your health. The exercise can be done:

- individually
- individually, followed by comparing results with other people
- as a group, pooling your ideas about what influences your health.

You are at the centre of the rings:
In the inner ring, write in factors that influence your health *and that are to do with yourself as an individual.*

In the second ring, write in factors that influence your health *and that are to do with your immediate social and physical environment.*

In the outer ring, write in factors that influence your health *and that are to do with your wider social, physical or political environment.*

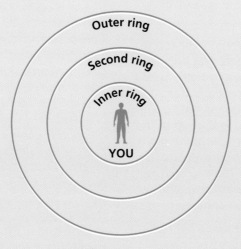

How do these factors influence your health – positively or negatively?

Which factors do you think are the most important?

Are there factors that you have not identified for yourself, but which may be important for other people?

Exercise 1.3 will have identified a huge range of factors which affect health. They are likely to include genetic make-up, gender, family, religion, culture, friends, income, advertising, social life, social class, race, age, employment status, working conditions, health services, self-esteem, self-confidence, access to leisure facilities and shops, housing, education, national food policy, environmental pollution and many more.

Case 1.1 – Salma[26]

This case study is taken from a research study of 16 Asian women in Bristol who had suffered from depression. The women were interviewed in depth in their own language.

Salma had been widowed twice, and now believed that people were plotting against her. At the same time, she was in desperate straits, living with her four children in a small, crumbling, two-bedroomed terraced house. She had no money for repairs, and no husband to support her or help put things right. She says:

> 'When we moved here – from one pit to another – I left all my furniture behind. We live like animals here.'

There was little wallpaper in any of the rooms. The geyser was broken and there was only cold water in the bathroom. To have a bath, Salma had to heat water on the cooker downstairs and carry it up. The plumbing needed repair, and there was no water in the cold water tap of the washbasin. Salma slept with her daughter in one of the bedrooms and her three sons slept in the other. One of the downstairs rooms could not be used because it needed replastering, and the floor boards were dangerous in another.

> 'Yes, we've applied for a repair grant, but that was about a year and a half ago. They came and took pictures and didn't do anything about it. You know what these people are like, they just see us and turn away. I don't understand it. We've also applied for a council house, but they say it will take a long time.
>
> 'You ask about my health, where do I start? There's nothing wrong with me, just nerves… I feel like my life is being squeezed out of me.'

Then there was worry about her children. They could not play outside or go to the park 'because the English children fought with them', and the house was too small and dangerous to play in.

- What affects the health of Salma and her children?
- What is Salma's own view about her health?
- What should be done to improve and promote the health of Salma and her children?

Case 1.2 – Tracy and Catherine[27]

This case study is based on a feature headlined 'generation gap' in the *Independent* newspaper, although we have changed the names.

Tracy is 6 months pregnant and smokes 10 cigarettes a day.

> 'My great-grandma smoked stronger fags than I do, and more than me. She lived to be 91 and everyone says I'm just like her. If you're going to die, you're going to die. I started smoking ages ago, when I was 13, and I smoked at home. I used to stick my clothes along the crack at the bottom of my bedroom door and smoke out of the window.
>
> 'You're not meant to smoke when you're pregnant but people do and have bright children. It doesn't damage the children's lungs – they just manage with a bit less oxygen. The doctors just say the birthweight will be a bit lighter. My friend smoked all the time and her three kids are really bright.
>
> 'My mum is hypocritical. She used to smoke. Every time she tells me not to I want to smoke more. She makes me conscious of it. If she wasn't here, I wouldn't be smoking. I'd be watching the tele.
>
> 'If you're going to get cancer, you'll get it anyway. Lots of our family died of cancer. Roy Castle died of cancer and he never smoked. I think passive smoking is more dangerous. That way, the smoke reaching the baby isn't filtered, but my cigarettes are filtered. My lungs are healthy. I did that smoking test where you blow into a bag, and my lungs are really healthy. My baby is kicking because it's healthy.

'I'd give up just like that, but Mike can't, his job's too stressful. What's the point of me giving up if I'll be doing passive smoking from his? I could be worse – I could be taking drugs, but I don't because it makes me feel funny. And I don't drink, because drinking makes you feel bad about yourself, and that will make the baby feel bad. But all cigarettes do is calm me down, I could be hit by a bus tomorrow and I might as well die unstressed.'

Catherine is Tracy's mother. This is what she says:

'Tracy's grandparents both died very young of smoke-related illnesses – throat cancer and lung cancer – and so my children never knew those grandparents.

'You're given a beautiful child that you love and nurture for however many years, then she does this to herself. Her eyes are dull, her hair loses its sheen, her skin grows sallow. The smell is repulsive – her clothes reek.

'I stopped 25 years ago when I was first pregnant. My husband was a heavy smoker but he gave up completely before the children were born because I made him. We tried to set a good example. We never let anyone smoke at home when they were little.

'But Tracy has never seen anyone die – someone with bronchitis, then emphysema like her uncle. He can't breathe without a nebuliser. She's never seen anyone die because they couldn't breathe at all.

'She was so health-conscious when she was younger. She wrote a poem about not testing cosmetics on rabbits and here she is harming her own baby. I thought she'd have more sense. Also, cigarettes are an appetite suppressant and she wants to stay looking like a stick insect while she's pregnant.

'I'm worried about the baby. She knows that if she smokes, there is more likelihood of a cot death, or the baby being stillborn. If it's born alive, it'll weigh less, have more chest infections and be less intelligent. If it's any less intelligent than Tracy, it will probably start smoking itself. Her baby is kicking because it's fighting for breath.'

- What does Tracy believe about smoking and health – her own health, and her baby's? What influences her beliefs?
- What does Catherine believe about smoking and health – her own health, Tracy's and Tracy's baby? What influences her beliefs?
- What has influenced Tracy's attitude and behaviour about smoking?
- What has influenced Catherine's attitude and behaviour about smoking?
- Should the health workers seeing Tracy in her pregnancy and afterwards address the question of Tracy's smoking? If so, how do you think they should approach it?
- Should anything else be done about Tracy's smoking and the smoking habits of others like her?

The Role of Medicine

There has been much debate since the 1970s about the relative importance of these many and varied determinants of health. One of the central concerns has been an increasing awareness that medicine, as a professional practice, has had little effect on the nation's health, which is surprising and disappointing. The National Health Service has evolved as a treatment and care service for people who are ill (a 'National Illness Service'), not as the major means of improving public health.[28] Only about 5% of deaths in the UK are preventable through good medical treatment. Cancers and heart disease, for example, are the most significant causes of death, but medical care has little impact on the overall death rate from them.[29]

Some people have taken this argument further and claimed that the practice of Western medicine has, in fact, done considerable harm. Examples are the side-effects of treatment, complications that set in after surgery, and dependence on prescribed drugs. But more important, perhaps, is that control over health and illness has been taken away from people themselves, who become dependent on doctors and medicines, expecting a cure for every ill and losing their own ability to cope with sickness, disability and death. Aspects of life that may be difficult, such as adolescence, pregnancy, the menopause and old age, have been increasingly labelled 'medical', and the onus of responsibility shifted from the lay public to the medical profession. These arguments that medicine is, at best, a treatment and care service for the ill and, at worst, a means of undermining people's competence and confidence to improve their health, probably reached a peak around 1980 and are still relevant today.[30]

Inequalities in Health

Widespread concern about differences in the health status of different groups of people started in the 1970s, with a government working group on inequalities in health leading to the publication of The Black Report in 1980.[31] This showed that, for almost every kind of illness and disability, people in the upper socioeconomic classes had a greater chance of avoiding illness and staying healthy than those in the lower classes. It also showed differences in the risks to men and women, and variations in the apparent 'healthiness' of living in different parts of the country.

All this pointed to the fact that the major determinants of health were concerned with social class, occupation, economic conditions, geographical location and gender. Further evidence from the late 1980s onwards shows that these inequalities continued to grow. This means that, while overall health may have improved, the rate of improvement is not equal across all sections of society. The gap in the health status between the less well-off social groups and the better-off social groups continues to increase[32] because of social and economic disadvantage, which in turn is associated with poorer housing, unemployment, stress, poorer nutrition and less social support.[33]

Work comparing data across different countries has shown another slant on the issue of inequalities.[34] It is not the richest societies that have the best health, but those that have the smallest income differences between rich and poor. It is the *relative* difference in income levels which is crucial. The reason seems to be that small income differences across society mean an egalitarian society that has a strong community life and better quality of life in terms of strong social networks, less social stress, higher self-esteem, less depression and anxiety and more sense of control. All of this adds up to better health.

It poses the challenge of improving health by building *social capital*. Social capital is the term used to describe investment in the social fabric of society, so that communities have characteristics such as high levels of trust and many networks for the exchange of information, ideas and practical help.[35] Social capital is produced when, for example, there are neighbourhood schemes of child care and crime prevention, community groups and social activities that engage a wide range of interests and people.

Other work shows that differences in health experience are not just about differences in social class. There are important differences in rates of illness and death between ethnic groups, which may be related to differences in income, education and living conditions, cultural factors or genetic make-up.[36] There are also differences associated with age, sex, occupation, and where people live.[37]

Addressing the distribution of wealth in society, reducing the gap between rich and poor, and tackling socioeconomic disadvantage are clearly political issues, and there were well-informed proposals for action in the 1990s.[38]

In 1997 the newly elected Labour government took action. It set up an independent inquiry to examine inequalities in health which reported in 1998: The Acheson Report.[39] The recommendations of the 1980 Black Report were echoed in the Acheson Report, which made recommendations for action covering a huge range of issues: poverty, education, employment, housing and the environment, transport, nutrition, measures to improve child, adult and older people's health, ethnicity, gender, and the NHS. The government responded to the Acheson Report in the 1999 White Paper *Saving Lives: Our Healthier Nation*, and followed up the recommendations in the Acheson Report with the action report *Reducing Health Inequalities*.[40]

Saving Lives: Our Healthier Nation is discussed below, section on National Initiatives, and in Chapter 6.

Improving Health – Historical Overview

So far we have seen that 'health' is a complex concept, meaning different things to different people. We have also seen that the degree of 'healthiness' is linked up with people's ability to reach their full potential. This, in turn, is affected by a wide range of factors, which may be broadly classified as:

- lifestyle factors to do with individual health behaviour
- broader social, economic and environmental factors such as whether people live in an egalitarian society, what social support networks are available, and how they live in terms of employment, income and housing.

The emphasis of health promotion work – whether it is on individual health behaviour or socioeconomic factors – has changed over the decades. Early public health work in the first half of the 20th century concentrated on environmental reforms such as slum clearance, improved sanitation and clean air. Then in the 1950s and 1960s the focus shifted towards the need for changes in individual health behaviour about, for example, family planning, venereal disease (the old term for sexually transmitted infections), accident prevention, immunisation, cervical smear checks, weight control, alcohol consumption, and smoking. This emphasis on the 'lifestyle approach' meant a concentration of effort on health education.[41]

During the 1970s, this emphasis was heavily criticised because it distracted attention from the social and economic determinants of health, and tended to blame individuals for their own ill health. For example, people with heart disease could be blamed for it because they were overweight and smoked, but the reasons for being overweight and smoking were ignored. (Reasons may have included lack of education, no help available to stop smoking, eating and smoking used as a way of coping with stresses such as poor housing or unemployment, lack of availability of cheap nutritious foods, and so on.) This was known as 'victim-blaming'.[42]

In the 1980s the pendulum swung again, and there emerged the broader approach of health promotion and public health we see now; at the time it was often called 'the new public health'.[43] It encompassed health education but also political and social action to address issues such as poverty, employment, discrimination, and the environment in which people live. It also, importantly, focused on the grass-roots involvement of people themselves in shaping their own health destiny.

See Chapter 4 for information on people and organisations working to improve public health.

International Initiatives for Improving Health

We say more about the role of the WHO and other international organisations in Chapter 4. The WHO took a leading role in action for health promotion in the 1980s and 1990s. It stated in 1977, at the Thirtieth World Health Assembly, that 'The main social target of governments and WHO in the coming decades should be the attainment of all citizens of the world by the year 2000 of a level of health that will permit them to lead a socially and economically productive life'.[44] This was the beginning of what came to be known as the *Health for All* movement. It led to the development of a regional strategy for the WHO European Region in 1980.[45]

This regional strategy called for fundamental changes in the health policy of member countries, including a much higher priority for health promotion and disease prevention. It called for not only health services but all public sectors with a potential impact on health to take positive steps to maintain and improve health. Specific regional targets were published in 1985, and updated in 1991. They emphasised the following themes, which became widely quoted as '*Health for All* principles':

- reducing inequalities in health
- positive health through health promotion and disease prevention
- community participation
- cooperation between health authorities, local authorities and others with an impact on health
- a focus on primary health care as the main basis of the health care system.

A further milestone was the publication in 1986 of what became known as the *Ottawa Charter*[46] (because it was launched at a WHO international conference on health promotion held in Ottawa, Canada). This identified five key themes for health promotion:

- building a healthy public policy
- creating supportive environments
- developing personal skills through information and education in health and life skills
- strengthening community action
- reorienting health services towards prevention and health promotion.

A more recent milestone for WHO was the Jakarta Conference in 1997 when the Jakarta Declaration[47] reiterated the importance of the Ottawa Charter principles and added priorities for health promotion in the 21st century:

- promote social responsibility for health
- increase investment for health development
- expand partnerships for health promotion
- increase community capacity and empower the individual
- secure an infrastructure for health promotion.

The *Health for All* targets, which European governments and the WHO aimed to reach by 2000, were reviewed and evaluated at the end of the century.[48] Progress had been made on many fronts, but targets had not been reached, mainly because of political, social and economic difficulties.

In 1999 the WHO published a new policy framework, *Health 21*, which set out 21 targets for the European region.[49] The targets cover a wide range, including reducing health inequalities. Target 2 states: 'By the year 2020, the health gap between socio-economic groups within countries should be improving the level of health of disadvantaged groups.'[50]

Other *Health 21* targets cover better health for children and older people; reducing communicable and chronic diseases, injuries, and harm from alcohol, drugs and tobacco; developing better health care, policies and strategies for health; and partnership working.

National Initiatives

See Chapter 7, section on National Health Strategies, for more about national strategies for health and how they are implemented.

An important development for the UK in the early 1990s was the advent of national strategies for health: *The Health of the Nation* in England, and comparable strategies for Wales, Scotland, and Northern Ireland.[51] These were welcome, as they were the first national strategies to focus on health and health gain rather than illness and health services.

More national strategies were published later in the 1990s. In 2002, the most recent of these were:[52]

■ 1997: in Northern Ireland the Department of Health and Social Services published *Health and Wellbeing: into the Millennium.*
■ 1999: in England, the Department of Health published *Saving Lives: Our Healthier Nation.*
■ 1999: the Scottish Office published *Towards a Healthier Scotland.*
■ 2001: the National Assembly for Wales published *Improving Health in Wales: a summary plan for the NHS with its partners* and an action plan *Promoting Health and Wellbeing: Implementing the National Health Promotion Strategy.*

A further significant development was that in 2001 the government published national targets to reduce inequalities in England.[53] This welcome emphasis on reducing inequalities ensures that work to improve the health of the public will have inequalities in health at its core, at both local and national levels. The targets are:

■ By 2010, to reduce by at least 10% the gap in infant mortality rates (the death rates of children under the age of one) between manual workers and their families and the population as a whole.
■ By 2010, to reduce by at least 10% the gap between the fifth of health authorities with the lowest life expectancy at birth and the population as a whole.

Also in 2001, a long-awaited report was produced by the Chief Medical Officer, setting out the role for a stronger public health function to implement *The NHS Plan* and build on targets set in national health strategies such as *Saving Lives: Our Healthier Nation.*[54] The report identified major themes relevant to achieving a stronger public health function, including:

■ a wider understanding of health
■ a better and more coordinated public health function
■ partnership working
■ community development and public involvement
■ an increased and more capable public health workforce
■ increased health protection.

At the same time another report was produced: *The House of Commons Select Committee on Health's Second Report on Public Health.* This endorsed existing policies for improving health and reducing inequalities as set out in *The NHS Plan,* and accepted that the public health function should remain in the Department of Health. The government in turn responded to the Select Committee's report, reaffirming its programmes for a modern public health service to protect and improve the public's health and reduce the health gap.[55] The consensus was clear for the focus on health promotion and disease prevention programmes.

Where Are We Now?

The change of government in 1997 resulted in more emphasis on addressing inequalities in health and the social and economic factors that affect people's health. The Minister for Public Health said, soon after the election: 'We want to attack the underlying causes of ill health and to break the cycle of social and economic deprivation and social exclusion. This signals a major change in the nation's policies, to maximise good health, as well as treating sickness. You might call it being tough on the causes of ill health.'[56] The government's plans for reforming and developing the NHS have included improving public health and tackling inequalities.[57]

As we stand now at the beginning of the 21st century, we have developed considerable understanding about what affects people's health, and we have international and national strategies for health, which are reviewed and revised on an ongoing basis. There is a stronger national and local emphasis on prevention, health improvement and reducing inequalities, with health promotion playing a bigger part in the role of all the health, social welfare and teaching professions. Health issues feature more in public policy debate at both central and local government and in the health service.

But as yet it is too soon to see whether these positive developments will successfully narrow the health gap between more prosperous people and disadvantaged people in the UK today. The reality in the UK is that we are still faced with entrenched inequality in health status, and huge problems of poverty, unemployment and homelessness. This raises questions about the distribution of wealth in society and demonstrates the extent to which health is a political issue.

This chapter has discussed what 'health' is, what affects health, and the ways in which health issues have been addressed over the last few decades. Against this background, we look in the next chapter at what is meant by 'health promotion' and the principles and activities it encompasses.

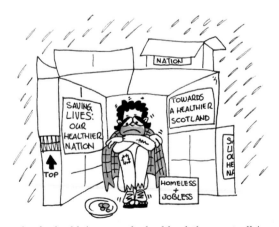

Do national strategies for health improve the health of the worst-off in our society today?

PRACTICE POINTS

- 'Health' and 'being healthy' mean different things to different people, and you need to explore and understand what they mean to you and to your clients.

- A wide range of factors at many levels influence and determine people's health.

- There are wide *inequalities* in the health of different groups of people: people from different social classes, ethnic groups, age groups, sexes, and people who live in different places.

- Improving people's health means addressing the social, environmental and economic factors that affect their health, as well as individual health behaviour and lifestyle.

- International and national strategies and movements have emerged to tackle the lifestyle, socioeconomic and environmental determinants of health, and to reduce inequalities in health.

Recommended Reading

On Concepts of Health

➤ Davey B, Gray A, Seale C (eds) 2001 Health and disease – a reader, 3rd edition Part 1, Cultural aspects of health, disease and healing. Buckingham: Open University Press

➤ Heller T, Muston R, Sidell M, Lloyd C 2001 Working for health. London: The Open University in association with Sage Publications. (A collection of thought-provoking readings on many aspects of the concept of health. Part 1 'Theory and Ideology' and Part 2 'Social Patterns of Health' are especially relevant)

➤ Helman C G 2000 Culture, health and illness, 4th edition. London: Arnold. (How culture influences concepts of health and illness)

➤ Katz J, Peberdy A, Douglas J (eds) 2000 Promoting health: knowledge and practice, 2nd edition. Chapter 2, What is health? Basingstoke: The Open University in association with Palgrave

➤ Naidoo J, Wills J 2000 Health promotion: foundations for practice, 2nd edition. Chapter 1, Concepts of health. London: Baillière Tindall

On Concepts of Health Among Minority Ethnic Groups in Britain

➤ Dickinson R, Bhatt A 1994 Ethnicity, health and control: results from an exploratory study of ethnic minority communities' attitudes to health. Health Education Journal, 53, 421–429

➤ Henley A, Schott J 1999 Culture, religion and patient care in a multi-ethnic society: a handbook for professionals. London: Age Concern Books. Available from Age Concern, Astral House, 1268 London Road, London SW16 4ER. (Deals with needs of people of all ages but has a special focus on the needs of older people. Covers an overview of culture, racial discrimination, illness and health care, generic issues about providing care in a multi-ethnic society, communication, dealing with specific health issues, and briefings on specific cultures and religions.)

➤ Smaje C 1995 Health, 'race' and ethnicity – making sense of the evidence. Chapter 6, section on health beliefs and knowledge. London: King's Fund Institute

On Concepts of Mental Health

➤ Health Education Authority 1997 Mental health promotion: a quality framework. London: Health Education Authority.

➤ Keeley P 2000 Mental health promotion. In: Kerr J (ed.) Community health promotion: challenges for practice, Chapter 4. London: Baillière Tindall

➤ Naidoo J, Wills J 1998 Practising health promotion: dilemmas and challenges. Chapter 13, Mental health promotion. London: Baillière Tindall

On Influences on Health

➤ Blaxter M 1990 Health and lifestyles. London: Tavistock Publications

➤ Davey B, Gray A, Seale C (eds) 2001 Health and disease – a reader, 3rd edition. Part 3, Influences on health and disease. Buckingham: Open University Press

➤ Daykin N, Doyal L (eds) 1999 Health and work. Basingstoke: Macmillan

➤ Graham H 1993 Hardship and health in women's lives. Hemel Hempstead: Harvester Wheatsheaf

➤ Katz J, Peberdy A, Douglas J (eds) 2000 Promoting health: knowledge and practice, 2nd edn. Chapter 3, Behavioural and environmental influences on health. Basingstoke: The Open University in association with Palgrave

➤ Naidoo J, Wills J 2000 Health promotion: foundations for practice, 2nd edn. Chapter 2, Influences on health. London: Baillière Tindall

➤ Squire A 2002 Health and well-being for older people: foundations for practice, Chapter 1. London: Baillière Tindall in association with the Royal College of Nursing

On Inequalities in Health

➤ Cooper H, Arber S, Fee L, Ginn J 1999 The influence of social support and social capital on health: a review and analysis of British data. London: Health Education Authority

➤ Department of Health 1998 Independent inquiry into inequalities in health. (The Acheson Report). London: The Stationery Office

➤ Department of Health 1999 Reducing health inequalities: an action report. London: Department of Health

➤ Douglas J 1997 Developing health promotion strategies with black and minority ethic communities which address social inequalities. In: Sidell M, Jones L, Katz J, Peberdy A (eds) Debates and dilemmas in promoting health, Chapter 27. Basingstoke: Macmillan/Open University Press

➤ Graham H (ed.) 2000 Understanding health inequalities. Buckingham: Open University Press

➤ Naidoo J, Wills J 1998 Practising health promotion: dilemmas and challenges. Chapter 4, Promoting equity in health promotion: health and poverty. London: Baillière Tindall

➤ Rogers A, Popay J, Williams G, Latham M 1997 Inequalities in health and health promotion: insights from the qualitative research literature. London: Health Education Authority

➤ Shaw M, Dorling D, Gordon D, Davey Smith G 1999 The widening gap: health inequalities and policy in Britain. Bristol: The Policy Press

➤ Townsend P, Whitehead M, Davidson N 1992 Inequalities in health. Harmondsworth: Penguin Books. (This volume contains The Black Report by Townsend and Davidson (first published in 1982) and The Health Divide (2nd edn) by Whitehead (first published in 1992) together in one volume.)

➤ World Health Organization 1999 Reducing inequalities in health – proposals for health promotion and action. Copenhagen: World Health Organization. http://www.who.int/

A Historical and Current Overview of Public Health Work in the UK

➤ Naidoo J, Wills J 2000 Health promotion: foundations for practice, 2nd edition. Chapter 9, Public health work. London: Baillière Tindall

Notes and References

1   See suggestions in Recommended Reading and four books from the Health Education Authority on how people view health and health issues:

Brynin M, Scott J 1996 Young people, health and the family. London: Health Education Authority

Hogg C, Barker R, McGuire C 1996 Health promotion and the family: messages from four research studies. London: Health Education Authority

Holland J, Mauthner M, Sharpe S 1996 Family matters: communicating health messages to the family. London: Health Education Authority

Prout A 1996 Families, cultural bias and health promotion. London: Health Education Authority

See also:
Aggleton P 1990 Health. London: Routledge and Kegan Paul

Jones L 1994 The social context of health and health work. Chapter 10, Health beliefs and health action. Basingstoke: Macmillan

Seedhouse D 1986 Health: the foundations for achievement. Chichester: Wiley

2   This exercise is adapted with kind permission, from:

Open University 1980 The good health guide. Harmondsworth: Pan Books, p. 16 (First published by Harper and Row.)

3 The idea for this analysis is based on the findings of an early French study on lay people's concept of health:

Herzlich C 1973 Health and illness. European Monographs in Social Psychology. London: Academic Press

4 For example, the Independent Magazine 19 January 2002 – the Sunday supplement of the Independent on Sunday newspaper – focused on health issues. The cover showed an image of an apple with the caption: 'Health: How to keep young and beautiful'

5 Pill R, Stott N 1982 Concepts of illness causation and responsibility; some preliminary data from a sample of working class mothers. Social Science and Medicine 16, 43–52

6 Blaxter M, Patterson L 1982 Mothers and daughters: a three generation study of health attitudes and behaviour. London: Heinemann Educational

7 Williams R 1983 Concepts of health: an analysis of lay logic. Sociology 17, 185–204

For another study on the health beliefs of older people:

Victor C R 1990 What is health? A study of the health beliefs of older people. Journal of the Institute of Health Education 28(1), 10–15

8 Paxton S J, Sculthorpe A, Gibbons K 1994 Concepts of health in Australian men: a qualitative study. Health Education Journal 53, 430–438

9 Donovan J 1986 We don't buy sickness, it just comes. Aldershot: Gower. (Quoted on p. 101 of Smaje C 1995 Health, 'race' and ethnicity – making sense of the evidence. London: King's Fund Institute.)

10 Backett K, Alexander H 1991 Talking to young children about health: methods and findings. Health Education Journal 50(1), 34–38

Pridmore P, Bendelow G 1995 Images of health: exploring beliefs of children using the 'draw-and-write' technique. Health Education Journal 54(4), 473–488

11 Pridmore P, Bendelow G 1995 Images of health: exploring beliefs of children using the 'draw-and-write' technique. Health Education Journal 54 (4), 473–488

Oakley A et al. 1995 Health and cancer prevention: knowledge and beliefs of children and young people. British Medical Journal, April 22, 1029–1033. (Study of 9–10-year-olds and 15–16-year-olds about knowledge of different types of cancer; beliefs about health; sources of information. Smoking, pollution and other environmental factors were seen as the dominant causes of cancer; television and media were the most important sources of information.)

12 Calnan M 1987 Health and illness – the lay perspective, Chapter 2. London: Tavistock

13 Calnan M 1987 Health and illness – the lay perspective. London: Tavistock

14 Backett K et al 1994 Lay evaluation of health and healthy lifestyles: evidence from three studies. British Journal of General Practice, 44, 277–280

15 On the difficult issue of measuring health status, see:

Bowling A (1997) Measuring health, 2nd edn. Buckingham: Open University Press

Naidoo J, Wills J 2000 Health promotion: foundations for practice, 2nd edition. Chapter 3, Measuring Health. London: Baillière Tindall

16 The issues of different lay and professional perceptions of health and illness, what causes illness and what should be done about it are dealt with extensively in literature on the sociology of health and illness. For example, see:

Davey B, Seale C (eds) 1996 Experiencing and explaining disease. Revised and updated edition. Buckingham: Open University Press. (A multi-disciplinary account of the factors influencing how states of wellness or illness are experienced by lay people and explained by professionals.)

Milburn K 1996 The importance of lay theorising for health promotion research and practice. Health Promotion International 11 (1), 41–46. (This paper argues that we should take more notice of lay people's thinking, which underpins their everyday health-relevant behaviour.)

Nettleton S 1995 The sociology of health and illness. Oxford: Polity Press

17 Aakster C 1993 Concepts in alternative medicine. In: Beattie A, Gott M, Jones L, Sidell M (eds) Health and wellbeing – a reader. Chapter 9. Basingstoke: Macmillan

18 World Health Organization 1948 Constitution

19 World Health Organization 1984 Health promotion: a WHO discussion document on the concepts and principles. Reprinted in: Journal of the Institute of Health Education 23 (1), 1985

20 Defining 'mental health', and the relationship between social, emotional and mental health, is a controversial area. For more on mental health and mental health promotion, see Recommended Reading and:

Tudor K 1996 Mental health promotion: paradigms and practice. London: Routledge

21 Naidoo J, Wills J 1998 Practising health promotion: dilemmas and challenges. Chapter 12, Sexual Health Promotion. London: Baillière Tindall

22 Aggleton P 1990 Health. London: Routledge

Seedhouse D 1986 Health: the foundations for achievement. Chichester: Wiley

23 Mansfield K 1977 Letters and journals. London: Pelican Books. (Katherine Mansfield discusses health in terms of becoming all that she is capable of becoming, which has become a much-quoted phrase.)

24 World Health Organization 1984 Health promotion: a WHO discussion document on the concepts and principles. Reprinted in: Journal of the Institute of Health Education 23 (1), 1985

25 The 'radiating circle' model is taken from:

Burkitt A 1982 Providing education about health. Nursing, June, 29–30. (Reproduced by kind permission of Medical Education (International) Ltd.)

26 Commission for Racial Equality 1993 The sorrow in my heart. Sixteen Asian women speak about depression. London: CRE. (Reproduced by kind permission of the CRE.)

27 The Independent Tabloid Monday 21.10.96. Generation gap: pregnant daughter, smoking gun. (Reproduced by kind permission of The Independent.)

28 Historically significant texts on how we have arrived at our current understanding of the determinants of health, especially the role of medicine and health services:

Cochrane A L 1972 Effectiveness and efficiency – random reflections on health services. London: Nuffield Provincial Hospital Trust

Illich I (1977) Limits to medicine – medical nemesis: the expropriation of health. Harmondsworth: Pelican Books. (Republished as Illich I 1995 Limits to medicine. London: Marion Boyers.)

McKeown T 1979 The role of medicine: dream, mirage or nemesis. Oxford: Blackwell

29 Jacobson B, Smith A, Whitehead M (eds) 1991 The nation's health: a strategy for the 1990s, revised edition. London: King Edward's Hospital Fund, p. 114

30 For further study of this critique of medicine, see:

Illich I 1977 Limits to medicine – medical nemesis: the expropriation of health. Harmondsworth: Pelican Books. (Republished as Illich I 1995 Limits to medicine. London: Marion Boyers.)

Horrobin D F 1978 Medical hubris. Edinburgh: Churchill Livingstone. (Horrobin's book is a reply to Illich's arguments in Limits to medicine.)

Inglis B 1981 Diseases of civilisation. London: Hodder & Stoughton

Kennedy I 1981 The unmasking of medicine. London: George Allen and Unwin

See also:

Bunker J P 2001 Ivan Illich and the pursuit of health. In: Heller T, Muston R, Sidell M, Lloyd C (eds) Working for health, Chapter 6. London: The Open University in association with Sage Publications

31 The original government report was:

Black D, Morris J, Smith C, Townsend P 1980 Inequalities in health: report of a research working group. London: Department of Health and Social Security

This book contains The Black Report by Townsend and Davidson – first published in 1982 – and The Health Divide (2nd edition) by Whitehead – first published in 1992 – together in one volume: Townsend P, Whitehead M, Davidson N 1992 Inequalities in health. Harmondsworth: Penguin

32 Shaw M, Dorling D, Gordon D, Davey Smith G 2000 The widening gap – health inequalities and policy in Britain. Bristol: The Policy Press

33 For more on inequalities in health, see Recommended Reading and:

Blane D, Brunner E, Wilkinson R (eds) 1996 Health and social organization. London: Routledge

Davey Smith G, Bartley M, Blane D 1990 The Black report on socioeconomic inequalities in health 10 years on. British Medical Journal 301, 373–377

Wilkinson R G (ed.) 1986 Class and health. London: Tavistock

34 Wilkinson R 1996 Unhealthy societies: the affliction of inequality. London: Routledge

Cooper H, Arber S, Fee L, Ginn J 1999 The influence of social support and social capital on health: a review and analysis of British data. London: Health Education Authority

Gillies P 1997 Social capital: recognising the value of society. Healthlines 45, 15–17

35 Wilkinson R 1996 Unhealthy societies: the affliction of inequality, Chapter 11. London: Routledge

Douglas J 1997 Developing health promotion strategies with black and minority ethic communities which address social inequalities. In: Sidell M, Jones L, Katz J, Peberdy A (eds) Debates and dilemmas in promoting health, Chapter 27. Basingstoke: Macmillan/Open University Press

36 Graham H 2000 (ed.) Understanding health inequalities. Buckingham: Open University Press. (Section on ethnicity and health.)

Health Education Authority 1994 Black and minority ethnic groups in England: health and lifestyles. London: Health Education Authority

Smaje C 1995 Health, 'race' and ethnicity – making sense of the evidence. London: Kings Fund Institute

37 Department of Health 1995 Health of the nation: variations in health – what can the Department of Health and the NHS do? London: Department of Health. (On differences by social class, sex, region and ethnicity.)

Dennehy A, Smith L, Harker P 1997 Not to be ignored: young people, poverty and health. London: Child Poverty Action Group. (On the connection between poverty and the health of young people.)

38 Association for Public Health 1996 Policy statement on poverty and health. London: APH

Benzeval M, Judge K, Whitehead M (eds) 1995 Tackling inequalities in health: an agenda for action. London: The King's Fund

Dennehy A, Smith L, Harker P 1997 Not to be ignored: young people, poverty and health. London: Child Poverty Action Group

39 Department of Health 1998 Independent inquiry into inequalities in health (The Acheson Report). London: The Stationery Office

40 Department of Health 1999 Saving lives: our healthier nation. London: The Stationery Office

Department of Health 1999 Reducing health inequalities: an action report. London: Department of Health

41 The first major government statement on health education clearly reflects the 'lifestyle approach':

Department of Health and Social Security 1976 Prevention and health – everybody's business. London: HMSO

42 For discussion and illustration of the individualistic 'victim-blaming' approach, see:

Rodmell S, Watt A (eds) 1986 The politics of health education – raising the issues. London: Routledge and Kegan Paul (especially Chapters 1 and 2).

For research-based argument that classic lifestyle factors (smoking, alcohol, diet and exercise) are important for health, but that social circumstances are more important than lifestyle habits, see:

Blaxter M 1990 Health and lifestyles. London: Tavistock

43 For further reading on the 'new public health', see:

Ashton J, Seymour H 1988 The new public health. Oxford: University Press

Martin C, McQueen D (eds) 1989 Readings for a new public health. Edinburgh: University Press

44 WHO resolution WHO30.43, quoted in:

WHO Regional Office for Europe 1985 Targets for Health For All. Geneva: World Health Organization, p. 1.

45 WHO Regional Office for Europe 1985 Targets for Health For All. Geneva: World Health Organization

For further reading on how health strategies have developed in different countries, see:

Nutbeam D, Wise M 1996 Planning for Health for All: international experience in setting health goals and targets. Health Promotion International 12 (1), 9–19

46 World Health Organization 1986 The Ottawa Charter for Health Promotion. Geneva: WHO (The Ottawa Charter is on the WHO website. http://www.who.int/hpr/hpr/documents/ottawa.html)

47 World Health Organization 1997 The Jakarta Declaration on Leading Health Promotion in to the 21st Century. Geneva: WHO. Can be found at http://www.who.int/hpr/hpr/documents/jakarta/english.html

48 Tones K, Tilford S 2001 Health education: effectiveness, efficiency and equity, 3rd edn. Chapter 1, section on The Meaning of Health Promotion. Cheltenham: Nelson Thornes.

Katz J, Peberdy A, Douglas J (eds) 2000 Promoting health: knowledge and practice, 2nd edn. Chapter 4. Basingstoke: The Open University in association with Palgrave

49 WHO Europe 1999 Health 21 – Health for All in the 21st century. Copenhagen: WHO Regional Office for Europe

Katz J, Peberdy A, Douglas J (eds) 2000 Promoting health: knowledge and practice, 2nd edition. Basingstoke: The Open University in association with Palgrave. (Chapter 4, section 4.4, lists the 21 targets.)

50 World Health Organization 1999 Reducing inequalities in health – proposals for health promotion and action. Copenhagen: World Health Organization. (http://www.who.int/)

51 Department of Health and Social Services 1991 A regional strategy for the Northern Ireland Health & personal social services 1992–1997. London: HMSO

Scottish Office 1992 Scotland's health: a challenge to us all. Edinburgh: HMSO

Secretary of State for Health 1992 The health of the nation: a strategy for health in England. London: HMSO

Welsh Office 1989 Strategic intent and direction for the NHS in Wales. Cardiff: Welsh Office NHS Directorate: The Welsh Health Planning Forum

52 England:
Department of Health 1999 Saving lives: our healthier nation. London: The Stationery Office. Cm 4386. (Full

and summary versions are available: www.official-documents.co.uk)

Scotland:
The Scottish Office 1999 Towards a healthier Scotland: London: The Stationery Office. Cm 4269 (www.scotland.gov.uk/library/documents)

Wales:
The National Assembly for Wales 2001 Improving health in Wales: a summary plan for the NHS with its partners. Cardiff: National Assembly for Wales

The National Assembly for Wales, Health Promotion Division 2001 Promoting health and wellbeing: implementing the national health promotion strategy, Cardiff: National Assembly for Wales. (www.wales.nhs.uk/pubs.cfm)

Northern Ireland:
Department of Health and Social Services 1997 Health and wellbeing: into the next millennium. Belfast: DHSS. (Full and summary version available from: Department of Health and Social Services, Belfast. Department of Health, Social Services and Public Safety (DHSSPS) website: www.dhsspsni.gov.uk)

53 See Department of Health website: www.doh.gov.uk/healthinequalities/targets.pdf

54 Department of Health 2001 The report of the Chief Medical Officer's project to strengthen the public health function. London: Department of Health

Secretary of State for Health 2000 The NHS Plan. London: The Stationery Office.

55 Secretary of State for Health 2001 Government response to the House of Commons Select Committee on Health's second report on public health. London: The Stationery Office

56 Department of Health Press Release, 7 July 1997, headlined 'Public health strategy launched to tackle root causes of ill health'.

57 Secretary of State for Health 1997 The new NHS – modern, dependable. London: The Stationery Office

2 What is Health Prom

SUMMARY

We start this chapter by discussing the definition of 'health , the terms health education, health gain, health improvement and development. We continue with a discussion on the movement towards multi-disciplinary public health. After this we outline the scope of health promotion work and provide frameworks for activities for health gain and for health promotion. We set out the broad areas of practice covered by professional health promoters and the core competencies needed, and outline the framework for national occupational standards in public health. Exercises are included to help you explore the range of health promotion activities, and the extent of your own health promotion work.

The previous chapter focused on health; we now move on to consider the meaning of health promotion.

Defining Health Promotion

Health promotion is about raising the health status of individuals and communities. Too often the word *promotion*, when used in the context of health promotion, is associated with sales and advertising, and taken to mean a propaganda approach dominated by use of the mass media. This is a misunderstanding. By *promotion* in the health context we mean improving health: advancing, supporting, encouraging and placing it higher on personal and public agendas.

We have seen that major determinants of health are social, economic and environmental, aspects that are often outside individual or even collective control. Therefore a fundamental aspect of health promotion is that it aims to empower people to have more control over aspects of their lives that affect their health.

These twin elements – improving health and having more control over it – are fundamental to the aims and processes of health promotion. The World Health Organization's definition of health promotion[1] neatly encompasses this:

Health promotion is the process of enabling people to increase control over, and to improve, their health.

This definition has become widely adopted. As discussed in the previous chapter, the WHO goes on to say:

This perspective is derived from a conception of 'health' as the extent to which an individual or group is able, on the one hand, to realize aspirations and satisfy needs; and, on the other hand, to change or cope with the environment. Health is, therefore, seen as a resource for everyday life, not the objective of living; it is a positive concept emphasizing social and personal resources, as well as physical capacities.

pt of Health Gain

Health gain, **health improvement** and **health development** are terms we often employ nowadays when we are describing the process of working to improve people's health. They tend to be used when we are referring to a broad range of activities, not just health promotion, with a focus on both individuals and populations.

In the UK, the term **health gain** emerged from the work of the Welsh Health Planning Forum.[2] In 1991, the World Health Organization Collaborative Centre for European Health Policy announced that the 1990s were 'the decade of health gain', and the first of a series of Health Gain Standing Conferences was held in Belfast. In 1992 the national health strategy *The Health of the Nation*[3] was published in England and 'health gain' began to be widely used in relation to the debate about improving health. However, as with the term 'health promotion', the meaning of health gain is a matter for debate. One useful definition is:

A measurable improvement in health status, in an individual or population, attributable to earlier intervention.[4]

This is very similar to the definition used in the *Introductory Guide to the National Occupational Standards for Professional Activity in Health Promotion and Care*, which states that health gain is:

A measurable improvement in the status of health and social well-being, in an individual or a population, which is attributable to an earlier intervention.[5]

Measurable means that it should be possible to put a value, usually a numerical value, on to health status, in order to demonstrate that a change has occurred.

Attributable means proving that the change in health status is the result of the intervention. It is very difficult to do with complete confidence. For example, it can be difficult to be certain that a particular programme to reduce smoking has been effective, because so many other influences can affect smoking habits.

An **intervention** means a planned activity designed to improve health. It could be treatment, a care service or a health promotion activity.

The role of public health workers in assessing health needs, deciding on priorities, setting objectives and targets, allocating resources, and monitoring and reviewing outcomes, has given a much clearer focus to health policy. This may be referred to as the **health gain cycle** (Figure 2.1).[6]

It is now widely accepted that health gain is a useful concept. It focuses attention on health outcomes and on how different choices or priorities can be compared by considering the extent to which they contribute to health gains for individuals or groups.

There is more about these standards later in this chapter.

From Health Education to Multi-disciplinary Public Health

Health Education and Health Promotion

See also Chapter 1, Improving Health – Historical Overview.

In the 1970s, the term **health education** was used to describe working with people to give them the knowledge to improve their own health and working towards individual attitude and behaviour change. But in the 1980s there was much debate over the use of

Fig 2.1 **The Health Gain Cycle**

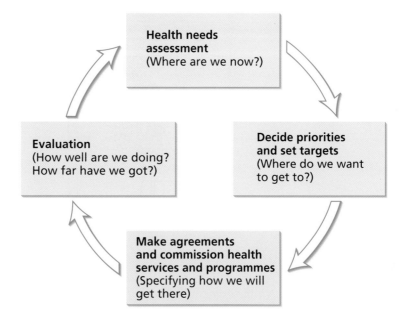

the terms health education and health promotion because the range of activities under-taken in the pursuit of better health diverged from traditional health education.

With rising criticism that the health education approach was too narrow, focused too much on individual lifestyle and could become 'victim-blaming', more work was done about wider issues. Examples are:

- political action to change social policies
- putting employee health on the agenda of employers
- engaging in community development work for health.

Such activities went beyond the scope of traditional health education, and **health promotion** became widely used as the umbrella term to encompass all these activities. Health education is seen as an important element in health promotion.

We subscribe to the view that using health promotion as an umbrella term for a range of activities is a useful and practical way forward. However, to avoid misunder-standings and time-consuming arguments about the meaning of words, we need to identify clearly the range of activities which are included in health promotion. This is the subject of the section 'The Scope of Health Promotion', later in this chapter.

Before moving on, it is important to note that there is no clear, widely adopted consensus of what is meant by 'health promotion'. Some definitions focus on activities, others on values and aims. The WHO definition we have adopted defines health pro-motion as a *process* but implies an *aim* ('enabling people to increase control over, and improve, their health') with a clear philosophical basis of self-empowerment.

Multi-disciplinary Public Health

Public health work focuses on health and disease in populations or communities as a whole, rather than on the health of individual people. It has been defined as:

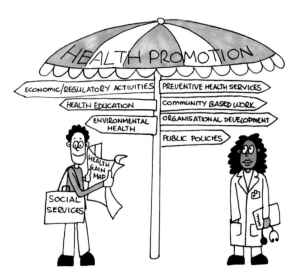

Health promotion is an umbrella term for a range of activities

The science and art of preventing disease, prolonging life and promoting health through the organised efforts of society.[7]

Important aspects of public health include measuring the distribution and determinants of health and disease in communities and controlling the spread of disease.

Public health and health promotion activities overlap, and public health information is vital for the work of health promoters and for evaluating the success of health promotion initiatives. Public health has broadened out from public health *medicine* and increasingly needs a wider range of skills, many of which are being developed by health promoters. This has led to the recognition that public health is more than the practice of public health medicine by medically qualified people; it is a multi-disciplinary activity involving people from many professions and backgrounds.

Recent national and local policy focuses on multi-disciplinary public health.[8] Key questions are about how to develop more capacity and capability in public health, where health promotion obviously has a huge contribution to make. In this book, we use the terms **health promotion** and **health promoters** to describe the range of activities and people who are working towards better health for individuals and communities. Sometimes we use the terms **public health** and **public health workers** when we are discussing work which aims to develop better health in populations, rather than at the level of working with individuals.

We now move on to more practical matters: how you can think about health promotion in a functional way, as activities you undertake.

The Scope of Health Promotion

Exercise 2.1 aims to start you thinking about the range of activities that may be included in health promotion.

The questions in the exercise give examples of the wide range of activities that may be classified as health promotion. Answering 'yes' to each one indicates a broad view of what may be included: mass media advertising, campaigning on health issues, patient

Exercise 2.1   Exploring the Scope of Health Promotion

Consider each of the following activities and decide whether you think each is, or is not, health promotion:

		Yes	No
1.	Using TV advertisements to encourage people to be more physically active.	☐	☐
2.	Campaigning for increased tax on tobacco.	☐	☐
3.	Explaining to patients how to carry out their doctor's advice.	☐	☐
4.	Setting up a self-help group for people who have been sexually abused as children.	☐	☐
5.	Providing 'lollipop' people to help children across the road outside schools.	☐	☐
6.	Raising awareness of how poverty affects health.	☐	☐
7.	Giving people information about the way their bodies work.	☐	☐
8.	Immunising children against infectious diseases such as measles.	☐	☐
9.	Protesting about a breach in the voluntary code of practice for alcohol advertising.	☐	☐
10.	Running low-cost gentle exercise classes for older people at local leisure centres.	☐	☐
11.	Providing 'healthier' menu choices at workplace canteens.	☐	☐
12.	Teaching a programme of personal and social education in a secondary school.	☐	☐
13.	Providing support to people with learning disabilities living in the community.	☐	☐

What were your reasons for saying 'yes' or 'no'? Can you identify the criteria you are using for deciding whether an activity is 'health promotion'?

education, self-help, environmental safety measures, public policy issues, health education about physical health, preventive and curative medical procedures, codes of practice on health issues, health-enhancing facilities in local communities, workplace health policies and social education for young people. Answering 'no' indicates that you identify criteria that exclude these activities from the realms of 'health promotion'. For example, you may have said 'no' to Item 2 because increasing tobacco taxation would place a heavier burden on smokers in poor financial circumstances, thus putting their health even more at risk.

The many attempts to provide frameworks for classifying health promotion activities have helped to clarify the issues.[9] Drawing on these, we propose to start by focusing on identifying the activities that contribute to health gain (Figure 2.2).

Figure 2.2 maps out all those activities which aim to improve people's health. The first point to note is that there are two sets of activities: those about providing services

Fig 2.2   **Activities for Health Gain**

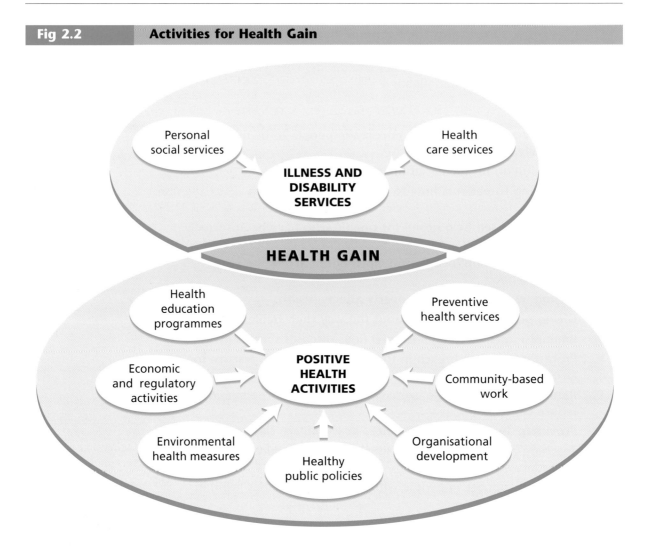

for people who are ill or who have disabilities, and positive health activities, which are about personal, social and environmental changes aiming to prevent ill health and develop healthier living conditions and ways of life. These two sets of activities overlap, because they both contribute to health gain, and they are often closely related in practice. We identify nine categories of activities, comprising two illness and disability services and seven types of positive health activities, as follows.

Illness and Disability Services

Personal social services This includes all those social services aimed at addressing the needs of sick people and people with disabilities whose health (in its widest sense) is improved by those services. This includes, for example, community care of mentally ill people and home help services.

Health care services This includes the major work of the health services: treatment, cure and care in primary care and hospital settings.

We now need to address a difficult issue: if all effective illness and disability services improve health (i.e. produce varying amounts of health gain; which they obviously do), are they all called 'health promotion'? For example, is taking out someone's appendix, or placing a child in a foster home 'health promotion'?

This is not just a quibble about words. It is an important question when considering the boundaries of service provision by health promotion agencies, of the many courses designed to educate health promoters in the necessary skills and knowledge, and, indeed, of this book.

It is helpful to go back to our definition of health promotion, 'enabling people to increase control over, and improve, their health'. Things that need to be done to people (like taking out their appendix or placing them in foster homes) are excluded from this definition, so are generally not considered to be health promotion activities (although they are health gain activities). But those aspects of care and treatment that are about enabling people to take control over their health and improve it (such as educating patients in the skills of self-care, or educating foster parents in the skills of parenting) are legitimate areas of health promotion. So is creating a health-promoting environment by, for example, modifying a home to make it suitable for a person with disabilities or providing affordable housing for homeless people with health problems.

Positive Health Activities

Health Education Programmes

These are planned opportunities for people to learn about health, and to undertake voluntary changes in their behaviour. Such programmes may include providing information, exploring values and attitudes, making health decisions and acquiring skills to enable behaviour change to take place. They involve developing self-esteem and self-empowerment so that people are enabled to take action about their health. They can happen on a personal one-to-one level such as health visitor/client, teacher/pupil, in a group such as a smoking cessation group or exercise class, or reach large audiences through the mass media, health fairs or exhibitions.

See Chapters 10–14 for detailed help on carrying out these health promotion activities.

As we have already discussed, health education programmes may also be a part of health care and personal social services, and because of this it is useful to understand the concepts of primary, secondary and tertiary health education.

Primary health education is directed at healthy people, and aims to prevent ill health arising. Most health education for children and young people falls into this category, dealing with such topics as hygiene, contraception, nutrition, and social skills and personal relationships, and aiming to build up a positive sense of self-worth in children. Primary health education is concerned not merely with helping to prevent illness but with positively improving the quality of health and thus the quality of life.

Secondary health education There is also often a major role for health education when people are ill. It may be possible to prevent ill health moving to a chronic or irreversible stage, and to restore people to their former state of health. This is known as secondary health education – educating patients about their condition and what to do about it. Restoring good health may involve the patient in changing behaviour (such as stopping smoking) or in complying with a therapeutic regime and, possibly, learning about self-care and self-help. Clearly, health education of the patient is of great importance if treatment and therapy are to be effective and illness is not to recur.

Tertiary health education There are, of course, many patients whose ill health has not been, or could not be, prevented and who cannot be completely cured. There are also people with permanent disabilities. Tertiary health education is concerned with educating patients and their carers about how to make the most of the remaining potential for healthy living, and how to avoid unnecessary hardships, restrictions and complications. Rehabilitation programmes contain a considerable amount of tertiary health education.

However, it is not always easy to see where people fit into this primary, secondary or tertiary framework because a person's state of health is open to interpretation. For example, is educating an overweight person who appears to be perfectly well, despite being overweight, primary or secondary health education?

Preventive Health Services

These include medical services that aim to prevent ill health, such as immunisation, family planning and personal health checks, as well as wider preventive health services such as child protection services for children at risk of abuse.

Community-based Work

This is a 'bottom-up' approach to health promotion, working with and for people, involving communities in health work such as local campaigns for better facilities. It includes community development, which is essentially about communities identifying their own health needs and taking action to address them. The sort of activities that may result could include forming self-help and pressure groups, and developing local health-enhancing facilities and services.

See Chapter 15, Working with Communities.

Organisational Development

This is about developing and implementing policies within organisations to promote the health of staff and customers. Examples include implementing policies on equal opportunities, providing healthy food choices at places of work, and working with commercial organisations to develop and promote 'healthier' products such as leaner meat, lower fat spreads and cheeses, low and non-alcoholic drinks, and biodegradable packaging.

See Chapter 16, Changing Policy and Practice.

Healthy Public Policies

Developing and implementing healthy public policies involves statutory and voluntary agencies, professionals and the public working together to develop changes in the conditions of living. It is about seeing the implications for health in policies about, for example, equal opportunities, housing, employment, transport, and leisure. Good public transport, for example, would improve health by reducing the number of cars on the road, decreasing pollution, using less fuel, and reducing the stress of the daily grind of travelling for commuters. It could also reduce isolation for those who do not own cars and enable people to have access to shopping and leisure facilities, all measures that improve well-being.

See Chapter 16, Changing Policy and Practice.

Environmental Health Measures

Environmental health is about making the physical environment conducive to health, whether at home, at work or in public places. It includes traditional public health meas-

See Chapter 16, Changing
Policy and Practice.

ures such as providing clean food and water and controlling pollution, as well as working on newer issues such as smoke-free areas in pubs, and controlling the use of environmentally damaging chemicals.

Economic and Regulatory Activities

These are political and educational activities directed at politicians, policy makers and planners, involving lobbying for and implementing legislative changes such as food labelling regulations, pressing for voluntary codes of practice such as those relating to alcohol advertising or advocating financial measures such as increases in tobacco taxation.

See Chapter 16, Changing
Policy and Practice.

A Framework for Health Promotion Activities

We propose the framework shown in Figure 2.3 for health promotion activities.

There are two important points to make about the use of this framework. The first is that activities do not always fall tidily into categories. For example, would a health visitor who was supporting a local women's health group be engaged in a health education programme because she provided health information to the group and set up stress management sessions, or in community-based work because some members of the group had got together to lobby their local health services for better sexual health advice clinics for young people? Would an environmental health officer concerned about air pollution levels on a factory site be engaged in organisational development because she was working towards healthier working conditions for the staff, or in environmental health measures because she aimed to achieve cleaner air for the local community?

Fig 2.3   **A Framework for Health Promotion Activities**

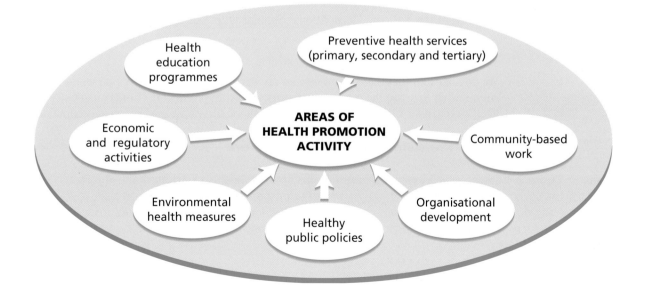

Obviously areas of activity overlap, but this is not important. What *is* important is to appreciate the range of activities encompassed by health promotion, and the many ways in which you can contribute to improvements in health status.

The second point about using this framework is to note that we are talking about planned, deliberate activities, and it is important to recognise that a great deal of health promotion happens informally and incidentally. For example, portrayal of damage caused by excessive drinking on a television 'soap', provision of low-cost exercise classes by a local entrepreneur and an advertising campaign to promote wholewheat breakfast cereals are all health promotion activities which are not likely to be planned with specific health promotion aims in mind. They may, however, be significant influences for change.

See Chapter 11, section on mass media.

Exercise 2.2 is designed to help you to identify your own contribution to health promotion.

Developing Competence in Health Promotion

Having mapped out the activities the health promoter may be engaged in, we now look at the skills and methods used when those activities take place; in other words, we are considering the competencies that health promoters need to develop (by 'competencies' we mean the specific combination of knowledge, attitudes and skills needed to do a particular job[10]).

It is useful to think that there are broadly two aspects of your work to consider. One is the technical/specialist aspect: immunising a child, taking a cervical smear test, recording blood pressure, undertaking microbiological tests for food hygiene purposes, enforcing legislation, building safer roads, interpreting welfare rights legislation or damp-proofing a home. All of these are the subject of specialist training, and outside the scope of this book.

The other aspect of your work is about working with people to promote health in many different situations with a variety of different aims. To do this, you need to have knowledge of particular methods and acquire special skills; in other words, to have public health competencies. First, we look at the range of competencies you need, and then at the National Occupational Standards that have been developed.

Core Competencies

We do not claim that these competencies are exclusive to health promotion work, but we suggest that they are the core competencies of health promotion. ('Core competence' is a term used to refer to competencies that are common to a number of different occupations.)

Exercise 2.2	Identifying your Health Promotion Work

Look at Figure 2.3 again, which identifies seven major areas of health promotion activity. By each of the seven headings, note down any parts of your work you think come into that category. (If you are not sure what each category includes, look back at the explanations.) Then think about each category again, and consider whether there is scope for developing your work within each category.

Managing, Planning, and Evaluating

All these are addressed in Part 2: Planning and Managing for Effective Practice, Chapters 5–9.

Managing resources for health promotion, including money, materials, oneself and other people, is crucial. Systematic planning is needed for effective and efficient health promotion. All health promotion work also requires evaluation, and different methods are appropriate for different approaches.

Communicating

Communication is addressed in Chapters 8–11.

Health promotion is about people, so competence in communication is essential and fundamental. A high level of competence is needed in one-to-one communication and in working with groups in various ways, both formal and informal.

Educating

Education is addressed in Chapters 11–14.

Educating about health requires good communication, but it also requires additional educational competence so that health educators can work in different settings such as formal lecturing or informal group work, and select and use appropriate strategies for different educational goals.

Educational competence is obviously used in health education programmes, but it is also used when undertaking other kinds of activities. For example, patient education is an integral part of preventive health services, education on policy implementation (such as a healthy food policy) is part of organisational development, public education is part of implementing an environmental health measure and educating members of statutory organisations may be a key part of political action for social change.

Marketing and Publicising

Marketing and publicising are addressed in Chapter 11.

This requires competence in, for example, marketing and advertising, using local radio and getting local press coverage of health issues. It may be used when undertaking any health promotion activities that would benefit from wider publicity.

Facilitating and Networking

Facilitating and networking are addressed in Chapters 9, 13 and 15.

By this we mean helping others to promote their own and other people's health, using various means such as sharing skills and information and building up confidence and trust. These competencies are particularly important when working with communities. They are also vital for working with other agencies and forming partnerships for health that cross barriers of organisations and disciplines.

Influencing Policy and Practice

Influencing policy and practice is addressed in Chapter 16.

Health promoters are in the business of influencing policies and practices that affect health. (By 'policies' we mean broad plans of action, which set the direction for detailed planning.) These can be at any level, from national (such as policies set by government or political parties about, for example, housing, transport and future directions for the NHS) to the level of day-to-day work of a health promoter (such as what sort of health promotion programmes will be run in a GP practice, or what resources will be devoted to specific health promotion activities in an environmental health department).

In order to influence policy and practice, you need to understand how power is distributed and exercised between people at any level, from a group of colleagues to those in positions of great authority or influence. You need to be able to use that knowledge to affect decisions. This includes working with statutory, voluntary and commercial organisations to influence them to develop health-promoting policies for their staff and to produce health-enhancing products and services. It also includes working for healthy public policies and economic and regulatory changes requiring lobbying and taking political action.

These six clusters of competencies are not exhaustive. As health promotion work grows and develops, and as it is practised in a variety of innovatory ways, there will be many more methods adopted and skills required. This is to be welcomed; what we aim to do here is to identify current core competencies and help you to acquire them.

It is clearly unrealistic to expect all health promoters to be highly competent in all aspects of health promotion. A practice nurse, for example, will work predominantly in health education and preventive health services, needing a high level of competence in communication and education. However, she also needs other competencies in order to plan and evaluate her work, market her health promotion programmes to her patients, facilitate change in her patients and be able to refer them to a network of helpful contacts. She will also need to be able to influence the development of health promotion policy in her practice.

All six competency areas identified here are fundamental to health promotion activities, but you will probably find that you need some to a greater degree than others. They will be acquired in a variety of ways, including your life experience outside work, basic training, in-service training and work experience.

National Standards in Health Promotion and Public Health

National standards (or national occupational standards, as they are often called) are nationally agreed statements of best practice. The first national occupational standards for health promotion and care[11] were launched in 1997 and these are now being used to improve the quality of health promotion training and work and to assist allocation of resources.[12] The national occupational standards describe performance – what people are expected to do in their jobs. They are derived from the values, ethics and principles on which good practice in the health and social care sector is based. They thus provide a specification, agreed nationally, of what should be achieved in health promotion and care work.

See Chapter 3, section on values and principles of good practice.

More recently, standards for specialist practice in public health have been developed by Healthwork UK[13] on behalf of the Tripartite Steering Group (a group comprising the Faculty of Public Health Medicine, the Multi-disciplinary Public Health Forum, and the Royal Institute of Public Health and Hygiene), together with the health departments of the four UK countries. In the light of government policy, which is focused on multi-disciplinary public health, these standards are a useful development, and probably more useful than the 1997 standards developed specifically for health promotion. We summarise the standards in Box 2.1.

Levels and Standards of Involvement in Public Health

See also Chapter 1, section on national initiatives for more about this report.

An important report published in 2001 – *The Report of the Chief Medical Officer's Project to Strengthen the Public Health Function of England*[15] – identified three levels of involvement in public health:

Box 2.1	**Overview of the National Standards for Specialist Practice in Public Health[14]**

AREA 1:   Surveillance and assessment of the population's health and well-being

This covers:

See Chapter 6. The management, analysis, interpretation and communication of information, knowledge and statistics applied to:
1. The determinants of health.
2. Health status and inequalities in health status.
3. Health needs assessment.
4. Health outcomes.
5. Ongoing surveillance and prediction.

AREA 2:   Promoting and protecting the population's health and well-being

This covers:

See Chapters 5–7 and 16.
1. Plan, monitor, evaluate and apply health promotion strategies to improve individual and population health and well-being.
2. Plan, implement, monitor and evaluate disease prevention and screening programmes to improve individual and population health and well-being.
3. Protect the population's health and well-being, including managing outbreaks, incidents and emergencies related to communicable and non-communicable disease agents and hazards.

AREA 3:   Developing quality and risk management within an evaluative culture

This covers:

See Chapter 7.
1. Assess evidence of effectiveness of health interventions and health care and apply this to practice.
2. Improve the quality of health interventions and health care through audit and evaluation.
3. Manage risk to the public's health and well-being.

AREA 4:   Collaborative working for health

This covers:

See Chapters 4, and 9–14.
1. Develop and sustain cross-sectoral collaborative working for health.
2. Advise organisations on health and health issues.
3. Communicate effectively with the public and others.

AREA 5:   Developing health programmes and services and reducing inequalities

This covers:

See Chapters 5–8.
1. Develop, implement and evaluate health programmes and services.
2. Facilitate the reduction of inequalities in health.

AREA 6:   Policy and strategy development and implementation

This covers:

See Chapter 16.
1. Shape and influence the development of health and health care policy.
2. Implement strategies for putting health and health care policies into effect.
3. Assess the health impact of policies.

AREA 7:   Working with and for communities

This covers:

See Chapter 15.
1. Involve the public and communities as active partners in planning, development, implementation and evaluation.
2. Empower communities to improve their own health.
3. Advocate for the health of communities.

AREA 8:   Strategic leadership for health

This covers:

See Chapters 8 and 13.
1. Develop, sustain and implement a vision and objectives for health.
2. Lead teams and individuals to improve health and reduce inequalities.

AREA 9:   Research and development

This covers:

See Chapter 7.
1. Appraise, plan and manage research.
2. Develop and implement research findings in practice.

AREA 10:   Ethically managing self, people and resources

This covers:

See Chapters 3, and 5–9.
1. Manage the development and direction of work.
2. Deliver effective services, the aim of which is to improve health.
3. Develop capacity and capability to improve health.

1. People such as teachers, social workers, voluntary sector staff and health workers. They all have a role in health improvement, but need to adopt a public health 'mind set' with greater appreciation of how their work can make a difference to health and well-being, and of where more specialist support can be obtained locally.
2. A smaller number of hands-on public health professionals, such as health visitors and environmental health officers, who spend a major part, or all, of their time in public health practice working with communities and groups.

The roles of all the people who contribute to health promotion work are discussed in Chapter 4.

3. A still smaller group of public health specialists from medical and other professional backgrounds, who work at a senior level with responsibility to manage strategic change and lead public health initiatives. This group includes health promotion specialists and medically qualified public health doctors.

The standards developed for specialist practice in public health are applicable (at least in part) to practitioners engaged in public health work at all three levels of the Chief Medical Officer's classification. It is useful to examine these standards and to

Exercise 2.3	Mapping your Health Promotion Work Against the Standards for Specialist Practice in Public Health[16]

Study the areas identified as specialist public health practice and tick the level of activity you are involved in. (Look back at Box 2.1 for details of the work covered by each area of activity.)

Note the areas you work in and the areas that are outside your current job responsibilities or which you are not trained to do.

Compare this mapping with that of colleagues or other health workers.

Area of public health practice	Very high level of activity	High level of activity	Fair level of activity	Some level of activity	No activity in this area
Area 1: Surveillance and assessment of the population's health and well-being.	☐	☐	☐	☐	☐
Area 2: Promoting and protecting the population's health and well-being.	☐	☐	☐	☐	☐
Area 3: Developing quality and risk management within an evaluative culture.	☐	☐	☐	☐	☐
Area 4: Collaborative working for health.	☐	☐	☐	☐	☐
Area 5: Developing health programmes and services and reducing inequalities.	☐	☐	☐	☐	☐
Area 6: Policy and strategy development and implementation.	☐	☐	☐	☐	☐
Area 7: Working with and for communities.	☐	☐	☐	☐	☐
Area 8: Strategic leadership for health.	☐	☐	☐	☐	☐
Area 9: Research and development.	☐	☐	☐	☐	☐
Area 10: Ethically managing self, people and resources.	☐	☐	☐	☐	☐

think about the areas of health promotion work you are involved in and which standards are important for your work. It is also important to recognise the areas you do *not* use in your work and to think about the implications for working collaboratively with other professionals when health development work requires that input. Exercise 2.3 is designed to help you to think about your health promotion work and how it contributes to the wider public health. It will also help you to think about the differences between health promotion and public health.

Ways in Which the National Standards Can be Used

Broadly speaking there are three uses for the national standards:

1. Employers and managers can use the standards to improve the quality of the performance of their staff. An organisation can map what it is trying to achieve against the areas and sub-areas of practice. It can then look at its service specifications and its management of human resources through job specifications, staff appraisal and performance review. The standards could also be used as the basis for auditing a service (checking whether it meets quality standards).

   We discuss audit in more detail in Chapter 7.

2. Individuals can use the standards to improve their competence through identifying their key areas of work, assessing their own performance, identifying their learning needs and defining the learning outcomes needed to meet the national standards.

   For more about how to do this, see Chapter 12.

3. Education and training providers may wish to look at the standards to see how they can modify their programmes to enable practitioners to achieve the standards, or use the standards as the basis of their programme design.

PRACTICE POINTS

- It is important for you to think about what *you* mean by health promotion, to identify the full scope of your health promotion work and to see how this fits with the work of your organisation or employer and the wider remit of public health.

- The national standards for specialist practice in public health provide a map which can be used by organisations, managers, education and training providers and individuals to improve the quality of public health and health promotion work.

- You can use this book as a guide to your own health promotion development and to assist you in assessing how well you are doing.

Recommended Reading

On the Historical Development of Health Education and Health Promotion

➤ Katz J, Peberdy A, Douglas J (eds) 2000 Promoting health: knowledge and practice, 2nd edn. Basingstoke: The Open University in association with Palgrave. (Chapter 4, The rise of health promotion and Chapter 10, Educating for health.)

➤ Naidoo J, Wills J 2001 Health promotion: foundations for practice, 2nd edition. Chapter 4, Defining Health Promotion. London: Baillière Tindall

➤ Parish R 1995 Health promotion – rhetoric and reality. In: Bunton R, Nettleton S, Burrows R (eds) The sociology of health promotion, Chapter 2. London: Routledge

An Analysis of the Concept of Health Promotion and the Implications for Professional Practice

➤ Tones K 2001 Health promotion: The empowerment imperative. In: Scriven A & Orme J (eds) Health promotion: professional perspectives, 2nd edn. Chapter 1. Basingstoke: Macmillan/The Open University

On the Meaning of Health Promotion and Current Models of Health Promotion

➤ Learmonth A 2001 The role of specialist health promotion services. In: Scriven A & Orme J (eds) Health

promotion: professional perspectives, 2nd edn. Chapter 6. Basingstoke: Macmillan/The Open University

An Analysis of the Changing Role of Specialist Health Promoters

➤ Seedhouse D 1997 Health promotion: philosophy, prejudice and practice, Chapters 1 and 2. Chichester: Wiley

Notes and References

1 World Health Organization 1984 Health promotion: a WHO discussion document on the concepts and principles. Reprinted in Journal of the Institute of Health Education, 23(1), 1985

2 See:
Welsh Health Planning Forum 1989 Strategic intent and direction for the NHS in Wales. Cardiff: Welsh Office
Welsh Health Planning Forum 1990 Protocol for investment in health gain – cancers. Cardiff: Welsh Office

3 Secretary of State for Health 1992 The health of the nation: a strategy for health in England. London: HMSO

4 Quoted in:
Simnett I 1995 Managing health promotion: developing healthy organisations and communities. Chichester: Wiley, p. 4

5 Care Sector Consortium 1997 National occupational standards for professional activity in health promotion and care – introductory guide. London: Local Government Management Board

6 The health gain cycle is adapted from the leaflet:
Health Gain, Glaxo Pharmaceuticals UK Ltd, 1993.

7 Secretary of State for Social Services 1998 Public health in England: report of the Committee of Inquiry into the future development of the public health function. London: HMSO

8 Department of Health 1999 Saving lives: our healthier nation. London: The Stationery Office
Department of Health 2001 Chief Medical Officer's report to strengthen the public health function of England. London: Department of Health

9 Some of these are summarised in:

Naidoo J, Wills J 2000 Health promotion: foundations for practice, 2nd edn. Chapter 5, Models and Approaches to Health Promotion. London: Baillière Tindall

10 For a model of the different aspects of competence, see:
Mansfield B, Mitchell L 1996 Towards a competent workforce. London: Gower

11 Care Sector Consortium 1997 National occupational standards for professional activity in health promotion and care – introductory guide. London: Local Government Management Board

12 For an example of how the standards are used in training, see:
Miller L et al. 2001 Health promotion competence in nurses and occupational therapists. Part 1: Using occupational standards to benchmark pre-registration programmes and gauge current competence. International Journal of Health Promotion and Education 39(2), 44–51
Miller L et al. 2001 Health promotion competence in nurses and occupational therapists. Part 2: Using occupational standards to identify training and development needs. International Journal of Health Promotion and Education 39(3), 68–75

13 Healthwork UK 2001 Standards for specialist practice in public health – consultation draft. London: Healthwork UK

14 Healthwork UK 2001 Standards for specialist practice in public health – consultation draft. London: Healthwork UK

15 Department of Health 2001 Chief Medical Officer's project to strengthen the public health function. London: Department of Health. (www.doh.gov.uk/cmo/phfunction.htm)

16 Healthwork UK 2001 Standards for specialist practice in public health – consultation draft. London: Healthwork UK

3 Aims and Values in Health Promotion

SUMMARY

In this chapter we identify and explore some key philosophical issues about aims and values in health promotion practice. We start with two fundamental questions about the aims of health promotion: whether we aim to change the individual or change society, and whether we aim to ensure compliance with a health promotion programme or to enable clients to make an informed choice. We provide a framework of five approaches to health promotion as a tool for analysing key aims and values, with two exercises and case studies. We discuss eight more ethical issues, set out a framework of questions to help health promoters to make ethical decisions, and provide an exercise on making ethical decisions. We finish with a discussion on the values base of occupational standards in health promotion, a sample code of practice in health promotion and another exercise.

In this chapter we tease out some of the key philosophical issues in health promotion. We encourage you to think deeply about why you are engaging in specific activities, what values are reflected in your work and what ethical dilemmas are presented. We consider guidelines on how to approach ethical decision-making and some key principles of practice.

Philosophical issues are important.[1] Health promotion work, if successful, will affect the lives of other people and it would be irresponsible to equip you with practical skills without also helping you to understand the values and ethics implicit in your work.

First, we look at the aims of health promotion.

Clarifying Health Promotion Aims

Aiming to Change the Individual or Change Society?

See section From Health Education to Multi-disciplinary Public Health in Chapter 2.

For decades there has been much debate over different approaches (often called 'models') of health education and health promotion.[2]

Much of the debate centres around the aims of the work. A key question is: should it aim to change individual behaviour and lifestyles or to change the socioeconomic and physical environment?

See Chapter 1 section Improving Health – Historical Overview.

As we discussed in Chapter 1, a great deal of traditional health education has aimed at changing the behaviour of individuals towards healthier lifestyles. In other words, it aims to change people to fit the environment, and has done little to make the environment a healthier place to live in. It has also resulted in 'blaming the victims' for their own ill health, which is an ethical issue health educators need to face. On the other hand, it can be argued that individuals often *can* do something to improve their own health, that they *want* to take responsibility for themselves and that health education is an essential tool in that process. It is also argued that sensitive health education can promote people's self-esteem and confidence, empowering them to take more control over their own health.

Proponents of the lifestyle change approach also argue that medical and health experts have knowledge that enables them to know what is in the best interests of their patients and the public at large, and that it is their responsibility to persuade people to adopt the 'healthiest' measures. Furthermore, society has vested that responsibility in them, and people often seek advice and help in health matters; it is not necessarily a matter of persuading clients against their will. Sometimes, too, individuals may not be in a position to take responsibility for themselves because they may be too young, too ill, or have severe learning difficulties.

There are several points to be taken into account if the lifestyle change aim is pursued.

- You cannot assume that lay people believe that 'experts' know best. The public perceives 'experts' to change their minds constantly. For example, whether jogging does more harm than good, whether eggs, chicken and beef are safe to eat or whether living near a nuclear power plant is hazardous to health. Sometimes the 'experts' are proved wrong.
- There is a danger of imposing alien values on a client. Frequently this is the imposition of middle-class values on working-class people. For example, a doctor may perceive that the most important thing is for a patient to lose weight and lower blood pressure, but drinking beer in the pub with friends may be far more important to the overweight, middle-aged, unemployed patient. Who is to say which set of values is 'right'? Whose life is it anyway?
- Linked to this, a health promoter advocating lifestyle changes can be seen as making a moral judgement on clients' failure to change, that it is 'their own fault' if, for example, the baby of a mother who smokes is born with low birth weight or dies a cot death.
- Pushing a lifestyle change approach may produce negative and counter-productive feelings: of guilt for failing to comply, or of rebelliousness and anger at being told what to do.
- We cannot assume that individual behaviour is the primary cause of ill health. This is a limited view, as we saw when looking at determinants of health and inequalities in health in Chapter 1. There is a danger that focusing on the individual distracts attention from the more significant (and, of course, politically sensitive) determinants of health such as the social and economic factors of racism, relative deprivation, poverty, housing and unemployment.

See Chapter 1 section What Affects Health?

- Finally, we also cannot assume that individuals have genuine freedom to choose 'healthy' lifestyles. Freedom to choose is often very limited. Economic factors may affect the choice of food because, for example, fresh fruit and wholemeal bread are relatively more expensive than biscuits and white bread. Social factors are also important: there is very little real freedom of choice about smoking for adolescents whose parents and friends all smoke, and who risk ridicule if they do not.

Also, how much freedom do people really have to change other health-demoting factors such as stressful working conditions and unemployment? It is easy to become 'victim blaming': blaming people for their own ill health when in fact they are the victims of their circumstances. In situations where resources of time, energy and income are limited, health choices become health compromises. What a health promoter may see as irresponsibility may actually be what the client sees as the most responsible action in the circumstances.[3] For example, chips are cheap, filling and enjoyed by children; if money for food is short, and cooking skills and facilities are limited, chips are a sensible choice for a mother with several hungry mouths to feed. Another example is the mother who smokes because it is the only way she knows of relieving her stress; it helps to stop her hitting her children when they drive her to breaking point.

It is crucially important that everyone engaged in health promotion should be aware of these ethical issues and have an opportunity to consider them in relation to their own work, particularly if they are engaged in health education with the aim of changing individual lifestyles. The following exercise is designed to help you to think through the issues.

Part 3 of this book is about how you can promote health in a way that is sensitive to these issues. Chapter 16 looks at what you can do to challenge and change health-related policies.

| Exercise 3.1 | Analysing Your Philosophy of Health Promotion[4] |

Consider the following statements A and B:

A. The key aim of health promotion is to inform people about the ways in which their behaviour and lifestyle can affect their health, to ensure that they understand the information, to help them explore their values and attitudes, and (where appropriate) to help them to change their behaviour.

B. The key aim of health promotion is to raise awareness of the many socioeconomic policies at national and local level (e.g. employment, housing, food subsidies, advertising, transport and health service policies) that are not conducive to good health, and to work actively towards a change in those policies.

1. **Taking Statement A:**
    ■ **list arguments in support of this view;**
    ■ **list any points about the limitations of this view, and any arguments against it.**
2. **Do the same with Statement B.**
3. **Do you think that the views in A and B are *complementary* or *incompatible*? Why?**
4. **Imagine these two views at either end of a spectrum:**
    A|. . . . .|. . . . .|. . . . .|. . . . .|. . . . .|B
        1   2   3   4   5

Indicate the two positions on the scale of 1 to 5 which most closely reflect (a) *what you actually do* in practice and (b) *what you would like to do* if you were free to work exactly as you would wish to.

Aiming for Compliance or Informed Choice?

Another key question about the aims of health promotion centres on what you aim to do with or for the client (whether the client is a single individual, a community, or an organisation). Is your aim to ensure that your client complies with your programme, using a mixture of education, publicity and persuasion as required? Or is it to enable your client to make an informed choice, and have the skills and confidence to carry that choice through into action, whatever that choice may be?

To take an example: supposing a health promoter is working with a client whose sexual behaviour is such that there is a serious risk of catching sexually transmitted infections, including HIV. If the aim is compliance it is more likely that the health promoter will be persuasive, will stress the risks to the client, and will consider the session a failure if the client does not choose to behave differently. If, on the other hand, the health promoter's aim is to enable the client to make an informed choice, the health promoter will ensure that the client understands the facts and the risks, will put a lot of effort into encouraging and supporting the client and accept that if the client chooses not to change his behaviour this choice will be respected. It would not be interpreted as a failure, because the client made an informed choice.

The same issues arise with health promotion work on a larger scale. For example, is the aim of a campaign to promote 'natural' food untouched by additives, chemical fertilisers and pesticides to persuade people to a particular point of view or to give them the information on which to make up their own minds? This is a difficult question. Most health promoters are doing their jobs because they believe that the action they are advocating is in the best interests of individuals, and of society as a whole. It raises questions about how far to go in imposing your own values and ideas of what is 'good' and 'right' on other people.

While considering this question it is also worth noting that it raises the issue of defining 'success' in health promotion. In the first example (about sexual health behaviour) if the aim is to change behaviour then success is likely to be measured in terms of rates of sexually transmitted infections and unplanned pregnancies. But if the aim is solely to educate, success will be measured in terms of changes in people's knowledge of health risks.

Analysing Your Aims and Values: Five Approaches

In our view there is no one 'right' aim for health promotion, and no one 'right' approach or set of activities. We need to work out for ourselves which aim and which activities we use, in accordance with our own professional code of conduct (if there is one), our own carefully considered values and our own assessment of our clients' needs.

Different models of health promotion and health education are useful tools of analysis, which can help you to clarify your own aims and values. We identify a framework of five approaches to health promotion, and suggest some of the values implicit in any particular approach.

1. The Medical Approach

The aim is freedom from medically defined disease and disability, such as infectious diseases, cancer and heart disease. The approach involves medical intervention to prevent or ameliorate ill health, possibly using a persuasive or paternalistic method – persuading, for example, parents to bring their children for immunisation, women to use family planning clinics and middle-aged people to be screened for high blood pressure.

This approach values preventive medical procedures and the medical profession's responsibility to ensure that patients comply with recommended procedures.

2. The Behaviour Change Approach

The aim is to change people's individual attitudes and behaviours, so that they adopt a 'healthy' lifestyle (as defined by you or your employing organisation). Examples include teaching people how to stop smoking, education about 'sensible' drinking, encouraging people to be more physically active, look after their teeth, eat the 'right' foods and so on.

Those using this approach will be convinced that a 'healthy' lifestyle is in the best interests of their clients, and will see it as their responsibility to encourage as many people as possible to adopt the 'healthy' lifestyle they advocate.

3. The Educational Approach

The aim is to give information, ensure knowledge and understanding of health issues, and to enable well-informed decisions to be made. Information about health is presented, and people are helped to explore their values and attitudes and to make their own decisions. Help in carrying out those decisions and adopting new health practices may also be offered. School health education programmes, for example, emphasise helping pupils to learn the skills of healthy living, not merely to acquire knowledge.

Those favouring this approach will value the educational process, will respect individuals' right to choose their own health behaviour, and will see it as their responsibility to raise with clients the health issues which they think will be in the client's best interests.

4. The Client-centred Approach

The aim is to work with clients to help them identify what they want to know about and take action on, and make their own decisions and choices according to their own interests and values. The health promoter's role is to act as a facilitator, helping people to identify their concerns and gain the knowledge and skills they require to make changes happen. Self-empowerment of the client is seen as central.[5] Clients are valued as equals, who have knowledge, skills and abilities to contribute, and who have an absolute right to control their own health destinies.

5. The Societal Change Approach

The aim is to effect changes on the physical, social and economic environment, to make it more conducive to good health. The focus is on changing society, not on changing the behaviour of individuals.

Those using this approach will value their democratic right to change society, and will be committed to putting health on the political agenda at all levels and to the importance of shaping the health environment rather than shaping the individual lives of the people who live in it.

Table 3.1	**Five Approaches to Health Promotion – Summary and Example**			
	Aim	**Health promotion activity**	**Important values**	**Example – smoking**
Medical	Freedom from medically defined disease and disability	Promotion of medical intervention to prevent or ameliorate ill health	Patient compliance with preventive medical procedures	*Aim* – freedom from lung disease, heart disease and other smoking-related disorders *Activity* – encourage people to seek early detection and treatment of smoking-related disorders
Behaviour change	Individual behaviour conducive to freedom from disease	Attitude and behaviour change to encourage adoption of 'healthier' lifestyle	Healthy lifestyle as defined by health promoter	*Aim* – behaviour changes from smoking to not smoking *Activity* – persuasive education to prevent non-smokers from starting and to persuade smokers to stop
Educational	Individuals with knowledge and understanding enabling well-informed decisions to be made and acted upon	Information about cause and effects of health-demoting factors. Exploration of values and attitudes. Development of skills required for healthy living	Individual right of free choice. Health promoter's responsibility to identify educational content	*Aim* – clients will have understanding of the effects of smoking on health. They will make a decision whether or not to smoke and act on the decision *Activity* – giving information to clients about the effects of smoking. Helping them to explore their own values and attitudes and come to a decision. Helping them to learn how to stop smoking if they want to
Client-centred	Working with clients on their own terms	Working with health issues, choices and actions that clients identify. Empowering the client	Clients as equals. Clients' right to set agenda. Self-empowerment of client	Anti-smoking issue is considered only if clients identify it as a concern. Clients identify what, if anything, they want to know and do about it

	Aim	Health promotion activity	Important values	Example – smoking
Societal change	Physical and social environment that enables choice of healthier lifestyle	Political/social action to change physical/ social environment	Right and need to make environment health-enhancing	*Aim* – make smoking socially unacceptable, so it is easier not to smoke than to smoke *Activity* – no-smoking policy in all public places. Cigarette sales less accessible, especially to children, promotion of non-smoking as social norm. Banning tobacco advertising and sports' sponsorship

Table 3.1 summarises and illustrates these five approaches to health promotion. We have used this framework because it is a simple one that helps health promoters to appreciate that there are many ways of tackling health promotion, and that these different ways reflect differing viewpoints and values. Our framework has rightly been questioned and challenged, and this is part of a healthy debate as the theory and practice of health promotion continue to develop.[6] There are other well-known models.[7]

Exercise 3.2   Identifying Your Aims and Values

Select two or three specific health promotion activities you are engaged in, such as a group health education programme, a publicity campaign, a patient education scheme, an immunisation programme, a one-to-one meeting with a client, a community activity or working on a health policy. Select different kinds of activities if you can.

With reference to Table 3.1, identify which approach you are using for each activity (you may find that you will identify more than one approach).

For each activity, define the aim and the important values implicit in your work (you may find it helpful to look at Case Studies 3.1 and 3.2).

Discuss your findings with a partner or in a small group.

Some More Ethical Dilemmas

There are many more difficult questions for health promoters to get to grips with. The following are some of the more common ones you are likely to encounter.

Case studies 3.1 and 3.2	Approaches A and B

Case study 3.1 Approach A

Jill is a hospital nurse running a programme of rehabilitation for patients who have had heart attacks. She decides that she is working with an educational approach, aiming for her patients to make informed decisions and have knowledge and skills about taking exercise, modifying their diet, etc. She accepts that some patients will choose not to do so. She thinks that sometimes she may be working in a behaviour change model, because she sincerely believes that her patients would be better off if they changed their behaviour and she finds that she sometimes really wants to persuade them. In the end, she decides that it is their choice and their life, and that she will not pressure them into doing what they do not want to do. Jill is aware, though, that some of her colleagues (who favour the behaviour change approach) think she should be tougher and shock the patients into complying by horror stories of what may happen to them if they do not.

Case study 3.2 Approach B

Terry is a community worker, based in a deprived housing estate. Facilities for recreation, exercise and buying good food (among other things) are poor. He decides that he is working with a mixture of client-centred and societal change approaches, because people in the community have identified that they want a better diet, and he is helping them to set up a food cooperative and help each other to learn new cooking skills. He is also helping them to lobby their local councillor for better green spaces on the estate where the children can play.

Bottom-up or Top-down?

There is a key issue of control and power at the heart of health promotion work: who decides what work will be done; who sets the agenda? Is it 'bottom-up', set by people themselves identifying issues they perceive as relevant, or is it 'top-down', set by health promoters who have the power and resources to make decisions and impose their own ideas of what should be done?

Put this way, it appears to be a straightforward polarised choice. In practice, of course, it is not simple. The issue can be considered at different levels.

At the level of individual health promoters there is a spectrum of possible positions they could take: at one end coercion or persuasion, then giving advice, then a more neutral position of giving the facts but leaving the client to decide. The position at the other end of the spectrum is the health promoter who listens, gives information when asked and supports the client but never offers advice or even an opinion.

The client, too, could be at any point along the spectrum. Ideally, the health promoter and client will adopt compatible positions: for example, with the health promoter giving information and the client happy to make up his own mind what to do about it. Problems can arise when positions are not compatible. An example is a client who wants to be told what to do and a health promoter who wants to empower him with information and confidence to make his own decision.

At a national level, governments identify certain health promotion priorities with the advice of professionals. These programmes are then imposed on the population, who may or may not perceive them as relevant. But ultimately the decision to implement these programmes is that of the government elected by the people in a democratic society; so we come full circle.

There is also a danger that, when the public is involved in health promotion at a local level, local people can be manipulated into changing their agenda to match that of the health promoters. Community development should be about empowering the public to work on their own agendas of health issues, even if these are radically different from the agendas of those working for health in a professional capacity. But health promoters have a responsibility to raise awareness of health issues, provide information about them and create demand for change: so where does this process differ from manipulating the community into wanting what the health promoters wanted in the first place?

See Chapter 15.

Perhaps one way forward is to be aware of the necessity to be absolutely honest and open about your aims and the limitations of your freedom to act on other people's priorities.

Just Widening the Inequalities?

See section on inequalities in health in Chapter 1.

As discussed in Chapter 1, there are wide differences in the health status of different groups of people; generally those in poorer social and economic conditions are the least healthy, with the gap between the health status of rich and poor becoming ever wider.

Some ways of working with those most in need, and often hardest to reach, are discussed in Chapter 15.

There is a danger that health promotion activities only reach better-off people, who have the time, money and education to make use of health information and take health action. Those who are trapped in poor financial circumstances and who struggle to survive are less likely to be in a position to change their lifestyle or devote their energies to lobbying for social or political changes.[8] There is clearly a need to be sensitive to this.[9]

We also need to be aware that efforts to change people's environments may have a negative effect. Evaluation of some schemes to regenerate run-down urban areas has revealed a mixed impact on health, with increased relative poverty and harmful effects on social networks. For example, private landlords may increase rents in regenerated areas, and properties may become eligible for higher council tax banding.[10]

The Health Promoter: A Shining Example?

Consider the cases of an overweight dietitian, a nurse who smokes and an environmental health officer whose own kitchen is unhygienic. All three are in a position where they need to address these issues as part of their work and may be asked for advice which they clearly do not follow themselves.

Few health promoters would claim that they are perfect examples of healthy living, but we suggest that they have a responsibility to consider their own health, and think of ways in which it could be improved and in which they could contribute to a healthier environment. Health promoters are teaching by example, and the examples discussed above convey silent messages that it is okay to be overweight, to smoke, or to risk health by cooking unhygienically. It is probably best to be open and honest in situations where health promoters' own lifestyles are at odds with the health-promoting ways they are advocating. Personal experience can also be turned to good advantage: for example, if the dietitian has a constant struggle to control her own weight, she can use that experience to develop a greater understanding of her clients' difficulties.

Facts, Fads or Fashions?

A common complaint from the public is that experts keep changing their minds. There are many examples to illustrate this, such as controversy about the safety of beef in

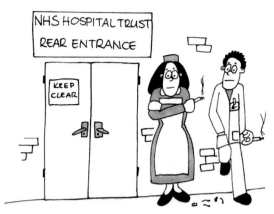

Few health promoters would claim that they are perfect examples of healthy living

the light of 'scares' about 'mad cow disease', and changes in guidelines about sensible drinking.[11] Health issues go in and out of the news, and the public may see them as fads or fashions with little solid foundation in fact, and certainly with low credibility.

A difficulty is that research continuously turns up new information. This is often controversial and not accepted as generally 'received wisdom' until it has been independently confirmed from new sources, which may take many years. But media attention focuses on the new and controversial, so the public is alerted to the debates.

At what point do you decide that the evidence is sufficiently convincing to begin publicising a new message, or to campaign to change an aspect of health policy or legislation? If you have insufficient knowledge or experience to judge questions that may be medically or technically complex, on what basis do you make your decision? Is it more appropriate to discuss the conflicting views openly and just air the debate more widely?

Health or Healthism?

In their enthusiasm for improving health, there is a danger that health promoters come to see health as the be-all and end-all: as an end in itself, not as a means to the end of enabling people to fulfil their potential and live life to the full. This ideology of health as the ultimate goal incorporating all life is sometimes called 'healthism'.

What 'being healthy' means to different people is discussed in Chapter 1.

The danger is that this may lead to a lack of acceptance that health means different things to different people, shaped by their various values and experiences. Health may become a stereotyped image of the health promoter's own idea of perfection, leading to a prescription of what people should and should not do. This is clearly contrary to the concept that health promotion is about enabling people to increase their control over their health and improve it in ways they see fit.

Health Information: an Insensitive Blunderbuss?

All health promotion should be sensitive to the social, ethnic, economic and cultural background of the people it is working with and for. Sadly, this is often not the case. Because of insensitivity, ignorance or the need to produce materials on a large scale for economic reasons, health information, and indeed entire health promotion programmes, are frequently aimed at an 'average' person, or the largest client group. So they often, for example, portray only white people, are available only in English, or assume a level of income above the poverty line. Frequently those with greatest needs are in the minorities and are therefore ignored.

Awareness of this issue is growing, but there is still a long way to go before health promotion can truly claim to practise equal opportunities.

To Professionalise or Empower the People?

Health promotion requires special competencies, some of which are the subject of this book. It is a whole or part of the work of very many professions, including health, education and community work. As health promotion becomes increasingly specialised, with its own body of knowledge based on research, and its own academic qualifications, there is a danger that health promotion 'experts' will exclude other workers and the public from the business of health promotion.

This would be a mistake. Health promotion, as we have said often, is about empowering people to take more control over their own health. Health promotion specialists therefore need to seek to share their knowledge and experience with lay people, to learn from them, and to see them and other workers as valued partners in health promotion.[12]

Health for Sale?

With a scarcity of resources available for health promotion and in a climate of market economy and income generation, some health promotion activities are sponsored by commercial companies. One pitfall is the issue of perceived endorsement of products. For example, an NHS organisation could be seen as advocating that patients should take vitamins if it accepted sponsorship of appointment cards printed with the name of the sponsoring vitamin manufacturer.

There is also a move to involve commercial companies in promoting products in a way that also promotes health. For example, food manufacturers may be involved in special promotions for lower fat products. There are dangers here, the most obvious one being that the interests of the company may not be in harmony with those of the health promoter, who will be perceived as endorsing the product. There is also a possibility that the independent credibility of the health promoter is compromised, with the public thinking 'they're just trying to sell me something' instead of perceiving an unbiased credible health message.

Another pitfall is that health promotion, which should be a fundamental part of the free national health service, is seen as a potential money maker. Basic services, such as health information materials, health teaching, and giving advice to commercial companies on health promotion for employees, become subject to charges.

There is a clear need to develop policies and guidelines on these issues.[13]

Making Ethical Decisions

We have identified many areas of ethical concern, and have raised difficult issues that do not present easy resolutions or 'right' answers. The following set of questions is designed to help you to think through some of the dilemmas you face, and to make decisions about ethical questions when faced with alternative courses of action.[14]

1. Questions Fundamental to Decisions About Health

- Will I be creating autonomy in my clients, enabling them to choose freely for themselves and direct their own lives?
- Will I be respecting the autonomy of my clients, whether or not I approve of what they are doing?
- Will I be respecting persons equally, without discrimination?
- Will I be serving basic needs before any other wants?

2. Questions About Duties and Principles

- Will I be doing good and preventing harm?
- Will I be telling the truth?
- Will I be minimising harm in the long term?
- Will I be honouring promises and agreements?

3. Questions About Consequences

- Will I be increasing individual good?
- Will I be acting for my own good?
- Will I be increasing the good of a particular group?
- Will I be increasing the social good?

4. Questions About External Considerations

- Am I putting resources to best use: what is the most effective and efficient thing to do?
- What is the degree of risk involved?
- Is there a professional code of practice that has a bearing on this?
- How certain am I of the evidence for the facts of the matter?
- Are there any disputed facts?
- Are there legal implications? If so, do I understand them?
- What are the views and wishes of other relevant people?
- Can I justify my actions in terms of the evidence I have before me?

These questions are tools to help clear thinking and moral reasoning. They are not substitutes for personal judgement, but they help you to think through the issue, weigh up the pros and cons and come to a reasoned decision. Not all the questions will be relevant, but they act as a useful checklist. Some questions may reveal that, on the surface, a 'wrong' action is being taken (such as not telling the truth or being discriminatory) but using the checklist ensures that careful consideration is given to the action and that it is justified. For example, a painful truth may be withheld from a seriously ill patient, or it may be necessary to discriminate between working with one group of people or another because there are insufficient resources to work with both.

Exercise 3.3 is designed to help you to think about ethical decision making.

Towards a Code of Practice

Many professions have codes of practice, which are broad principles and guidelines on how professionals should and should not act. They reflect the values accepted as

Exercise 3.3   Ethical Decisions in Health Promotion

You may find it helpful to use the questions in the section above on making ethical decisions to identify the issues relevant to each situation, and to decide what you would do.

Case A

A group of local people, led by a woman whose son died of a heroin overdose, have got together because they are concerned about drug misuse in the neighbourhood. They are afraid for the safety of their teenagers and younger children: drugs seem to be an established part of the teenage social scene, are easily available in the neighbourhood, and needles and syringes are found in local alleyways.

The group has decided that the best way to combat drugs is to go into local schools and scare the children off drugs with horror stories of bad 'trips' and addiction. They have recruited a former drug addict who is prepared to tell his story. They have asked the school nurse to help by getting them supplies of leaflets and supporting them in their approach to the schools.

The school nurse believes that the 'shock-horror' approach the group proposes has been shown by research into drug education to be ineffective. At best it will do no good, and at worst it could glamorise the drug scene and a make a hero out of the ex-addict. She believes that the local schools' approach is best: education on the facts of drug-taking and how to minimise harm from taking drugs, coupled with building up self-esteem, social skills and confidence for young people to deal with drug situations. The parents think this is far too soft, and believe that their idea for a hard-hitting approach will work for their children.

- Identify the ethical issues in this situation.
- What do you think the school nurse should do, and why?

Case B

An environmental health officer (EHO) wants to undertake some research into the impact of air pollution on asthma rates in a neighbourhood that straddles a main road. Town planning colleagues have told the EHO that they expect this road to become even busier soon because it will become the feeder road to a new bypass leading to a massive new out-of-town office development. The EHO has a well worked out research proposal and has the cooperation of local GPs, which will enable him to see if there is any correlation between traffic flow, air pollution levels and asthma rates. If he can show a correlation, it will help to put health issues on the agenda of the council's Planning Committee, so that the health impact of planning decisions will be taken into account in future.

He needs to secure a research grant to pay for the additional pollution measurements and traffic flow counts, and to collect and process the data from the GPs. If he does not start within the next month, he will miss the chance to collect vital baseline measurements before the expected increase in traffic when the bypass opens.

Despite applications to many sources, the only offer of research money he has received has come from a research trust which specialises in the impact of environmental pollution on respiratory disease. It is funded primarily by the tobacco industry. The trust assures the EHO that that they will not interfere with the research in any way, and the grant will be given with 'no strings attached'. The EHO is unhappy about accepting money from the tobacco industry, but this is now his only chance to get the research under way.

- Identify the ethical issues in this situation.
- What do you think the EHO should do, and why?

| Box 3.1 | **National Occupational Standards for Professional Activity in Health Promotion and Care, July 1997**[16] |

Values and Principles of Good Practice

Professional standards from a number of different professional bodies were analysed to identify the values and principles on which the national occupational standards for professional activity in health promotion and care should be based. The *values* identified are respect for:

- the human condition and its complexity
- our essential humanity
- the wealth of human experience
- the holistic nature of health and social well-being
- diversity.

The National Occupational Standards for Professional Activity in Health Promotion and Care have been built on ten *Principles of Good Practice*:

1. Balancing people's rights with their responsibilities to others and to wider society and challenging those that affect the rights of others.
2. Promoting values of equality and diversity, acknowledging the personal beliefs and preferences of others and promoting anti-discriminatory practice.
3. Maintaining the confidentiality of information, provided that this does not place others at risk.
4. Recognising the effect of the wider social, political and economic contexts on health and social well-being and on people's development.
5. Enabling people to develop to their full potential, to be as autonomous and self-managing as possible, to have a voice and to be heard.
6. Recognising and promoting health and social well-being as a positive concept.
7. Balancing the needs of people who use services with the resources available and exercising financial probity.
8. Developing and maintaining effective relationships with people and maintaining the integrity of these relationships through setting appropriate role boundaries.
9. Developing oneself and one's own practice to improve the quality of services offered.
10. Working within statutory and organisational frameworks.

National occupational standards are explained in Chapter 2.

underpinning sound professional practice. We suggest that readers make sure they are familiar with the codes of practice of their own professional bodies.[15]

The values and principles on which the National Occupational Standards for Health Promotion were based are set out in Box 3.1.

The principles of practice in Box 3.2 have been produced by the Society of Health Education and Health Promotion Specialists (SHEPS). SHEPS intend them for use by health education/promotion specialists and others working in the fields of health education, health promotion and public health, as they cover areas that all health promoters may find helpful to consider. They consider issues similar to those in the national occupational standards, but focus more specifically on health promotion activities.

Exercise 3.4 asks you to think about the values and principles that underpin your own health promotion work.

| Box 3.2 | **Society of Health Education and Health Promotion Specialists Principles of Practice, July 1997[17]** |

Relationship to Client/Recipient

1. Adequate needs assessment, consultation with and involvement of the client or target group is essential to the effective planning, implementation and reviewing of health promotion activities.
2. The promotion of self-esteem and autonomy amongst client groups/recipients should be an underlying principle of all health promotion practice.
3. Health promotion should encourage people to value others whatever their gender, age, race, class, religion, culture, sexuality, ability or health status, and should attempt to counter prejudice and discrimination wherever it occurs.

Social and Environmental Influences

4. Health promotion programmes should be relevant and sensitive to the nature of the intended client group; for example, the social, economic and cultural framework of the group.
5. Health promotion work should include recognition of and action focused on the social, economic and environmental determinants of health.
6. Health promotion work should aim to empower and enable people to exercise informed choice and influence structures and systems that have an impact on health.
7. Health promotion programmes that focus on specific issues should always be set in the wider political, social, economic, geographical, psychological and environmental contexts, which have a bearing on health.
8. The sustainability of health promotion interventions needs to be considered within the context of the aims of any programme of activity. Health promotion interventions should aim to have a positive impact on both the immediate recipients and future generations of people.

Health Promotion Practice

A. An aim of health promotion practice is to bring about change in the social and economic environment to improve health and to reduce or eliminate inequalities in health at a local, national and international level.
B. Appropriate research and evaluation is an essential component of health promotion activity. Practitioners should endeavour to disseminate results and findings.
C. Practitioners have a responsibility for ensuring an accurate and appropriate information flow between the public, professionals, local and national agencies, and for taking the initiative and responding accordingly.

D. Practitioners will endeavour to provide services or information that they have at their disposal that would, in the light of current theory and/or evidence, maintain and promote health. They will endeavour to keep their knowledge of current developments in health promotion up to date.

E. Practitioners will have due regard to the confidentiality of information to which they have access, bearing in mind the requirements of the law.

F. Health promotion work should encourage all services and organisations to develop their health promotion role and to adopt the above principles of practice.

G. Health promotion activity is by its nature a collaborative endeavour. Practitioners should seek to collaborate actively with colleagues and others to promote health.

H. The methods and process of health promotion should be health promoting.

Exercise 3.4   **Developing a Code of Practice**

Work in small groups of three or four.

Consider the points in the *National Occupational Standards for Professional Activity in Health Promotion and Care – Values and Principles of Good Practice* and the *Society of Health Education and Health Promotion Specialists – Principles of Practice*, reproduced in Box 3.1 and 3.2 above.

- **To what extent do you think you take account of these values and principles in your work?**
- **Do you encounter any difficulties in putting these values and principles into practice?**
- **Are there any values and principles you would like to amend?**
- **Are there any values and principles you would like to add?**

PRACTICE POINTS

- You need to recognise the range of approaches to health promotion that reflect different aims and values.

- Ethical issues and dilemmas are inherent in health promotion practice.

- You need to think through the process of how you will make ethical decisions.

- Professional codes of practice can help you to be clear about the underlying principles of your work, and you should be familiar with the code of professional practice of any profession to which you belong.

- Good practice in health promotion means working to the specific values and principles of practice. The Society of Health Education and Health Promotion Specialists *Principles of Practice* provide helpful guidelines.

Recommended Reading

Critical Overviews of Models of Health Promotion

➤ Katz J, Peberdy A, Douglas J (eds) 2000 Promoting health: knowledge and practice, 2nd edn. Chapter 5, Theories and models in health promotion. Basingstoke: The Open University in association with Palgrave.

➤ Naidoo J, Wills J 2000 Health promotion – foundations for practice, 2nd edn. Chapter 5, Models and Approaches to Health Promotion. London: Baillière Tindall

➤ Squire A 2002 Health and well-being for older people: foundations for practice. London: Baillière Tindall in association with the Royal College of Nursing. (Chapter 2, on the scope, goals and values of health promotion with older people.)

Client-centred and Empowerment Approaches to Health Promotion

➤ Kendall S 1998 Health and empowerment. London: Arnold

➤ Kerr J 2000 Community Health Promotion: Challenges for Practice. London: Baillière Tindall. (Empowerment is a theme throughout this book, which discusses approaches and examples of health promotion work with a variety of client groups and different settings.)

➤ Raeburn J, Rootman I 1998 People centred health promotion. Chichester: Wiley

On Ethical Issues in Health Promotion

➤ Duncan P 1999 Making sense of morality: a qualitative study of practitioners' writing about ethical problems of health promotion. Health Education Journal 58, 249–258. (Study that identifies key themes underpinning moral dilemmas for health promotion practitioners.)

➤ Katz J, Peberdy A, Douglas J (eds) 2000 Promoting health: knowledge and practice, 2nd edn. Chapter 6, Ethical issues in health promotion. Basingstoke: The Open University in association with Palgrave

➤ Naidoo J, Wills J 1998 Practising health promotion: dilemmas and challenges, Part 2: Dilemmas in Practice. London: Baillière Tindall

➤ Naidoo J, Wills J 2000 Health promotion – foundations for practice, 2nd edn. Chapter 6, Ethical Issues in Health Promotion. London: Baillière Tindall

➤ Naidoo J & Wills J (eds) 2001 Health Studies: an introduction. Basingstoke: Palgrave. (Chapter 8, Ethics and the Law, explores a range of issues and dilemmas about, for example, the value of life, and the relationship between legal obligation and ethical and moral duty.)

➤ Seedhouse D 1998 Ethics: The heart of health care, 2nd edn. Chichester: Wiley

Notes and References

1 Some further reading on philosophy and ethics – see Recommended Reading and:

Downie R S, Tannahill C, Tannahill A 1996 Health promotion: models and values, 2nd edn. Part 2. Oxford: University Press

Hunt G (ed.) 1994 Ethical issues in nursing. London: Routledge. (Deals with specific nursing issues but also general themes applicable to a wide range of health promoters, such as professional responsibility.)

Pike S, Forster D (eds) 1995 Health promotion for all. Chapter 5, Values and ethical issues. Edinburgh: Churchill Livingstone. (Discusses ethical issues in health promotion, particularly as applied to nurses.)

Seedhouse D 1997 Health promotion – philosophy, prejudice and practice. Chichester: Wiley

2 See Recommended Reading for current views on models of health promotion and:

Maben J, Macleod Clark J 1995 Health promotion: a concept analysis. Journal of Advanced Nursing 22(6), 1158–1165. (On nurses' concepts of health promotion.)

Tones K, Tilford S 2001 Health education: effectiveness, efficiency and equity, 3rd edn. Chapter 1. Cheltenham: Nelson Thornes

For a historical view, see these articles and readings on models of health education/promotion in the 1980s and early 1990s:

Burkitt A 1983 Health education. In: Clark J, Henderson J (eds) Community health. Edinburgh: Churchill Livingstone

Catford J, Nutbeam D 1984 Towards a definition of health education and health promotion. Health Education Journal 43 (2 & 3), 38

Draper P 1983 Tackling the disease of ignorance. Self Health 1, 23–25

French J 1990 Boundaries and horizons, the role of health education within health promotion. Health Education Journal 49(1), 7–10

French J, Milner S 1993 Should we accept the status quo? Health Education Journal 52(2), 98–101

Tannahill A 1985 What is health promotion? Health Education Journal 44(4), 167–168

3   For discussion about the 'lifestyle approach' and the impact of social factors on health, see:

Blaxter M 1990 Health and lifestyles. London: Tavistock

Burrows R, Bunton R, Nettleton R (eds) 1995 Towards a sociology of health promotion. London: Routledge

Edmondson R, Kelleher C (eds) 2000 Health promotion – new discipline or multi-discipline? Dublin: Irish Academic Press

Graham H 1993 Hardship and health in women's lives. Hemel Hempstead: Harvester Wheatsheaf

4   This exercise is based on an idea in the training manual for the Schools Health Education Project 5–13, published by the Health Education Council, London, and reproduced here by kind permission of the Council.

5   For a description of an 'empowerment' model of health education, see:

Tones K, Tilford S 2001 Health education: effectiveness, efficiency and equity, 3rd edn. Chapter 1, pp. 49–55; Chapter 2, pp. 101–107. London: Chapman & Hall.

6   See Recommended Reading on critical overviews of models of health promotion.

7   One of the best known is Tannahill's model of three overlapping circles, which together form health promotion. The three circles comprise prevention, health education and health protection:

Tannahill A 1985 What is health promotion? Health Education Journal 44(4), 167–168

Downie R S, Tannahill C, Tannahill A 1996 Health promotion: models and values, 2nd edn. Chapter 4, Health Promotion. Oxford: University Press

8   Graham H 1993 Hardship and health in women's lives. Hemel Hempstead: Harvester Wheatsheaf. (Chapter 8, Making Ends Meet, shows that many families are living on incomes that make it hard to survive, and looks at how low-income families spend their limited budget and at the strategies that mothers develop to keep their family in health and out of too much debt. Such strategies often include mothers going without food, heating and other basic necessities themselves so that their children can have them.)

9   For some examples of successful health promotion initiatives in reaching 'hard-to-reach' groups, see:

Edmondson R, Kelleher C (eds) 2000 Health promotion: new discipline or multi-discipline? Dublin: Irish Academic Press

Kerr J 2000 Community health promotion: challenges for practice. London: Baillière Tindall. (Section 2 includes chapters on work with homeless women, ethnic minority groups, people with HIV, older people.)

Percy-Smith J 2000 Policy responses to social exclusion. Buckingham: Open University Press

Power R et al 1999 Promoting the health of homeless people. London: Health Education Authority

10   Papers presented at UKPHA Conference, Bournemouth, April 2001: Ambrose P Urban Regeneration by Area-base Initiatives – how much health gain? Ward O Report on the Bryson House Project.

11   In 1997, government-backed Health Education Authority publicity promoted the notion of 'daily benchmarks' of 2–3 units of alcohol a day for women, and 3–4 units a day for men. This replaced guidelines which advocated a weekly sensible drinking limit of 14 units for women, 21 for men in:

Department of Health 1995 Sensible drinking: the report of an inter-departmental working group. London: Department of Health

12   A good example of lay people working in partnership with professionals is the successful experience of using non-professional volunteer mothers working with disadvantaged first-time mothers to develop their parenting skills:

Johnson Z, Howell F, Molloy B 1993 Community mothers' programme: randomised controlled trial of non-professional intervention in parenting. British Medical Journal 36, 1449–1452

Other examples can be found in:

Freeman R et al 1997 Community development and involvement in primary care. London: Kings Fund

Geddes M 1998 Local partnership: a successful strategy for social cohesion? Bristol: The Policy Press

Higgins JW 1999 Citizenship and empowerment. Community Development Journal 34(4), 287–307

Myers F 1996 Power to the people? Involving users and carers in needs assessment and care planning. Health and Social Care in the Community 4(22), 88–95

13   This question is addressed in:

The Society of Health Education and Health Promotion Specialists 1996 Income generation – moral threat or marvellous opportunity? Principles of Practice Standing Committee, Briefing Sheet No. 2

14   The questions in this section (reproduced by kind permission of John Wiley & Sons) are based on the work

of Seedhouse, which is recommended for further study:

Seedhouse D 1988 Ethics – the heart of health care. Chichester: Wiley

15 For example, professional bodies such as the Community Practitioners' and Health Visitors' Association.

16 Care Sector Consortium 1997 National occupational standards for professional activity in health promotion and care – introductory guide. London: Local Government Management Board

17 This is reproduced with the kind permission of the Society of Health Education and Health Promotion Specialists. It is the Principles of Practice part of the Principles of Practice and Code of Professional Conduct for Health Education and Promotion Specialists, July 1997.

4 Who Promotes Health?

SUMMARY

In this chapter we identify the major agents and agencies of health promotion, and discuss their role. We cover international and national organisations, the government, the Health Development Agency (and sister organisations in Scotland, Wales and Northern Ireland), the NHS, local authorities, local groups and many others. We include an exercise on identifying key local health promoters. We end the chapter with suggestions and an exercise about how you can improve your own health promotion role.

In Chapter 1 we discussed *what* affects people's health; in this chapter we review *who* has a role in promoting people's health: the people and organisations that help, support and encourage better health.

To some extent everyone is a health promoter, because everyone discusses health matters and gives advice and guidance to others from time to time. This usually happens informally, for example when parents are reminding children to clean their teeth, or when friends are discussing their experiences. Health promotion may also occur incidentally: for example, the availability of a wide variety of cheap fruit and vegetables in the summer means that it is easier for people to choose a healthy diet, so the greengrocer is unwittingly promoting health. These informal and unplanned sources of health promotion are very significant. Our aim here, however, is to identify the agents and agencies through which planned, deliberate programmes and policies are channelled.

The Developing Public Health System in the United Kingdom

We discuss the role of the main agencies of health promotion in more detail later in this chapter.

Many organisations at national and local level are recognised as having a role in improving public health. Box 4.1 identifies organisations at national, regional and local level. (Box 4.1 applies to England and most of it also applies to other parts of the UK. Wales has the Welsh Assembly, and Scotland has a separate parliament and legal system.)

The organisations identified in Box 4.1 support the key across-the-board themes of the government at the beginning of the 21st century:

■ Modernisation: using up-to-date streamlined methods of management and communication.

Box 4.1	**The Developing Public Health System**[1]

National

Key government departments:

- Health
- Education and Skills
- Environment, Food and Rural Affairs

- Cabinet Office
- Home Office
- International Development

- Culture, Media and Sport
- Lord Chancellor's Office
- Trade and Industry

- Social Security
- Treasury
- Transport, Local Government and Regions

Examples of key health-related units:

- Neighbourhood Renewal
- Social Exclusion
- Teenage Pregnancy

Other health-related national organisations and bodies:

- Health Development Agency
- Modernisation Agency

- Commission for Health Improvement
- Audit Commission

- Food Standards Agency
- Voluntary Sector and Professional Bodies

- National Institute for Clinical Excellence
- Local Government Association

Regional

Regional government:

- Regional Director of Health and Social Care
- Government Office for the Regions
- Health Development Agency regional support

Other health-related regional and sub-regional organisations:

- Public Health Observatory
- Strategic Health Authorities
- Learning and Skills Council

Local

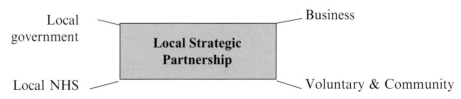

Key strategies:

- Health Improvement and Modernisation Plan
- Community Strategy
- Neighbourhood Renewal Strategy

- Equity and inequalities: equal opportunities for everyone and reducing inequalities between different social groups.
- Social and economic regeneration: addressing poverty, unemployment, poor living conditions and social exclusion (a sense of not being a part of a community, of not belonging).
- Democratic renewal: ensuring that the process of democracy is applied through all levels of public service.
- Public involvement: getting people involved with decisions and actions that affect them, such as consulting people about proposed changes to local health services.

Two other organisations concerned specifically with public health are the UK Public Health Association and the Public Health Institute of Scotland (PHIS).

The UK Public Health Association (UKPHA)[2] was launched in 1999. It is an independent voluntary organisation bringing together two other organisations: the Public Health Alliance and the Association for Public Health. The UKPHA aims to be a unifying and powerful voice for the public's health and well-being in the UK, focusing on the need to eliminate inequalities in health, promote development that does not damage the environment and combat anti-health forces.

The Public Health Institute of Scotland (PHIS)[3] was established in 2001. It is an NHS organisation, created for the public health community in Scotland within the NHS and beyond. Its aims are to strengthen the public health information and evidence base (especially by developing a database for public health) and to support the development of public health skills.

Agents and Agencies of Health Promotion

Figure 4.1 identifies a wider range of the most important agents and agencies of health promotion. Most have a variety of health promotion roles. For example, environmental health officers in local authorities are involved in formal health education through educating caterers about food handling in kitchens, but they are also involved in environmental measures such as control of air pollution. And they have important duties related to the enforcement of laws such as food hygiene regulations and health and safety at work legislation.

See Chapter 9, section Working in Partnership with other Organisations.

An increasing number of agencies are working together in collaborative partnerships, which make them more effective than working in isolation. In 1993, as part of the first national strategy for health in England (*The Health of the Nation*), the Department of Health produced guidance on how agencies could work together for better health.[4] Subsequent documents produced in 1998 (*Partnership in Action*)[5] and the next national strategy in 1999 (*Saving Lives – Our Healthier Nation*)[6] reaffirmed the importance of partnership working for better health. Since then, government strategies and guidelines have continued to focus on the importance of partnerships for health between agencies and, most importantly, across government departments.

Fig 4.1   Agents and Agencies of Health Promotion

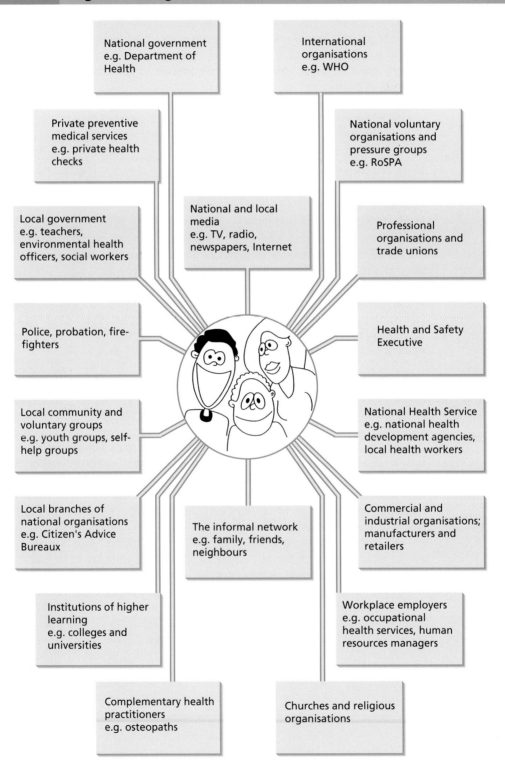

International Organisations

The European Community

The European Community is increasingly making an impact on health by, for example, setting standards for beach pollution and through directives regulating permitted food additives. In 2000 a new public health strategy was developed, *Communication on the Health Strategy of the European Union*, adopting a programme of community action.[7] Through the framework of the *Community Action Programme on Health Promotion, Information, Education and Training*, the European Commission funds projects in the member states and produces directories of concise information about projects, networks and other activities. The aim is to improve people's knowledge about preventing ill health and to encourage healthy lifestyles.

The World Health Organization (WHO)

The WHO's role in promoting health is discussed in Chapter 1.

The WHO has a role in guiding European health policy. It has issued many statements in the form of Declarations and Charters addressing important areas of policy in relation to, for example, young people, nursing and midwifery, health promotion, transport, environment, water and health. It coordinates European networks such as Health Promoting Schools and Hospitals, and Healthy Cities.

Other International Organisations

We discuss these initiatives in settings such as schools and hospitals in Chapter 16.

The International Union for Health Promotion and Education (IUHPE)

The IUHPE is an independent professional association of individuals and organisations, established over 50 years ago. It provides a link between organisations working in health promotion and education and ensures a world-wide exchange of experience and knowledge, promoting scientific research and informed public opinion on 'healthful living.'[8] There are currently 42 members, drawn from 25 countries.

European Public Health Alliance

This is a network of 80 non-governmental organisations (NGOs – organisations that are independent of government control) and other agencies actively involved in protecting and promoting public health.[9]

World Federation of Public Health Associations (WFPHA)

The WFPHA provides a medium through which NGOs can work more effectively with their partners in health agencies, to promote community and individual health. It supports public health professionals through exchanging information and facilitating collaborative initiatives to improve health and health services.[10]

The Government

Government departments, particularly the Department of Health but also the Department of Social Security, the Department for Education and Skills, the Department of the Environment, Food and Rural Affairs and the Department of Transport, Local Government and the Regions, have an interest in, and responsibility for, health promotion, through the impact of legislation and economic and fiscal policies on health.

The government's national strategies for health in the 1990s signalled a major change towards the pursuit of improved health and a reduction in health inequalities, rather than focusing almost exclusively on treatment services and health care. Key units for neighbourhood renewal and social exclusion were set up; they produced national strategies to be implemented locally by partnerships of health services, local authorities, and voluntary and community organisations.[11]

The government has also taken a lead in tackling health issues such as drug misuse[12] and teenage pregnancy.[13] In relation to drug misuse, for example, its aims are to increase the safety of communities from drug-related harm, to reduce the acceptability and availability of drugs to young people and to reduce the health risks and other damage related to drug misuse. Multi-agency drug action teams produce local plans, coordinate work and bring together a wide range of people and agencies to work at a local level.

See Chapters 1 and 7 for more on national strategies for health.

Other National and Local Organisations

National Voluntary Organisations and Pressure Groups

There are many national organisations concerned with health promotion, some of which have regional and/or local branches. An example of an organisation that has no local network is The Advisory Council on Alcohol and Drug Education (TACADE). Organisations with local branches include the National Childbirth Trust (NCT), the National Association for Mental Health (MIND) and the Citizens Advice Bureaux. Most of these organisations produce educational material, and some run training courses for professionals and/or the public. Some organisations act primarily as pressure groups, for example Friends of the Earth.

See also UK Public Health Association in the section above, The Developing Public Health System in the United Kingdom.

Professional Associations

Professional associations, such as the British Medical Association (BMA), the Royal College of Nursing (RCN), the Community Practitioners' and Health Visitors' Association (CPHVA), the Royal College of General Practitioners, the Chartered Institute for Environmental Health (CIEH) and the Faculty of Public Health Medicine (FPHM), have been influential in policy making, in pressing for legislative changes and in the practice and training of their members in health promotion.

Trade Unions

Trade unions are active in promoting health and safety at work, both through negotiating workplace conditions and through their health and safety representatives. The Health and Safety Executive also oversees the implementation of health and safety at work legislation.

Commercial and Industrial Organisations

These have a role in safeguarding public health. Examples include companies providing water, refuse removal companies, and the transport industries. In recent years, many facilities with a public health protection function have been privatised, which has produced new problems. For example, should water companies have the right to cut off supplies to consumers who do not pay their bills, when a possible consequence of this is the occurrence and spread of infectious diseases such as dysentery?

Manufacturers and Retailers

Manufacturers are increasingly taking the health and safety aspects of their products into account. These include manufacturers of children's clothes and toys, food manufacturers, producers of 'green' household products, and pharmaceutical companies. Large supermarket chains have made an increasingly wide range of 'healthy' options available to the public, such as fat-reduced and low-sugar foods. These trends are due to increased consumer demands, reflecting heightened awareness of health issues.

The Mass Media

See Chapter 11 for more about mass media in health promotion.

Health education is undertaken by national and local mass media, such as television, radio, newspapers and magazines. Through the Internet many people now have easy access to a huge range of health information.

Churches and Religious Organisations

Churches and religious organisations play an important part in developing values, attitudes and beliefs that affect health. Some provide training in skills, such as meditation, which can improve mental, emotional and spiritual health.

The National Health Service (NHS)

The Structure of the NHS

Before we look at the role of the many different agencies and professionals in the NHS, it is helpful to review how the NHS is organised. There has been so much reorganisation since the late 1980s that people are often unsure about the current structure. We describe the structure as it is in 2002; there may, of course, have been more changes since the time of writing.[14]

The NHS was established in 1948. The way it was organised was changed in the 1970s, when health authorities were established at regional, area and district level and some of the public health functions of local authorities (such as health visiting and district nursing) came under the NHS. Further changes followed, but the most significant and fundamental reorganisation happened in the 1990s, starting with the 1990 *National Health Service and Community Care Act* reforms.

During the 1990s a key feature was the 'internal market': the NHS was divided into *purchasers* and *providers*. Local health authorities were the purchasers, who decided what health care was required and purchased it, setting and monitoring contracts with provider local hospitals and community services. These providers became NHS trusts, in competition with one another to win contracts from the purchasers.

The election of the Labour government in 1997 brought a new approach, with an emphasis on replacing the competitive 'market place' with 'integrated care', and working in a spirit of cooperation.[15] *The New NHS: Modern, Dependable* set out the government's plan for the health service, with partnership, quality and performance at the heart of the NHS, a focus on improving health and well-being, and tackling the root causes of ill health and inequalities.[16] In a shift towards a 'primary care-led NHS', *primary care groups* (PCGs) were set up in the late 1990s. These were basically groups of GP practices that worked closely with local authorities, especially social services, to assess local health needs and develop local health services. *The NHS Plan*[17] (2000) set out a further programme for reform, investment and expansion of the NHS: Chapter 13 ('Improving health and reducing inequality') outlined a central role for the wider public health function, including health promotion.

See below for information on primary care trusts and care trusts.

Shifting the Balance of Power Within the NHS – Securing Delivery,[18] published in 2001, set out further change with a power shift to 'front-line staff'. Primary care groups were given additional responsibilities to run services; they developed into *primary care trusts* (PCTs) or *care trusts*. (PCTs work closely with social services; care trusts go one step further by being formed from a merger of local authority social services with NHS primary care services.)

Twenty-eight larger strategic health authorities replaced the existing 95 smaller health authorities in 2002 in England. Strategic health authorities in England cover an average population of about 1.5 million; their role is to support the PCTs and NHS trusts in delivering *The NHS Plan*, to build capacity and support performance improvement, ensuring that all NHS organisations work together to meet government targets.

Also in 2002, the Department of Health was refocused; the NHS Executive and its Regional Offices were abolished and replaced by four new Regional Directors of Health and Social Care.[19]

The structures in England, Scotland, Wales and Northern Ireland differ. In the interests of keeping the text in this book short and simple, we use the terms applicable in England (Strategic Health Authorities, PCTs, etc.) but readers in all countries will need to familiarise themselves with the structure in the country where they work – see Exercise 4.1 (page 73).[20]

National Health Promotion Agencies

The Health Development Agency (HDA)

The HDA was launched in June 2000; it drew on the resources of the Health Education Authority, which was abolished in April 2000. As a special health authority, the HDA has a remit to raise the quality of public health work in order to improve the health of people in England.[21] It does this by:

- maintaining a database of research evidence about what works to improve health
- providing information about the effectiveness of health improvement programmes
- supporting, setting and implementing standards of public health work
- acting as a national resource for developing the public health workforce.

| Fig 4.2 | **The Structure of the NHS in England in 2002** |

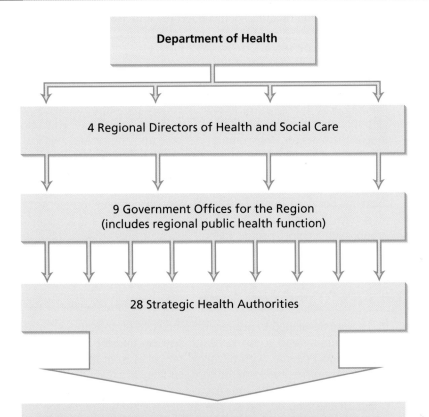

Department of Health

4 Regional Directors of Health and Social Care

**9 Government Offices for the Region
(includes regional public health function)**

28 Strategic Health Authorities

Many local **NHS Trusts** providing hospitals and specialised services such as mental health and ambulance, and many local **Primary Care Trusts** and **Care Trusts** providing GP and community-based health services and commissioning all acute and specialised services for their populations.

The HDA's performance is reviewed annually by the Secretary of State for Health and priorities are decided in consultation with other government departments. Regional HDA posts ensure that the work is delivered at regional and local levels.

During its first few years the HDA has supported people in the NHS and other statutory and voluntary agencies working to reduce health inequalities. Particularly strong links have been developed with the regional Public Health Observatories.[22] Building on the *Health at Work in the NHS* project initiated by the Health Education Authority, the HDA has produced advice and guidance focusing specifically on the primary care sector.[23]

See also Chapter 16 for more about the Health at Work initiative.

The Health Education Board for Scotland (HEBS)

The HEBS is the national agency responsible for health education in Scotland.[24] As a special health board it organises programmes, projects, training, research and evaluation at the national level, and supports 15 health boards and local education authorities with their own health education.

The **Health Promotion Agency for Northern Ireland** and the **Health Promotion Division of the National Assembly for Wales** are bodies performing similar functions for Northern Ireland and Wales.[25]

Regional Workforce Development Confederations

Workforce Development Confederations (WDCs) were established in April 2001[26] in each region in England, replacing the education purchasing consortia. Their role is to support health care organisations in recruiting and retaining staff to meet the needs of patients, in partnership with colleagues in social care, educational institutions, the independent sector, the voluntary sector and the prison service. Sub-groups ensure effective involvement by partner agencies at a local level, focusing on, for example, continuing professional development or care groups and policies such as the National Service Frameworks for mental health, coronary heart disease and older people.[27] (National Service Frameworks are national documents that set out the pattern and level of service – standards – which should be provided for a major care area or disease group, such as older people, mental health or heart disease.) For health promotion and public health specialists it is important to be aware of the local WDC in order to ensure that opportunities for education and development are maximised.

Primary Care Trusts (PCTs) and Care Trusts

PCTs were developed to become the lead NHS organisations for assessing local health needs, planning and securing health services and for improving health.[28] Led by doctors and local people, with devolved power to front-line staff, they work closely with local communities and local authorities. They are responsible for preparing and implementing the local Health Improvement and Modernisation Plans (HIMPs – previously called Health Improvement Programmes) – annual plans for improving health and developing health services.[29] They have a responsibility for public health through the Director of Public Health and the public health team, and they link into broader public health networks across the area served by their strategic health authority.

Improving the health of the local community involves PCTs in programmes of community development, health promotion and education. Membership of Local Strategic Partnerships – partnerships of all the local NHS organisations, local authorities, voluntary and community groups and local businesses – ensures that priority is given to shared plans and integrated multi-agency programmes.[30] Examples are *Sure Start* (a government scheme in areas of high health need, which aims to support parents and children under 4 years), community safety programmes, teams dealing with young offenders, *Quality Protects* (services for children in need, including vulnerable children in local authority care) and regeneration programmes aimed at improving social and economic conditions in run-down areas.[31] PCTs also have responsibility for all primary care services (pharmacy, dental, medical and optical) as set out in the government's *NHS Plan*.

For more detail, see Chapter 7, section Local Health Strategies and Initiatives.

The Local Government Act 2000 and the Health and Social Care Act 2001 brought about further integration of health and social care. Some care trusts have been created to provide improved 'joined-up' health and social care services.[32]

NHS Trusts

NHS trusts provide patient-centred hospital services based on local agreements and national standards; some trusts provide specialised services such as mental health services or ambulance services. NHS trusts are expected to take account of patients' views as they plan their services, and to ensure that local people are involved in decisions about service planning. NHS trusts have a part to play in health promotion, particularly health education and preventive health work with patients, their carers and families.

Local Specialist Health Promotion Services

Specialist Health Promotion Services are an NHS service and since 2002 most have been located within the public health directorate in PCTs. Health promotion specialists are broadly responsible for the provision of expert advice, leadership, partnership development, training, programme development (including strategy and policy) and resources to support local health promotion initiatives.[33] They liaise with other health promotion agents and agencies, both within and outside the NHS, to ensure that activities, wherever initiated, are coordinated and supported.

Primary Health Care Teams

The WHO International Conference on Primary Health Care in Alma-Ata (1978) defined primary health care as:

> *Essential health care ... made universally accessible to individuals and families in the community ... It forms an integral part both of the country's health system, of which it is the central function and main focus, and of the overall social and economic development of the community.*

Primary health care teams are the first point of contact with the NHS. *The NHS Plan* confirmed the government's vision of robust primary care services, with GPs and PCTs taking a lead in meeting people's needs.[34] To do this, the primary care role has been enhanced, with policies and investment to improve services through, for instance, more flexible agreements about the way GPs can provide services, NHS Direct (a national telephone helpline staffed by specially trained nurses) and NHS walk-in centres (a service offering advice, information and treatment for health problems from specially trained nurses, with no appointment necessary). Some roles are being developed, so that, for example, there are nurse practitioners who are able to undertake some tasks previously done by doctors, including examining and assessing some patients, and providing treatment, including prescribing certain medication. There is also a move to encourage GPs to develop special areas of expertise (in skin diseases, for example) so that other GPs can refer patients to them rather than to a hospital specialist.

In Britain, the work of primary health care is shared by a team. The exact membership of each primary health care team varies but it usually includes the following.

General Practitioners

GPs provide a comprehensive range of medical services – diagnosis and treatment – for patients registered with their practice, and for those outside the practice in an emergency. They refer patients to other health workers as necessary, for example to counsellors, practice nurses, health visitors, physiotherapists or consultants specialising in a particular disease area. Some GPs also play a central role in PCTs as members of the PCT management structure.

Practice Managers

These are key people in enabling the smooth running of practices. They have overall responsibility for ensuring that patients are efficiently, confidentially and caringly received at the practice. They have an important role in health promotion because they can control access to health information for patients.

Receptionists

The uniqueness of the receptionist's role and its inherent challenges have been recognised and courses are available within colleges of further education. These emphasise the roles of the receptionist in health promotion and provide training in communication skills.

Community Nurses

The role of community nurses in improving the health of the local population was emphasised in the Department of Health policy paper *Making a Difference*, published in 1999.[35] PCTs depend on the contribution of a range of community nurses to achieve their objectives; their work in health promotion and in assessing health needs of the local population is particularly important.[36] There is a range of nursing roles and professions within community nursing, notably including:

- district nurses
- health visitors
- school nurses
- community mental health nurses
- community midwives[37]
- practice nurses
- others, such as diabetes specialist nurses.

Other Health Professions

Many other health professionals, such as hospital nurses, dentists, hospital and retail pharmacists, opticians and the professions allied to medicine (such as chiropody and dietetics) have a part to play in health promotion, especially in patient education.

Patient Advice and Liaison Services and Community Health Councils

Until 2001 Community Health Councils (CHCs) were regarded as 'the patient's watchdog', representing patients' interests when NHS policies and plans were discussed. They could influence health promotion policies and plans, and sometimes carried out health education as part of their work. In 2000, *The NHS Plan* introduced far-reaching reforms to bring citizens more closely into decision making processes. It also announced the establishment of Patient Advice and Liaison Services (PALS) and the abolition of CHCs.[38]

Health Services Outside the NHS

Complementary Health Practitioners

These include homoeopaths, chiropractors, osteopaths, acupuncturists, reflexologists, practitioners of herbal medicine, yoga, massage and shiatsu, amongst others. These practitioners can play a part in promoting health and relieving health problems, often using a more holistic approach than conventional medicine. They are also known as alternative or natural health practitioners. Therapies may be available on the NHS, either by a member of the primary care team or through referral to a complementary practitioner. General interest in the use of complementary therapies is increasing.[39]

Private Agencies

Some private agencies are funded through insurance schemes and offer a range of health checks and preventive medical services.

Local Authorities

Many local authorities have health committees and full-time health policy officers responsible for promoting liaison and consultation between all departments of the council, and with other bodies, on matters related to health. In 1996 the Health Education Authority commissioned and published an audit of health promotion work in local authorities[40] and a guide on developing health strategy in local authorities.[41] Towards the late 1990s the emphasis on partnership working led to some joint posts between health and local authorities, particularly social services. As PCTs and care trusts become more developed, with pooled budgets and integrated services, the links are likely to become stronger.

See also Chapter 9 section Working in Partnership with Other Organisations.

A host of initiatives has been developed over the last decade to promote and improve economic, social and environmental well-being, through regeneration and partnership working. These include the Neighbourhood Renewal Strategy and Fund,[42] New Deal for Communities,[43] Sure Start,[44] the Children's Fund, Community Strategies[45] and Local Strategic Partnerships,[46] and Action Zones for health, education and employment.[47] Health promoters from both local authorities and health services have been key to their development and success.

For more detail see Chapter 7, section Local Health Strategies and Initiatives.

Environmental Health Officers

The measures necessary to deal with the physical factors in the environment that threaten health, in the widest sense, constitute what is known as 'environmental health'. The organisation of environmental health services is mainly the function of local authority environmental health departments, but may be combined with other departments such as housing, community development and leisure. National and local legislation gives these departments power to take advisory and legal action on behalf of people who visit, live, or work in an area. The scope for health promotion by these departments is wide and constantly growing, along with new threats to the environment. Many departments appoint specialist officers to work on specific health issues, such as home safety, community safety or recycling.

The Local Education Authority

LEAs have responsibility for health education in schools and further education colleges through the work of teachers and lecturers.[48] They may also have advisors with specific responsibility for health education, and other staff who provide advice, support and training in health education for teachers. There have been considerable developments in school health education over the last 20 years: many major curriculum-development projects have taken place, resulting in significant progress.[49]

Social Services

Social services staff, including social workers, staff of residential homes and home helps, are often concerned with improving the health of clients. With the policy of providing care in the community rather than hospital, the role of social services departments in promoting the health of vulnerable groups such as older people, people with mental health problems and people with learning difficulties has increased greatly.

Many other local authority staff have a role in health promotion, such as recreation and leisure officers, housing officers, regeneration, youth and community workers, trading standards and community safety officers.

Other Local Organisations and Groups

There are numerous individuals and groups at local level who help to promote particular aspects of health. Some notable ones are described here.

Institutions of Higher Education

Universities are responsible for the basic training of professionals with health promotion roles. They are also becoming increasingly involved in post-basic and continuing education for health promoters, including running Health Education Certificate Courses, postgraduate diplomas and masters'-level courses. Some health promotion postgraduate courses are now offered through a Master's in Public Health (MPH). The Open University has been very active, both in developing degree courses in health (especially useful to professionals without a first degree) and in producing community education material on health issues for the general public.[50]

Local Voluntary and Community Groups

A huge range of local voluntary and community groups exists, many of which undertake educational work on health matters. Patients' associations, self-help groups, environmental action groups and youth groups are just a few examples.

Employers

Employers can be active in developing health-promoting policies and conditions in the workplace. Personnel officers and occupational health staff, in particular, are vital to implement workplace policies and to promote the well-being of staff.

Police and Probation Officers

The police protect the public from crime and violence, take action to prevent misuse of drugs and alcohol and help to ensure road safety. Prison officers and probation officers are involved in the health and well-being of prisoners and their families, and may be

Exercise 4.1   What's on Your Patch? Finding out About your Local NHS and Agents and Agencies of Health Promotion

1.   **Find out about the structure of the NHS in the area where you work**

   ■ What is the name and function of the local organisation with responsibility for public health? (This will be your local primary care trust/care trust or its equivalent in Scotland, Wales or Northern Ireland. Try www.nhs.uk for information.)
   ■ What regional and/or national organisations are responsible for public health where you work?

2.   **Find out about the agencies and people on your patch**

   ■ Think of the geographical patch where you work, and identify its boundaries as clearly as you can. It could be the area served by a GP practice, the catchment area of a hospital, the population of a primary care trust/care trust or the geographical patch that is your responsibility as an environmental health officer or community worker.
   ■ Identify as many health promotion agents and agencies on your patch as you can, using Figure 4.1 and the information about agents and agencies in health promotion in this chapter as checklists.

It is likely that you will know some very well and others not at all. Identify those you would find it helpful to know more about and plan to find out about them. If there are some you know nothing about, such as the community groups on your patch, identify people who are likely to know about them (such as local health visitors or health promotion specialists) and contact them to find out more.

involved in initiatives such as health-promoting prisons, health education about HIV/AIDS, and educational programmes on sensible drinking for drink/drive offenders.

Fire Fighters

The fire service has a key role to play in preventing injuries at home and on the roads; they may run innovative projects such as schemes inviting people to bring in electric blankets for a safety check.

Exercise 4.1 is designed to help you to find out how your local NHS is organized and to identify the health promotion agents and agencies which are important for your work. There is much to gain by having good local knowledge of other people you can work with or refer people to.

The Informal Network

Finally, as we mentioned at the beginning of this chapter, it is essential to remember that the whole informal network of family, friends and neighbours is of great significance in shaping people's health beliefs and behaviour and in providing healthy living conditions.

Improving Your Health Promotion Role

A number of factors affect the development of the health promotion role of professionals. The need for improved training is recognised, but one of the difficulties is how to fit more into the already crowded curriculum of basic professional training courses. It may help to identify the core competencies health promoters need (such as basic communication skills) and to ensure that these are taught as part of basic professional training.

Post-basic courses such as Health Education Certificate courses, and postgraduate diplomas and master's degrees in health education, health promotion and public health are increasingly becoming available, often in a range of learning modes (such as full-time, part-time, college-based or open learning). It is now possible for students to accumulate 'credits', which they can use to contribute towards higher qualifications. Training is being developed to meet occupational standards of competence in the workplace, with the emphasis moving towards assessment of competencies: employees demonstrate whether they are competent to carry out particular activities.

See Chapter 2 for details of the national occupational standards relevant to health promotion and public health.

All these developments help to minimise the time students are 'off the job' for training, provide more flexible training opportunities, and help managers to assure the quality of their staff's work. In the fast-changing world of health and social care, ensuring that staff are competent to carry out new roles is an increasingly important focus of the work of managers.

A problem for students is that they use trained professionals as examples to follow ('role models'), but research has long since shown that trained professionals themselves may not have the necessary skills.[51] This is particularly true of health promotion skills in networking, joint working, facilitating, marketing and political skills, which have not traditionally been included in professional training.

Some professionals have too narrow a concept of health and what is meant by health promotion and health education. Therefore they may use only individual behaviour change approaches and fail to take advantage of opportunities for using alternative or complementary approaches. Lack of knowledge about which approaches to health promotion are likely to be effective in different circumstances is also a problem. Furthermore, the health promotion and health education needs of the professionals themselves may not have been met. They may be exhorted to be a good example but they are often not given the help they need to make health choices and carry these through.

In addition, resource constraints may hinder the professions from achieving their potential in health promotion. For instance, staff shortages and work overload may reduce the time available for long-term health promotion work.

On the positive side, there is ample evidence that people want more information and welcome health education from, for example, GPs.[52]

In summary, some strategies have proved very useful in improving the role of professionals in health promotion. But overall education and training for professionals remains an underdeveloped area, particularly the training of policy makers and managers and training in the skills of networking, joint working, facilitation, marketing and influencing policy and practice.

The following exercise is designed to help you identify factors that help and hinder you in carrying out health promotion work, and what you might do to improve the situation.

| **Exercise 4.2** | **What Helps and Hinders Your Health Promotion Work?** |

This exercise is designed to help you identify helping and hindering forces in your own situation.

In a stable system, the forces for producing changes are balanced by forces opposed to change. It is essential to pinpoint all the possible helping and hindering forces, so that you can take steps to increase the power of helping forces and decrease the power of the hindering forces. The disruption of the balance results in progress towards change.

For your own situation:

■ Make a list of forces that *help you* in your health promotion work.
■ Make a list of forces that *hinder you* in your health promotion work.
■ Identify ways of *increasing the helpful forces*.
■ Identify ways of *decreasing the hindering forces*.

→   health   ←

helping forces   →   promotion   ←   hindering forces

→   work   ←

→

Direction you want to go

PRACTICE POINTS

■ It is important to appreciate the whole range of agents and agencies with a health promotion role: informal and formal, local, national and international.

■ Think about how you can best work with other people and agencies.

■ Ensure that you are clear about your role in health promotion.

■ Consider how you could improve your health promotion role, through education and training or through identifying what helps and hinders your health promotion work and how the situation could be improved.

Recommended Reading

Health Promotion by a Range of Different Professionals in a Variety of Settings

➤ Kerr J 2000 Community health promotion: challenges for practice. London: Baillière Tindall. (Has chapters about health promotion for a range of client groups and in different settings, including youth health promotion in the community, homeless women and primary health care, neighbourhoods.)

➤ Naidoo J, Wills J 1998 Practising health promotion: dilemmas and challenges. London: Baillière Tindall. (Chapter 7, Health Promotion in a Primary Care Led NHS, is a detailed discussion of health promotion in NHS primary care.)

➤ Naidoo J, Wills J 2000 Health promotion: foundations for practice, 2nd edn. London: Baillière Tindall. (Chapter 13 discusses implementation in schools, workplaces and primary health care.)

➤ Scriven A, Orme J (eds) 2001 Health promotion: professional perspectives, 2nd edn. Basingstoke: Palgrave/Open University. (Has chapters on health promotion in different settings: health service, local authority, education and youth organisations, voluntary sector and workplace.)

➤ Squire A 2002 Health and well-being for older people: foundations for practice. London: Baillière Tindall in association with the Royal College of Nursing. (Chapter 3 discusses who promotes the health of older people.)

➤ Tones K, Tilford S 2001 Health promotion: effectiveness, efficiency and equity, 3rd edn. London: Stanley Thornes. (Has chapters on health promotion in schools, health care settings, workplace and community.)

Classic Studies on Informal Sources of Health Education, and the Role of Women in Family Health

➤ Blaxter M, Paterson E 1982 Mothers and daughters: a three generational study of health attitudes and behaviour. London: Heinemann

➤ Doyal L 1995 What makes women sick – gender and the political economy of health. Basingstoke: Macmillan Press.

➤ Graham H 1984 Women, health and the family. London: Wheatsheaf Books

➤ Roberts H (ed.) 1990 Women's health counts. London: Routledge

➤ Roberts H (ed.) 1992 Women's health matters. London: Routledge

Further Reading on Health Promotion Training Needs and Evidence-based Practice

➤ Naidoo J, Wills J 2001 Health studies. Basingstoke: Palgrave

➤ Simnett I, Lawrence T 1996 The role of health professions in health promotion: a review of current practice, training needs and training provisions. Journal of the Institute of Health Education 34(3), 86–88

➤ Simnett I, Perkins E, Wright L (eds) 1999 Evidence-based health promotion. Chichester: John Wiley.

Notes and References

1   Adapted from the chart 'The developing public health system'. In: Summary of activities 2001–2002. Health Development Agency 2001. Reproduced by kind permission.

2   UK Public Health Association, 7th Floor, Holborn Gate, 330 High Holborn, London, WC1V 7BA. Tel: 0870 0101930. Email: info@ukpha.org.uk Website: www.ukpha.org.uk

3   Public Health Institute of Scotland, Clifton House, Clifton Place, Glasgow G3 7LS. Tel: 0141 300 1010. www.show.scot.nhs.uk/phis

4   Department of Health 1993 Working together for better health. London: Department of Health

5   Department of Health 1998 Partnership in action (new opportunities for joint working between health and social services) a discussion document. London: The Stationery Office

6   Department of Health 1999 Saving Lives – Our Healthier Nation. London: The Stationery Office

7   For further information about the work of the European Community on health promotion see www.europa.eu.int/health/ph/programmes/

8   International Union for Health Promotion and Education: www.iuhpe.nyu.edu

9   European Public Health Alliance: www.epha.org

10 World Federation of Public Health Associations: www.wfpha.org

11 For further information on Neighbourhood Renewal and Social Exclusion see:
   ■ www.cabinet-office.gov.uk/seu/2001/Action_Plan/default.htm
   ■ www.regeneration.dtlr.gov.uk/neighbourhood/index.htm
   ■ www.socialexclusionunit.gov.uk

12 Department of Health 1998, reprinted 2001 Tackling drugs to build a better Britain – the government's 10 year strategy for tackling drug misuse. London: The Stationery Office

13 Social Exclusion Unit 1999 Teenage pregnancy. Cm 4342. London: Teenage Pregnancy Unit

   For information on the Teenage Pregnancy Unit and Report see: www.teenagepregnancyunit.gov.uk and www.cabinet-office.gov.uk/seu/1999/teenpreg.pdf

14 We suggest that readers check websites for more up-to-date information, including information about NHS structures in Scotland, Wales and Northern Ireland: www.nhs.uk

15 The Queen's speech at the opening of the new parliament following the general election in 1997 included 'My Government will improve the National Health Service ... They will bring forward new arrangements for decentralisation and cooperation within the service and for ending the internal market.'

White Papers setting out the government's intentions were published in December 1997: Secretary of State for Health 1997 The new NHS: modern, dependable. London: The Stationery Office

A separate White Paper was published for Scotland:

Department of Health/Scottish Office 1997 Designed to care: renewing the National Health Service in Scotland. London: The Stationery Office

16 Department of Health 1999 Modernising health and social services. National priorities guidance 2000/01–2002/03. London: The Stationery Office

The inequalities agenda was further highlighted in a report by Sir Donald Acheson in 1998: Independent inquiry into inequalities in health. London: The Stationery Office

17 Department of Health 2000 The NHS Plan. A plan for investment. A plan for reform. London: The Stationery Office

18 Department of Health 2001 Shifting the balance of power within the NHS – securing delivery. London: The Stationery Office

19 Department of Health 2001 Department of Health, focusing on delivery. (The major changes followed a review in spring 2001 of the Department and its regional offices. The changes created a Department of Health with fewer priorities, a top team working across health and social care, open involvement of stakeholders and partners and decentralisation of activity and authority.)

20 This information can be found on the NHS website: www.nhs.uk

21 Health Development Agency 2000 Health Development Agency corporate plan 2000–03.

For more details see:
Annual report 2001. Health Development Agency, Holborn Gate, 330 High Holborn, London, WC1V 7BA. Tel: 020 7430 0850. www.hda-online.org.uk

22 Each NHS region in England established a Public Health Observatory (PHO) to undertake two roles outlined in Saving lives – our healthier nation. The first is to strengthen the availability and use of information about health at a local level, the second is to strengthen public health input into the cross-government initiatives for improving health and reducing inequalities.

For further information see Public Health Observatories in England: progress and prospects 2000/01 and visit the national website at: www.pho.org.uk

23 Health Development Agency 2001 Workplace health in small practices: issues for GPs and their staff. London: Heath Development Agency.

24 Health Education Board for Scotland (HEBS): www.hebs.scot.nhs.uk

25 Health Promotion Agency for Northern Ireland: www.healthpromotionagency.org.uk

Health Promotion Division of the National Assembly for Wales: www.hpw.wales.gov.uk

26 For further details of the objectives and procedures of the workforce development confederations see: www.wdconfeds.org./WDCGuidance.htm

27 Department of Health 1999 National service framework for mental health. London: Department of Health

Department of Health 2000 National service framework for coronary heart disease. London: Department of Health

Department of Health 2001 National service framework for older people. London: Department of Health

28 Department of Health 1999 Primary care groups: taking the next steps. HSC 1999/246: LAC (99)40. London: Department of Health

Department of Health 2001 Shifting the balance of power within the NHS – securing delivery. London: Department of Health

See also: www.doh.gov.uk/pricare/pcts.htm

29 Department of Health 1998 Health improvement programmes: planning for better health and better health care. London: The Stationery Office

For further information on HIMPs see: www.doh.gov.uk/hrforhimps

30 Department for the Environment, Transport and the Regions 2000 Local strategic partnerships: consultation document. London: DETR

For further information see: www.local-regions.dtlr.gov.uk/index.htm

31 Useful website addresses:

■ Primary care trusts: www.doh.gov.uk/pricare/pcts.htm
■ Health improvement and modernisation plans: www.doh.gov.uk/hrforhimps
■ Local strategic partnerships: www.local-regions.dtlr.gov.uk/index.htm
■ Sure Start: www.surestart.gov.uk
■ Community safety and crime reduction: www.crimere duction.gov.uk

- Quality Protects: www.doh.gov.uk/qualityprotects
- Regeneration: www.regeneration.dtlr.gov.uk

32 Department of Health 2001 Care trusts: emerging framework. London: Department of Health Publications. Email: doh@prolog.uk.com

33 For a review of the role of health education officers/health promotion specialists until the early 1990s, see:

Ewles L 1993 Paddling upstream for 50 years: the role of health education officers. Health Education Journal 52/3, 172–181

For a more recent review see:

Learmonth A, McMenamin M, McBride M, Watts C 2000 Health promotion and a public health approach in primary care: the role of specialist health promotion services. (A SHEPS Briefing Paper. Available from SHEPS, 64 Terregles Avenue, Pollockshields, Glasgow G41 4LX.)

See also:
Learmonth A 2001 The role of specialist health promotion services. In: Scriven A, Orme J (eds) Health promotion: professional perspectives, 2nd cdn. Basingstoke: Palgrave/Open University

34 Department of Health 2001 Primary care, general practice and the NHS plan, London: Department of Health

35 Department of Health 1999 Making a difference. Strengthening the nursing, midwifery and health visiting contribution to health and healthcare. London: The Stationery Office (www.doh.gov.uk/nurstrat)

36 For an analysis of the current role of community nurses see:

Wright C 2001 Community nursing: crossing boundaries to promote health. In: Scriven A, Orme J (eds) Health promotion: Professional perspectives 2nd edition. Basingstoke: Palgrave/Open University

37 See: Crafter H 1997 Health promotion in midwifery: principles and practice. London: Hodder Arnold

38 For further details of the reforms see: Department of Health 2000 The NHS Plan: a plan for investment, a plan for reform. Chapter 10, Changes for patients. London: The Stationery Office

39 Department of Health 2000 Complementary medicine information pack for primary care groups. London: Department of Health

Health Education Authority 1994 HEA guide to complementary therapies. London: HEA

An example of an innovative project in the primary care setting is the Hartcliffe and Withywood Complementary Therapies Project in Bristol, run by Hartcliffe Health and Environment Action Group (HHEAG) and Health Promotion Service Avon. For further details contact HHEAG, Gatehouse Centre, Harclive Road, Hartcliffe, Bristol.

40 Moran G 1996 Promoting health and local government. London: Health Education Authority and Local Government Management Board

41 Health Education Authority and Local Government Management Board 1997 Health on the agenda? A guide to health strategy development for local authorities. London: HEA

42 Social Exclusion Unit 2001 A new commitment to neighbourhood renewal. National strategy action plan. London: Cabinet Office. (www.cabinet-office.gov.uk/seu/2001/Action_Plan/default.htm)

43 For further information see: www.regeneration.dtlr.gov.uk/ndc.htm

44 For further information see: www.surestart.gov.uk

45 Department for the Environment, Transport and the Regions 2000 Preparing community strategies. Government guidance to local authorities. London: DETR. For further information see: www.local-regions.dtlr.gov.uk/index.htm

46 Department for the Environment, Transport and the Regions (2000) Local strategic partnerships: consultation document. London: DETR. For further information see: www.local-regions.dtlr.gov.uk/index.htm

47 For further information see: www.haznet.org.uk/; www.dfes.gov.uk/index.htm; www.dfee.gov.uk/employmentzones/map/map.htm

48 For further reading on health promotion in educational settings, see:

Cale L 1997 Health education in schools: in a state of good health? International Journal of Health Education 35(2), 59–62. (Argues that school health education is not in good health, and must fight for its survival and growth in a rapidly changing educational climate.)

Simnett I 1996 How to become a health promoting college. Healthlines, July/August, 18–19

49 Department for Education and Employment 1999 The national curriculum handbook for primary teachers in England. Key stages 1 and 2. London: The Stationery Office

Department for Education and Employment 1999 The national curriculum handbook for secondary teachers in England. Key stages 3 and 4. London: The Stationery Office

There is now a large and growing number of curriculum development materials, teachers' guides and classroom materials for health education in schools. These cover both broad health education programmes and work in specific subject areas such as alcohol, drugs, smoking, dental health, preventing heart disease and preventing child abuse. There are materials for primary, secondary and special schools and colleges, for use during initial teacher training, in-service training of teachers, and with school governors.

50 For details of the Open University Community Education materials, contact: Department of Community Education, The Open University, Walton Hall, Milton Keynes, MK7 6AA. Tel: 01908 653743.

51 Mitchinson, S 1995 A review of the health promotion and health beliefs of traditional and Project 2000 student nurses. Journal of Advanced Nursing 21, 356–363

52 See, for example:

Office for Public Management 1997 Achieving health gain through health promotion in a primary care-led NHS. London: Health Education Authority, p. 42

2 PLANNING AND MANAGING FOR EFFECTIVE PRACTICE

PART SUMMARY

Part 2 aims to provide guidance on how you can:

- Plan and evaluate your health promotion work using a basic framework.
- Identify the views and needs of the clients/users/receivers of health promotion, and set priorities for your work.
- Link your work to the efforts of colleagues and to local and national strategies.
- Use an 'evidence-based' approach, through using published research, doing your own research when necessary, and auditing your work, thus ensuring that your efforts are effective and provide value for money.
- Organise yourself and manage your work in order to be effective and efficient.
- Develop skills to work more effectively with colleagues and people from other organisations.

In Chapter 5 we set out a seven-stage planning and evaluation cycle, which will help you to clarify what you are trying to achieve, what you are going to do, and how you will know whether you are succeeding. We discuss the meaning of terms such as aims, objectives and targets, and provide guidance on how to specify them.

In Chapter 6 we consider what a 'need' for health promotion means, and describe the sources of information you require to identify the needs of a community, a group, or an individual. We provide guidelines on how to gather and apply information in order to assess needs and set priorities.

Chapter 7 provides guidance in greater depth on the knowledge and skills required to plan health promotion activities effectively, including how to find and use published research. We include guidance on how you can contribute to national and local public health strategic plans and complement what other people are doing. We discuss the meaning of 'evidence-based health

PART SUMMARY

promotion' and how you can carry out small-scale research, audit your activities and ensure value for money. We end with a description of the key steps required to undertake a health impact assessment.

In Chapter 8 we focus on how you can develop the skills to manage yourself and your work effectively, including managing information, writing reports, using time effectively, planning project work, managing change and working for quality.

Chapter 9 is about how to work with other people, including communicating with colleagues, coordination and teamwork, participating in meetings, and working in health partnerships with other organisations.

5 The Basic Planning and Evaluation Process

SUMMARY

In this chapter we outline a seven-stage planning and evaluation cycle useful in the everyday work of health promoters:

1. Identify needs and priorities.
2. Set aims and objectives.
3. Decide the best way of achieving aims.
4. Identify resources.
5. Plan evaluation methods.
6. Set an action plan.
7. Action!

We give examples of aims, objectives and action plans, and exercises on setting aims and objectives and using the planning framework to turn ideas into action.

This chapter is about planning and evaluation at the level of your daily work in health promotion. It provides a basic framework for you to use to plan and evaluate your health promotion activities, whether you work with clients on a one-to-one or group basis, or undertake specific projects or programmes.

The Planning Process

Planning is a process that ends up with a plan; at its very simplest, a plan should give you the answers to three questions:

- What am I trying to achieve?
- What am I going to do?
- How will I know whether I have been successful?

If you are really clear on these three issues you should be well on the way to effective and efficient health promotion work.

The first question ('What am I trying to achieve?') is concerned with identifying needs and priorities, then with being clear about your specific aims and objectives, which we discuss in more detail below.

The second question ('What am I going to do?') can be helpfully broken down into smaller steps:

- Select the best way of achieving your aims from a variety of possible ways.
- Identify the resources you are going to use.
- Set a clear action plan of who does what and when.

To answer the third question ('How will I know whether I have been successful?') you will need to include plans for evaluation in your overall plan. This highlights a very important point: evaluation is an integral part of your overall plan; it should not be tacked on as an afterthought. It is all too easy to plan a project, carry it out, and then think about evaluating it, often too late to capture the information you need.

Putting these together, we have a seven-stage flowchart (Figure 5.1).

There are three key points to note about using the flowchart. One is that the arrows on the flowchart lead you round in a circle. This is because, as you carry out your plan and evaluation, you will probably find things that make you re-think and change your original ideas. For example, things you might want to change could include: working on a client need you found you had overlooked; scaling down your objectives because they were too ambitious; or using different educational or publicity materials because you found that they were not as useful or effective as you had hoped.

The second point is that the main direction of the arrows is anti-clockwise, but in reality planning is not a tidy process. You may actually start at Stage 6, with a basic idea of something you would like to do. Thinking more about it may lead you to clarify exactly what your aims are (Stage 2). Next, you might think about what resources you are going to need (Stage 4) and realise that you do not have enough time or money

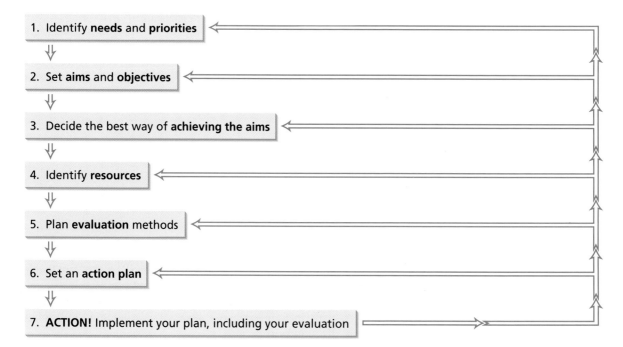

Fig 5.1   **A Flowchart for Planning and Evaluating Health Promotion**

1. Identify **needs** and **priorities**

2. Set **aims** and **objectives**

3. Decide the best way of **achieving the aims**

4. Identify **resources**

5. Plan **evaluation** methods

6. Set an **action plan**

7. **ACTION!** Implement your plan, including your evaluation

to do what you had in mind, so you go back to Stage 2 and modify your aims. Then you think about the best way of achieving your aims (Stage 3) and work out an action plan (Stage 6). After that, you start to think seriously about how you will know whether you are successful (Stage 5) and you put your evaluation plans into your action plan (Stage 6 again). This is not meant to imply that you are muddle-headed or 'doing it wrong'. On the contrary, you are continually reviewing and improving your plan, using the framework appropriately to help you keep on course.

The third point is that planning takes place at many levels. If you are embarking on a major project, you will need to take time to plan it in depth and detail. If you are simply planning a short one-to-one session with a client you will still need to plan, and to go through all the stages, but the process might take only a few minutes and may not even be written down.

For example, a chiropodist seeing a patient with a foot care problem may identify that the patient needs knowledge and skills in cutting toenails correctly. She decides that her aim is to give the patient basic information and training on this. She will know if she has been successful by getting feedback from the patient about how he managed next time she sees him. She identifies a leaflet that she can give the patient to reinforce what she says. She decides on an action plan of explanation, demonstration and then getting the patient to practise. She reviews the patient's toe-nail cutting skills next time she sees him, reinforcing or correcting as necessary. All this planning takes place inside the chiropodist's head, and is an integral part of her everyday professional practice.

We will now look at each stage of the planning and evaluation flowchart.

Stage 1. Identify Needs and Priorities

How do you find out what health promotion is needed? If you think you already know, what are you basing your judgement on? Who has identified the need: you, your clients or someone else? These questions begin to show that identifying need is a complex process, which we look at it in depth in the next chapter.

See Chapter 6.

You may have a long list of health promotion needs you would like to respond to, but you cannot do everything, so another question is how to establish your priorities. Again, we discuss this in detail in the next chapter. All there is to say now is that you must have a clear view about which needs you are responding to, and what your priorities are.

Stage 2. Set Aims and Objectives

This is the point where you ask yourself 'What exactly am I trying to achieve?' and go on asking it until you have the answer very clearly defined.

People use a whole gamut of words to describe statements of 'What I am trying to achieve?' – aims, objectives, targets, goals, mission, purpose, achievement, result, product, outcomes. Though there is no universal agreement about the precise meaning of these words, it can be helpful to think of them as forming a hierarchy (Figure 5.2). At the top of the hierarchy are words that tell you why your job exists, such as your job purpose or your mission. In the middle of the hierarchy are words that describe what you are trying to do in general terms, such as your goals or aims. At the bottom

Fig 5.2   **A Hierarchy of Aims**

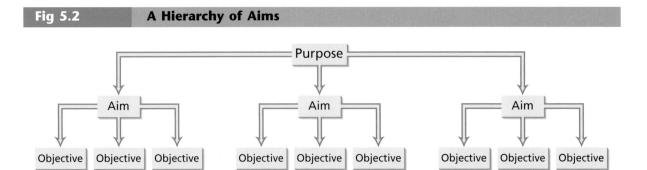

of the hierarchy are words that describe in specific detail what you are trying to do, such as targets or objectives.

It is worth noting that objectives can be of different kinds. *Health* objectives are usually expressed as the outcome or end state to be achieved in terms of health status, such as reduced rates of illness or death. However, in health promotion work objectives are often expressed in terms of a step along the way towards an ultimate improvement in the health of individuals or populations.

In health education work, *educational* objectives are framed in terms of the knowledge, attitudes or behaviour to be exhibited by the learner. Objectives can also be in terms of *other kinds of changes*, such as a change in health policy (e.g. introducing a no-smoking policy in a workplace) or health promotion practice (e.g. providing health information in minority ethnic languages or starting a coronary rehabilitation programme).

See the section below on setting educational objectives.

A further point is that the term 'targets' is increasingly used in health promotion. Targets usually specify how the achievement of an objective will be *measured*, in terms of quantity, quality, and time (the date by which the objective will be achieved). So *a health target* can be defined as a measurable improvement in health status, by a given date, which achieves a health objective. This is the approach used in national strategies for health, such as *Saving lives – our healthier nation*,[1] the *national service frameworks*[2] and *The NHS Plan*.[3] A summary of the targets and ways of measuring progress can be found in the *NHS Plan technical supplement on target setting for health improvement*.[4]

There is more about national strategies and targets in Chapter 7, section National Health Strategies.

The objectives are framed as *health objectives*, and the targets are framed as *health targets* (changes in rates of death or illness by a specific date), *behaviour targets* (such as changes in population rates of smoking or drinking by a specific date) or *progress measures* (such as the number of people attending a smoking cessation service and the number setting a date when they plan to stop smoking – a 'quit date').

We now turn to how the individual health promoter sets aims, objectives and targets.

When planning health promotion initiatives, it is the levels of aims, objectives and targets that we need to focus on. (We choose to use the words aims, objectives and targets in our discussion here, but, as we said above, many other terms are used, such as goals and outcomes.)

Your aims (or aim – there does not have to be more than one) are broad statements of what you are trying to achieve. Your objectives are much more specific, and setting these is a critical stage in the planning process.

Objectives are the desired end state (or result, or outcome) to be achieved within a specified time period. They are not tasks or activities. Objectives are:

- **Challenging**. The objective should provide you with a challenge. It should 'stretch' you.
- **Attainable**. On the other hand, it should be both realistic and achievable within the constraints of your situation.
- **As measurable as possible**. You should try to identify your objectives in terms that are as measurable as possible, for example specifying quantity, quality and a time when they will be achieved (i.e. you are clear about your *targets*). For example (using the example in Exercise 5.1), an objective of 'to improve access to health information through the use of videos...' has been improved by working out the appropriate number of videos and languages, and then specifying the target as 'to have ten videos in six languages...'
- **Relevant**. It should be consistent with the aims of the organisation and with the overall aims of your job.

It is often difficult to distinguish between aims and objectives and action plans. For example, a dietician who wants to improve the information she gives to patients may describe her aim as 'to produce an information leaflet' – but this is also her objective and her action plan. The answer is to think it through further, and ask 'Why produce a leaflet? What am I aiming to achieve by producing the leaflet?' It then becomes clearer that the aim is to improve patient compliance with dietary treatment, and one of the objectives is to improve patients' understanding of their dietary instructions. The action is to produce the leaflet. The importance of actually thinking through your aims and objectives in this way is that it helps you to be absolutely clear about *why* you are doing something, not just *what* you are doing. Failure to think through this stage means that health promoters waste time and energy ploughing ahead with 'a good idea' only to realise, too late, that what they are doing is not actually achieving what they want.

Exercise 5.1   **Clarifying Your Purpose, Aims and Objectives**

Think about this example of a health promoter's purpose, aims and objectives.

Mark is a health promoter working for a local authority. His *purpose* is to reduce inequalities in health in the population living and working in the borough. To do this, one of his *aims* is to improve levels of health knowledge of black and ethnic minority groups. One of his *objectives* is to improve access to health information through the use of videos. He sets a target of having a selection of ten health videos in six languages available in 25 shops within four months.

Now:

1. **Thinking of your own job, write down what you believe to be its mission or purpose.**
2. **Then give an example of one of the health promotion aims you are trying to achieve.**
3. **Finally, give an example of an objective you are trying to achieve, in fulfilment of the aim you selected.**

If you can't find a real-life example, make up an example of what you would like to do if you had the opportunity.

Setting Educational Objectives

If your health promotion activity is a health education programme, it is useful to plan in terms of *educational* objectives.

Educationalists traditionally often think of objectives (sometimes called 'learning outcomes') in terms of what the clients will gain. Furthermore, the objectives are considered to be of three kinds: what the educator would like the clients to *know*, *feel* and *do* as a result of the education. (In the language of the educationalist, these may be referred to as cognitive, affective and behavioural objectives.)

Objectives About 'Knowing'

These are concerned with giving information, explaining it, ensuring that the client understands it, and thus increasing the client's knowledge. For example, explaining the pros and cons of vaccination to a baby's parents has the objective that they will know what the advantages and disadvantages of vaccinations are.

Objectives About 'Feeling'

These objectives are concerned with attitudes, beliefs, values and opinions. These are complex psychological concepts, but the important feature to note now is that they are all concerned with how people feel. Objectives about 'feelings' are about clarifying, forming or changing attitudes, beliefs, values or opinions. In the example above, when a health educator is educating parents about vaccination, in addition to the 'knowledge' objective, there may be an objective about helping anxious parents to feel less worried about it.

Objectives About 'Doing'

These objectives are concerned with a client's skills and actions. For example, teaching a routine of physical exercises or teaching a diabetic how to give himself an injection has the objective that clients acquire practical skills and are able to do specific tasks.

In health education, educational objectives are rarely concerned exclusively with knowing, feeling or doing – a mixture is usually required. For example, when advising a mother about feeding her toddler, a health educator probably has several objectives in mind, which she may be planning to achieve within three home visits:

- The objective of ensuring that the mother knows which foods are nourishing for her child and which are best given in restricted amounts.
- The objective of changing the mother's erroneous belief that sugar is essential to give her child energy, and relieving her anxiety that her healthy child's 'food fads' may cause serious ill health.
- The objective that the mother learns what to do at meal times when her child has a tantrum about eating.

To summarise the key points about setting aims and objectives:

- The focus is on *what you are trying to achieve.*
- Be as specific as possible – avoid vague, woolly notions of what you want to achieve.

Exercise 5.2	Setting Aims and Objectives

Yewtree scheme

The three practices at Yewtree Health Centre have agreed to establish physical activity assessment sessions, backed up by a display in the shared waiting area, with the aim of reducing the incidence of coronary heart disease in the practice populations.

The detailed objectives are:

1.   To raise the users' awareness of the link between inadequate exercise and coronary heart disease, and the part which individuals can play in reducing their own vulnerability to the disease.
2.   To assess, and advise about, individuals' physical fitness levels and help them to prepare an appropriate exercise action programme based on those results.
3.   To monitor and evaluate, on a continuing basis, the effectiveness of the fitness testing, in respect of the resources involved and the reduction in vulnerability to heart disease.

Ask yourself the following questions:

1.   **Do the objectives match the characteristics of objectives described above? Are they challenging, attainable, as measurable as possible, and relevant?**
2.   **How would you suggest changing the objectives?**

- Express your objectives in ways that can be measured if possible – How much? How many? When?
- Do not get bogged down in terminology – it does not matter whether you talk about goals, aims, objectives, targets or outcomes. The key principle is *to be very clear about what you are trying to achieve.*

Stage 3. Decide the Best Way of Achieving the Aims

Occasionally, there might be only one possible way of accomplishing your aims and objectives. Usually, however, there will be a range of options. In Case Study 5.1, Jim has a number of options about how to achieve his objective of raising awareness with publicans of the feasibility and advantages of smoke-free areas in pubs. He could write to the breweries, he could drop leaflets in the pubs, he could lobby consumer groups to take up the cause, he could find out if there are any local meetings of publicans and ask to speak at them, he could conduct a campaign in the local media, he could write to the trade journals which publicans read, or he could try to meet each publican face-to-face. Or he could do two or more of these together.

You are therefore faced with the problem of how to identify the best option. There is no one 'best buy' for health promotion as a whole. Factors to consider include:

Case studies 5.1 and 5.2 — Aims and Objectives for Health Promotion Projects

Case Study 5.1

Jim is an environmental health officer. His project is to tackle the problem of smoky atmospheres in pubs. This fits in with the overall purpose of his job, which is to work for a health-enhancing environment. Jim works out that his **aim** is to work with local publicans to set up smoke-free areas in pubs. He researches the subject in detail, looking at the results achieved from similar projects and working out how much time and money it is likely to take. He then decides that it is reasonable to set his **objective** as:

■ within 6 months to have raised awareness of the feasibility and advantages of a smoke-free area with 10 publicans, and worked with at least five to set up smoke-free areas.

Case Study 5.2

Sue is a nurse specialising in coronary care. Her project is to run patient education programmes so that discharged patients know how to look after themselves. This fits in with the overall purpose of her job, which is to care for patients while they are in hospital, and maximise their chances of a healthy life afterwards.

Sue decides that her **aim** is that patients will have participated in a cardiac rehabilitation programme for post-heart-attack patients. Her **objectives** are:

■ That every patient, before leaving hospital, knows what they are advised to do about diet, exercise, smoking and stress control.
■ That every patient will be confident and competent to put this advice into practice.
■ That every patient, and their carers and relatives, will have had an opportunity to discuss questions and anxieties with a qualified member of the staff.

Sue's programme is a continuous course of group sessions each week, with each session focusing on a specific issue. So each individual session also has a set of objectives. Objectives for the session on 'Eating well when you go home', for example, include:

■ Patients will understand the basic principles of a healthy diet: low fat, low salt, low sugar and high fibre.
■ Patients will know which foods they can eat in unlimited amounts, which they should restrict and which they should avoid.
■ Patients will know what their ideal weight should be.
■ Patients who are overweight will have devised a personal weight-loss plan.

■ Which methods are the most appropriate and effective for your aims and objectives? (This is explored in more detail below.)
■ Which methods will be acceptable to the consumers?
■ Which methods will be easiest?
■ Which methods are cheapest?
■ Which methods are the most acceptable to the people involved?
■ Which methods do you find comfortable to use? (Bear in mind that you may feel uncomfortable with some methods at first, but that this can be overcome with experience to build your confidence.)

There is more about evidence for success, cost effectiveness and value for money in Chapter 7, and Part 3 of this book covers how to use these methods to develop the necessary competency.

Looking at the first of these questions (Which methods are most appropriate and effective for your aims?), there is an accumulated body of evidence that helps to identify effective methods for particular aims.[5] Table 5.1 identifies the range of aims, grouped into categories, and the appropriate and effective methods for achieving them. This provides a general guideline, to which there may be exceptions.

Table 5.1	Aims and Methods in Health Promotion
Aim	**Appropriate method**
Health awareness goal Raising awareness, or consciousness, of health issues	Talks Group work Mass media Displays and exhibitions Campaigns
Improving knowledge Providing information	One-to-one teaching Displays and exhibitions Written materials Mass media (including the Internet) Campaigns Group teaching
Self-empowering Improving self-awareness, self-esteem, decision-making	Group work Practising decision-making Values clarification Social skills training Simulation, gaming and role play Assertiveness training Counselling
Changing attitudes and behaviour Changing the lifestyles of individuals	Group work Skills training Self-help groups One-to-one instruction Group or individual therapy Written material Advice
Societal/environmental change Changing the physical or social environment	Positive action for under-served groups Lobbying Pressure groups Community development Community-based work Advocacy schemes Environmental measures Planning and policy making Organisational change Enforcement of laws and regulations

You may have decided on more than one of these categories of aims. For example, the inputs that contribute towards changing the behaviour of individuals can be complemented by societal changes, so that together they are more effective than either intervention alone. (This is known as 'synergy'.) So, for example, to reduce the over-consumption of alcohol by young people, you could:

■ Provide health education about alcohol as part of school personal and social education programmes.
■ Provide educational rehabilitation programmes for young drink–drive offenders.

- Work with young people to promote the social acceptability of drinking non-alcoholic drinks.
- Lobby for an increase in alcohol taxation.

The example in Figure 5.3 shows the range of aims and methods that might be used to promote healthy eating. We do not suggest that all of these would be used by a health promoter at any one time – they are given here to illustrate the range of possibilities.

Fig 5.3   Aims and Methods for the Promotion of Healthy Eating

AIM: Health awareness

Possible **methods:**
- articles in local newspapers
- exhibition on healthy eating and weight control, including weighing machine, height/weight charts, information on physical activity and healthy eating cookery demonstrations
- posters on nutritional themes in health service premises
- programmes on local radio

AIM: Social change

Possible **methods:**
- working with parents and teachers to encourage the sale of nutritious foods in school tuck shops
- working with NHS caterers to devise lower fat, higher fibre hospital food for patients and staff
- lobbying food manufacturers to include clearer information on food labels

AIM: Knowledge

Possible **methods:**
- nutrition teaching as part of science and health education in schools
- advice and help for patients from health professionals in clinical settings
- talks on aspects of nutrition to community groups

PROMOTION OF HEALTHY EATING

AIM: Behaviour change

Possible **methods:**
- groups for healthy eating and weight control
- individual support for patients on special diets
- groups and cooking clubs to develop skills and confidence in preparing healthier meals for families
- recipes and ideas for nutritious packed lunches for schoolchildren

AIM: Self-awareness, attitude change decision-making

Possible **methods:**
- informal group work with antenatal clients and pre-retirement groups
- work with individual clients on whether to lose weight, cut down on salt, or increase fibre

Stage 4. Identify Resources

What resources are you going to use? You need to clarify what resources are already available (which may be more than you think at first), what you are going to need, what additional resources you are going to have to acquire, and whether you will need money. A number of different kinds of resources can be identified.

You

Your experience, knowledge, skills, time, enthusiasm and energy are a vital resource.

People Who Can Help You

It helps to identify all the people with something to offer. This may include colleagues and other people with relevant expertise who can advise and help you make your plans, clerical and secretarial staff who can help with administration, technicians and artists who can help with exhibitions, displays and teaching/publicity materials.

Your Client or Client Group

These are another key resource. Clients may have knowledge, skills, enthusiasm, energy and time, which can be used and built upon. In a group, clients can share their knowledge and previous experience and in this way help each other to learn and change. An ex-client can be a very valuable resource too. For example, someone who has successfully lost weight, an ex-smoker or a person who has undergone a particular experience can be a great help to clients who are grappling with similar problems and experiences.

People Who Influence Your Client or Client Group

These may include clients' relatives, friends, volunteers, patients' associations and self-help groups. It may also be possible to harness the help of significant people in the community who are regarded as opinion leaders or trendsetters, such as political figures, religious leaders or pop stars.

Existing Policies and Plans

National and local plans, which your work could contribute to, are discussed in Chapter 7.

For example, if you are planning to do work on 'safer sex' to help prevent the spread of sexually transmitted infections and HIV and reduce unwanted pregnancies, find out if there is already a policy on promoting sexual health in your area. If there is, you can use it to back up the work you plan to do. Also find out whether your work fits into the national Strategy for Sexual Health and HIV.[6]

Existing Facilities and Services

Find out what facilities already exist and whether they are fully utilised; for example, sports centres offering facilities for exercise and local classes or groups on cooking for healthy eating.

Material Resources

These might include leaflets, posters, display/publicity materials – or, if you are planning health promotion involving group work, you need resources such as rooms, space, seats, audiovisual equipment and teaching/learning materials.

Stage 5. Plan Evaluation Methods

How will you know whether your health promotion is successful? And how will you measure success? There are no easy answers to these crucial questions about evaluation. On a large scale, sophisticated research is required. However, this should not deter health promoters; modest methods of evaluating the everyday practice of health promotion can, and should, be used routinely.

Defining Terms

What is meant by 'evaluation'? Simply, making a judgement about the value of something – in our case, about the value of a health promotion activity (whether it is a health education programme, for example, a community project or an awareness-raising campaign to change local policy). Evaluation is the process of assessing *what* has been achieved and *how* it has been achieved. It means looking critically at the activity or programme, working out what was good about it, what was bad about it, and how it could be improved.

The judgement can be about the *outcome* (what has been achieved): whether you achieved the objectives which you set. So, for example, you should judge whether people understood the recommended limits for alcohol consumption as a result of your 'sensible drinking' education, whether people in a particular community became more articulate about their health needs as a result of your community development work, whether you achieved media coverage for your campaign.

Judgement can also be about the *process* (how it has been achieved): whether the most appropriate methods were used, whether they were used in the most effective way, and whether they gave value for money. So, for example, you could consider whether the video-based discussion you used in your teaching programme was the best teaching method to use, whether the community development approach you chose was the most appropriate one in the circumstances, or whether you would have achieved more public awareness with less money if you had opted for a media 'stunt' with possible free news coverage rather than an expensive advertising and leaflet campaign.

Key terms often used in discussions about evaluation are defined in the Jargon Explained section at the end of this book.[7]

Why Evaluate?

You need to be clear about why you are evaluating your work, because this will affect the way you do it and the amount of effort you put in. Some reasons could be:

- To improve your own practice: next time you do something similar, you will build on your successes and learn from any mistakes.

- To help other people to improve their practice: if you tell people about your experiences, it can help them to improve their practice as well. It is vital to publicise failures as well as successes, to prevent other people reinventing square wheels.
- To justify the use of the resources that went into the work, and to provide evidence to support the case for doing this work in the future.
- To give you the satisfaction of knowing how useful or effective your work has been; in other words, for your own job satisfaction.
- To identify any unplanned or unexpected outcomes that could be important. For example, a publicity campaign to deter young people from taking drugs could have the opposite effect by unwittingly glamorising drug-taking and making it appear to be a more common activity than it really is.

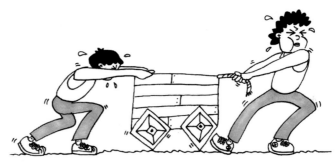

Publicise your failures as well as your successes, to prevent other people reinventing square wheels

Who For?

Who will be using your evaluation data? The answer to this affects what questions you ask, how much depth and detail you go into and how you present the information.

If you are solely assessing how well a health education session went, for your own benefit so you can change it appropriately next time you run a similar session, you will simply make a judgement on how you think it went based on your observation and the learners' reactions, and make a few notes. But if you are writing a report for your manager, or for a body that you want to fund the work, you need to think through what questions those people will expect to be answered, and how much detail they will want.

For example, a group of health visitors evaluating a pilot scheme for a telephone advisory service at evenings and weekends need an evaluation report after six months for their manager, who is funding the service. What will the manager need to know? At the very least, she will probably need a clear indication of the use made of the service (how many people used it, the characteristics of the users, e.g. whether they were first-time parents, how much it was used, what sort of issues people rang about?), what the clients gained from it, and how much it cost. It would be helpful for the health visitors to ask their manager what evaluation data will be required at the planning stage of the project, so that the appropriate data can be collected from the start.

Assessing the Outcome

Looking first at outcome measures, you need to go back to the objectives you set, and plan how you are going to get the answer to the question 'have I achieved these objectives?' Objectives are about changes you aim to make: changes in people's knowledge or behaviour, for example, or changes in policies or ways of working. Large long-term health promotion projects may also have objectives about changes in health status. The following list indicates the kinds of changes that may be reflected in your objectives, and what methods you might use to assess or measure those changes.

Changes in Health Awareness Can Be Assessed By:

- Measuring the interest shown by consumers, e.g. how many people took up offers of leaflets, how many people enquired about preventive services, how many people visited a website.
- Monitoring changes in demand for health-related services.
- Analysis of media coverage.
- Questionnaires, interviews, discussion, observation with individuals or groups.

Changes in Knowledge or Attitude Can Be Assessed By:

- Observing changes in what clients say and do: does this show a change in awareness and attitude?
- Interviews and discussions involving question-and-answer between health promoter and clients.
- Discussion and observation on how clients apply knowledge to real-life situations and how they solve problems.
- Observing how clients demonstrate their knowledge of newly acquired skills.
- Written tests, or questionnaires that require clients to answer questions about what they know. The results can be compared with those of tests taken before the health promotion activity or from a comparable group that has not received the health promotion.

Behaviour Change Can Be Assessed By:

- Observing what clients do.
- Recording behaviour. This could be regular records, such as numbers attending a health promotion clinic or bringing their children to be vaccinated. It could be a periodical inventory, such as a follow-up questionnaire or interview to check on smoking habits six and twelve months after attending a stop-smoking group. Records of client behaviour can be compared with those of comparable groups in other areas, or with national average figures.

Policy Changes Can Be Assessed By:

- Policy statements and implementation, such as increased introduction of 'environmentally friendly' products in everyday use, or healthy eating choices in workplaces and schools.
- Legislative changes, such as increased restriction on tobacco advertising.
- Changes in the availability of health-promoting products, facilities and services, such as low-cost recreational facilities or more smoking cessation advice.
- Changes in procedures or organisation, such as more time being given to patient education.

Changes to the Physical Environment Can Be Assessed By:

■ Measuring changes such as levels of pollutants in the air, traffic or pedestrian flows or the amount of open green space available to the public within a defined area.

Changes in Health Status Can Be Assessed By:

■ Keeping records of simple health indicators such as weight, blood pressure, pulse rates on standard exercise, or cholesterol levels.
■ Health surveys to identify larger scale changes in health behaviour or self-reported health status.
■ Analysis of trends in routine health statistics such as infant mortality rates or hospital admission rates.

Help with these is in Chapter 7, section Doing Your Own Small Scale Research, and Part 3 of this book.

It will be seen from this list that common methods are observation, asking questions, holding discussions and giving questionnaires.

Assessing the Process

Having looked at assessing the outcome, we now turn to assessing the process. This means looking at what went on during the process of implementation, and making judgements about it. Was it done as cheaply and quickly as possible? Was the quality as good as you wished? Were the appropriate methods and materials used? You may, for instance, achieve your objectives, but in a time-consuming, costly or inefficient way, so it is important to evaluate the process as well as identify whether you have achieved your desired outcome.

How are you going to assess the process? We suggest three key aspects: measuring the input, self-evaluation by asking yourself questions and getting feedback from other people.

Measuring the Input

This is essential if you are going to make judgements about whether the outcome was worthwhile. You need to record everything that went into your health promotion activity, in terms of time, money and materials. Then you can make an informed judgement about whether the outcome was worth the cost.

Self-evaluation

Ask yourself 'What did I do well?' 'What would I like to change?' and 'How could I improve that next time?' All kinds of health promotion can be subjected to this kind of process evaluation, whether it is one-to-one health education with a client, facilitating a self-help group, undertaking community work, developing and implementing policies, or lobbying for organisational changes.

An important point to note about self-evaluation is the value of emphasising the positive. It is all too easy to criticise oneself in a negative, destructive way, which is unhelpful because it erodes confidence. Always look for the positive, identify the things you feel pleased with, and look for constructive ways forward about things that could be improved.

Feedback From Other People

See section in Chapter 10
Asking Questions and
Getting Feedback.

Giving and receiving feedback is an essential skill for every health promoter. Getting feedback from a trusted colleague on your work performance is a valuable form of peer evaluation. Asking for, and getting, feedback from your manager should be part of the regular monitoring of your performance.

Obtaining feedback from the clients or users themselves should also be part of assessing the process of every intervention. The important thing is to encourage an atmosphere of openness and honesty, where problems can be confronted without people feeling blamed or judged as bad people. It can be done in many ways; simply observing clients and users accurately is an important tool. Do they look anxious or relaxed? Do they look interested and alert or bored and detached? You can also ask for feedback in various ways – through a suggestions box, through a sensitive and accessible complaints procedure, through noting any spontaneous verbal feedback you receive, or through asking questions.

Stage 6. Set an Action Plan

Now that you know:

■ what you are trying to achieve and have identified the best way to go about it
■ how to evaluate it
■ what resources you need

you can get down to planning in detail exactly what you are going to do. This means writing a detailed statement of who will do what, with what resources and by when.

It is helpful, especially if you are tackling a large project, to break down your plan into smaller, manageable elements ('bite-sized pieces'). One way of doing this is by thinking in terms of *key events*. Draw up a schedule showing the key events that are planned to happen at particular points in time. Key events plans specify deadlines that must be met by the people involved and can be useful in planning health promotion campaigns, for example.

For more discussion about
the skills of project
management, see Chapter 8,
section Managing Project
Work.

Another way of breaking down a large project is by *milestone* planning. This is different from key events planning: instead of listing events, it lists a series of dates at fixed intervals (the 'milestones') and shows what must have happened by each of them. Example 5.1 illustrates both types of plans.

Stage 7. Action!

This is the stage in which you actually *do* your health promotion, remembering to evaluate the process as you go along.

To summarise planning:

I once did meet six serving men (or women)
They served me well and true
Their names were what and why and when
And how and where and who!

Example 5.1	Action Plans

A **key events plan** drawn up by a health visitor who plans to set up a health stall in a local supermarket could look like this:

1. *Discuss with my manager* at October meeting.
2. *Identify support from colleagues* by November.
3. *Approach supermarket manager* (before Christmas rush); agree space and times.
4. *Convene planning group* of colleagues and health promotion officer in January to sort out who will do what and when, and evaluation plans, and identify the resources required.
5. *Set up first stall* in March.

A brief **milestone plan** for the early .stages of setting up a community health project could be like this, in a framework of three-monthly 'milestones':

January–March 2003	Steering group agrees job description for community health worker. Job advertised.
By end of June 2003	Interviews; appointment made. Community worker takes up post.
By end of September 2003	Community worker induction programme completed.
By end of December 2003	First progress report to Steering Group.

Exercise 5.3	Ideas Into Action: Planning a Health Promotion Project

Work alone or in a small group.

Think of an area of health promotion where there is an identified need, and it is within the remit of your job to meet that need. It could be an established area of work such as antenatal education, patient education, teaching food hygiene, or an area of new work you would like to tackle. (If you are not currently in a job which involves health promotion, think of a health-related project you would like to tackle in your personal life, or a project for any voluntary/community group you are associated with, or just imagine what you would like to do if you had the opportunity.)

Work through the following stages of the planning cycle. Start by writing each of the following headings at the top of a separate large sheet of paper, and then work through them:

1. **Aims and objectives**

   Ask yourself 'What am I trying to achieve?' Identify your broad aim, or aims, then be more specific and identify your objectives.

2. **The best way of achieving my aims**

   Think of all the ways in which you could achieve your aims and identify the best way.

3. **Resources**

Identify the resources you already have available and any extra ones you will need.

4. **Evaluation**

Ask yourself 'How will I know if I am succeeding?' Identify how you will evaluate both the process and outcome of your work.

5. **Action plan**

Identify who will do what, with what resources, and by when.

Be aware that when you are thinking about one section, it may have implications for the others, so you may find yourself going back to modify and refine what you have already written.

PRACTICE POINTS

- Health promotion work benefits from being planned and evaluated in a systematic way.

- The following seven-stage planning cycle can help you to do this:

  1. Identify needs and priorities: find out what your clients need, and work out your priorities.

  2. Set aims and objectives: be clear about exactly what you are trying to achieve, and by when.

  3. Decide the best way of achieving aims: think about which methods are likely to be effective, will be acceptable to your clients, will give value for money, and that you have the competence to use.

  4. Identify resources: people (their time, knowledge and skills), things (existing policies and plans, facilities, educational materials) and money.

  5. Plan evaluation methods: work out why you need to evaluate, who for, and what you will do.

  6. Set an action plan: who will do what, with what resources and by when.

  7. Action: this is the stage where you actually do your health promotion, remembering to evaluate as you go along.

Recommended Reading

On Planning

An outline and discussion of several models of programme planning:

➤ Naidoo J, Wills J 2000 Health promotion: foundations for practice, 2nd edn. Chapter 18, Planning health promotion interventions. London: Baillière Tindall

A framework for developing and assessing health promotion interventions:

➤ South and West Devon Health Authority 2000 A Seven Keys Framework for Effectiveness in Health Promotion. Dartington: S & WDHA and University of Bristol

On Evaluation of Health Promotion Activities

A useful discussion and guide to evaluating health promotion:

➤ Katz J, Peberdy A, Douglas J (eds) 2001 Promoting health: knowledge and practice, 2nd edn. Chapter 16, Evaluation in health promotion: why do it? and Chapter 17, Evaluation design. Basingstoke: Open University and Palgrave

A study of the theory and practice of evaluation, written by leading figures in the field of health promotion:

➤ Scott D, Weston R 1998 Evaluating health promotion. Cheltenham: Stanley Thornes

An in-depth look at questions of defining success, issues in evaluation research, indicators of success and measures of performance, which reviews effectiveness in different settings of schools, health care, workplace and communities, and the use of mass media:

➤ Tones K, Tilford S 2001 Health promotion: effectiveness, efficiency and equity, 3rd edn. Cheltenham: Nelson Thornes

On Planning and Evaluating Health Promotion with Older People

➤ Squire A 2002 Health and well-being for older people: foundations for practice. London: Baillière Tindall in association with the Royal College of Nursing

On Planning and Evaluation of Health Alliances

A useful framework for planning and evaluating health promotion work by alliances of agencies working together:

➤ Funnell R, Oldfield K, Speller V 1995 Towards healthier alliances: a tool for planning evaluating and developing healthy alliances. London: Health Education Authority

Examples of Health Promotion Work Planned, Implemented and Evaluated in a Range of Settings with Various Client Groups

➤ Kerr J 2000 Community health promotion: challenges for practice. London: Baillière Tindall. (Section 2 includes chapters on work around pregnant women and families, men's health, young people, homeless women, ethnic minority groups, people with HIV, older people)
➤ Naidoo J, Wills J 1998 Practising health promotion: dilemmas and challenges. London: Baillière Tindall. (Part 3 includes chapters on work around accident prevention, heart disease and stroke, cancer, sexual health, and mental health)

Notes and References

1 Department of Health 1999 Saving lives: our healthier nation. London: The Stationery Office. (www.doh.gov.uk/ohn.htm)

2 Examples of National Service Frameworks:

Department of Health 1999 The national service framework: mental health – Modern standards and service models. London: Department of Health (www.doh.gov.uk/nsf/mentalhealth)

Department of Health 2000 The national service framework for coronary heart disease. London: Department of Health. (www.doh.gov.uk/nsf/coronary.htm)

Department of Health 2001 The national service framework for older people. London: Department of Health. (www.doh.gov.uk/nsf/olderpeople.htm)

3 Department of Health 2000 The NHS plan (CM 4818–1). London: The Stationery Office. (www.doh.gov.uk/nhsplan)

4 Department of Health 2001 NHS plan technical supplement on target setting for health improvement. London: Department of Health statistics division and central monitoring unit. (www.doh.gov.uk/nhsplantechnicalsupplement)

5 For an in-depth overview and discussion of the effectiveness of health promotion see: Tones K, Tilford S 2001 Health promotion: effectiveness, efficiency and equity, 3rd edn. Cheltenham: Nelson Thornes

The Health Development Agency have an online database, which aims to provide access to the best available information on what works to improve health and reduce inequalities: www.hda-online.org.uk/evidence. They have also published a number of effectiveness reviews, which can be downloaded from their website.

Since the mid-1990s, a number of organisations and academic centres have published reviews of effectiveness that summarise evidence from research in specific topics or approaches. See Chapter 7, section Evidence-Based Health Promotion.

6 Department of Health 2001 The strategy for sexual health and HIV. London: Department of Health. (www.doh.gov.uk/jointunit/jip.htm)

7 We suggest that readers make themselves familiar with the following terms, which are often used when discussing evaluation: effectiveness, efficiency, input, outcome, process, impact, monitoring, qualitative, and quantitative. They are all defined in the Jargon Explained section at the end of this book.

6 Identifying Health Promotion Needs and Priorities

SUMMARY

We start with an analysis of the concept of need. We follow with a section discussing four factors for you to consider when identifying health promotion needs (the scope, reactive/proactive choices, putting the user at the centre and adopting a marketing philosophy), and an exercise on the 'user-friendliness' of services. In the next section, on finding and using health information, we identify types and sources of information and include exercises on gathering and applying information. There follows a framework for assessing health promotion needs, with a case study and an exercise. In the final section we focus on setting priorities, and include exercises on analysing the reasons for health promotion priorities and on setting priorities.

See Chapter 4 for information on the range of agencies with a public health and health promotion role, Chapter 7 for national and local health strategies, and Chapter 16 for making and implementing national and local health strategies.

Many organisations at different levels have a role in identifying public health needs, including those that can be addressed by health promotion work. These range from international organisations (such as the World Health Organization), organisations at a national level (such as government departments, the Scottish Parliament and the Welsh Assembly) down to a more local level.

In this chapter we focus on the level of work undertaken by health promoters working with individual clients, families, groups and communities.

Identifying the people who are intended to benefit from health promotion activities (sometimes called *target groups*) is a complex process. These people may be referred to as *users*, by which we mean those who use health promotion services such as smoking cessation groups, maternity services or pest control services. In some cases people receive help that they may or may not use, for example receiving advice and information. Alternatively, people may be called *consumers*, *customers*, *clients* or, of course, *patients* if they are receiving medical services. Sometimes it is as important to identify potential users as current users, because a service may not be accessible or attractive to some people. Positive action may be necessary to ensure that everyone has equal access to services and can benefit from them.

Going one stage further and identifying and prioritising people's needs is also a complex and difficult process. There is a bottomless pit of needs, and only finite resources available to meet them; difficult choices have to be made.

Before looking further at how we can meet the needs of the users and receivers of health promotion, it is worth considering what may be meant by a need.

Concepts of Need

It is useful to think of four kinds of need.[1]

1. Normative Need – Defined by the Expert

Normative need is need defined by experts or professionals according to their own standards; falling short of those standards means that there is a need. For example, a dietitian may identify a certain level of nutritional knowledge as the desirable standard for her client and defines a need for nutrition education if her client's knowledge does not reach that standard. This normative need is based on the value judgements of professional experts, which may lead to problems. One is that expert opinion may vary over what is the acceptable standard, and the values and standards of the experts may be different from those of their clients.

Some normative needs are prescribed by law, such as food hygiene regulations.

2. Felt Need – Wants

Felt need is the need that people feel; it is what they *want*. For example, a pregnant woman may feel the need for (want) information about childbirth. Felt needs may be limited or inflated by people's awareness and knowledge about what could be available; for example, people will not feel the need to know their blood cholesterol level or the sex of their unborn child if they have never heard that such a thing is possible.

3. Expressed Need – Demands

Expressed need is what people say they need; it is felt need that has been turned into an expressed request or demand. Commercial weight-control groups and exercise classes are examples of expressed need; they are provided in response to demand.

Not all felt need is turned into expressed need or demand. Lack of opportunity, motivation or assertiveness could all prevent the expression of a felt need. Lack of demand should not be equated with lack of felt need.

Expressed needs may conflict with a professional's normative needs. For example, a patient may express a need for a considerable amount of information on his medical condition, which may be far more than a nurse is able or willing to give. The converse may also happen, with the nurse wishing to tell the patient far more than he wants to know.

4. Comparative Need

Comparative need for health promotion is defined by comparison between similar groups of clients, some in receipt of health promotion and some not. Those who are not are then defined as being in need. For example, if Company A has health policies about smoking at work and provides 'healthy' food choices in the staff dining room and Company B does not, it could be said that there is a comparative need for health

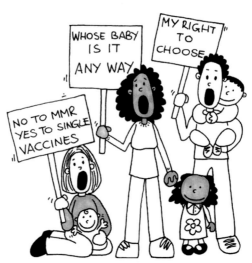

Expressed need is felt need turned into demand

promotion in Company B. This assumes that the health promotion in Company A is desirable and ideal, which of course it may not be.

To summarise:

Need, like beauty, is in the eye of the beholder.[2]

Need, Demand and Supply

In the last decade we have seen a dramatic increase in public debate over need, demand and supply of health services – and, indeed, other public sector services such as education. We are now aware that levels of service can vary across the country, and between GPs and hospitals even in the same neighbourhood. The 'need' for services may be similar or different, but it is clear that the supply is unevenly distributed.

It is also clear that demand often outstrips supply, which means that people do not always get the health care they want, or that health professionals believe they need. The health services and other public bodies are faced with demands they cannot meet because they have a finite pot of money to spend, so they have to prioritise. Sometimes this is called 'rationing': limiting the supply of health care and providing it only according to specified criteria. The issue of uneven provision of services also applies in prevention and health promotion, with different levels of provision in different areas.[3] However, comparative figures are unreliable because there is no clear definition of what constitutes health promotion and therefore 'counts'.

Measures to address the uneven supply of services in the health service include publication of national standards – National Service Frameworks – that set out the pattern and level of service which should be provided for major care areas such as mental health and disease groups such as cancer.[4] Local services are required to work towards these standards. National bodies also have a role in ensuring that the best value-for-money services and treatment are provided fairly wherever people live: the Commission for Health Improvement is responsible for ensuring good-quality services in the NHS, and the National Institute of Clinical Excellence oversees standards of clinical practice throughout the country.

Identifying Health Promotion Needs

How does a public health worker set about identifying people's needs? We suggest four key areas it is useful to think about first: the scope and boundaries of your job; the balance between being reactive and proactive in your work; the extent to which you are putting your clients first; and the usefulness of adopting a marketing philosophy. We address each of these in turn.

The Scope

For some workers the task of identifying needs has already been done to some extent. For example, dental hygienists working in a dental surgery with individual patients already have the clearly identified task of educating patients in oral hygiene. But they may want to think carefully about how they can make their service as person-centred and user-friendly as possible. And they will certainly have to identify and respond to the individual needs of each patient.

Other workers, however, have more choice and scope in the range of health promotion activities they can undertake. Health visitors and community workers may have considerable scope, but the degree of autonomy they have will vary according to the policy of their managers and the resources available. All health promoters will need some competency in being responsive to the health promotion needs of their clients, and will need to be clear about the boundaries of their work: which health promotion activities are within their remit to undertake and which are not, however desirable they may be. For example, a family planning nurse may be asked to undertake educational work with young people in schools, but is this within the boundaries of her job?

Reactive or Proactive?

It is useful to make an initial distinction between being *reactive* and being *proactive* when identifying needs. Being reactive means responding (i.e. reacting) to the needs and demands that other people make. Pressure from vested interest groups and the media may introduce bias into how needs are perceived, and produce pressure to react. Being proactive means taking the initiative and deciding yourself on the area of work to be done. It may include saying 'no' to the demands of other people if these do not fit existing policies and priorities.

See Chapter 3, section Analysing Your Aims and Values: Five Approaches.
Being reactive or proactive can be related to the approaches to health promotion, which were discussed in Chapter 3. Using a client-directed approach means being reactive to consumers' expressed needs, whereas using a medical or behaviour change approach probably means being proactive. This is particularly true of preventive medical interventions such as immunisation campaigns. In practice, there is usually a balance to be struck between being reactive and proactive.

Putting Users' Needs First

Whose needs should come first – the users' or the providers'? There may be conflict between the two; for example, users may want a family planning service to be open on Saturdays but providers are unable to supply this service because of difficulties in getting staff to work at weekends. However, several trends have emphasised putting the views and needs of users at the centre of health promotion provision:[5]

- The emphasis on users as unique people with their own individual needs.
- A more client-centred approach to health promotion, with self-empowerment of the client the key aim.
- Emphasis on improving the availability of, and access to, services that promote health, for example leisure and recreational services, and preventive health services. The growth of the consumer movement has led to shops and other services being available 24 hours a day, seven days a week, and people now expect services at times and locations that fit in with their lifestyle.
- The trend towards professionals working in partnership with lay people, with much more public participation in the planning and evaluation of health services, including health promotion activities. Service users are no longer passive patients and often expect (rightly) to have a say in the development of services.
- People are more knowledgeable, with information more readily available on computers and via the Internet, so that they are more likely to have requests and questions.
- A trend to give people more choice and flexibility; for example, if a person needs medical or health advice they can phone NHS Direct (a national NHS telephone help line staffed by specially trained nurses), go to an NHS Walk-in Centre (NHS service offering advice, information and treatment for health problems from specially trained nurses, with no appointment necessary) or go to their GP. New services such as NHS Direct have been marketed using techniques such as advertising and leafleting, which are used in commercial enterprises.

Adopting a Marketing Approach[6]

We referred to the growth of the consumer movement in health services and marketing above; *marketing* is a term frequently used in relation to health promotion.

Marketing is often associated solely with commercial businesses and making profits, and with the activities of sales and advertising. How, then, does it relate to health promotion, and, more specifically, to the question of identifying needs?

Usually health promoters work in the public or voluntary sector and are not generally required to make profits, and so they are different from commercial enterprises. But health promoters could be more effective and efficient if they adopted a marketing approach.[7] The fact that health is obviously a 'good thing' (which therefore does not need a 'hard sell') and that health promotion services often emphasise person-to-person involvement have tended to convince health promoters that they are in touch with their clients/users and that marketing may have nothing more to offer. However, there is increasing recognition that this is not so.

Although the phrase 'the customer is always right' originated in the service industries, there are many cases where this is patently not practised. For example, people are placing an increasing value on their time, and resent it if they are kept waiting because the health professional's time appears to be more valuable than their own.

What would 'adopting a marketing approach' mean in the context of health promotion? In general usage, marketing is the management skill of identifying opportunities for satisfying customers' requirements and, by doing so, maximising profits. In the context of health promotion, we suggest the following definition of marketing:

> *Marketing is the management skill of identifying opportunities for satisfying consumers/clients' requirements and, by doing so, maximising the protection and/or improvement of their health.*[8]

So the output is health, not profits. Fundamentally, marketing is an attitude of mind. It is about identifying consumer needs and satisfying them in the most efficient way, so that the maximum output is achieved in terms of people's health. Through adopting this approach, health promotion activities can benefit from greater effectiveness and efficiency, and from improved consumer satisfaction. In certain circumstances this may involve using specific marketing techniques, such as market research. It also means being much more responsive to the consumers' needs and wants, tailoring services to these rather than to the providers' ideas of what people should have. A marketing approach means making services 'user-friendly'. Exercise 6.1 provides a checklist to assess how user-friendly your health promotion services are.

We now return to the central questions: how can needs for health promotion be identified, and once identified, what criteria can the health promoter use to decide whether, and how, to respond?

Finding and Using Information

The starting point for defining health promotion needs is information of various kinds from a range of sources. If you are gathering information on a local area for the first

---

Exercise 6.1   How User-friendly are Your Services?[9]

Think of a health-related service you provide as part of your job, or if you can't, one which you use as a client (such as your family planning clinic, GP or dentist).

Below is a list of ten factors that may affect how users view the service. Rate the service on each factor using a scale from 1 (very poor) to 5 (excellent). The maximum score is 50. How does the service measure up?

1. **Availability of service** – do the times suit the user?
2. **Accessibility** – easy access by public transport? Easy car parking?
3. **Quality of service** – what are the standards, reliability, results?
4. **Speed of service** – do appointments keep to schedule?
5. **Friendly service** – a warm, welcoming atmosphere, continuity of relationship?
6. **Good environment** – safe, warm, clean, comfortable?
7. **Information about the service** – do local people know that there is such a service? Is information widely available, inviting, accurate, easy to understand?
8. **Reputation of the service** – do local people rate the service highly?
9. **Attitudes** – is there understanding and acknowledgement of the user's circumstances and feelings?
10. **Responsiveness of the service** – is the service relevant to local people? Does it reach all potential groups of users? Are suggestions encouraged and complaints handled sensitively?

time, it would be helpful to share the work, and the findings, with colleagues. For example, health visitors may have done a neighbourhood profile as part of their training, the local NHS health promotion department may have collected information, public health workers in the local primary care trust will probably have health data on the local population. Gathering and updating all these different kinds of information is an ongoing project for every health promoter and sharing the task makes sense. Working with colleagues needs to go hand in hand with developing good links with local people, in order to gear health promotion more effectively towards the active participation of users and receivers.

We will now look at the major kinds of information and how they may help to identify health promotion needs.

Epidemiological Data

Epidemiology is the study of the distribution and determinants of disease in communities. Epidemiological data indicate how many people are affected by a health problem, how many people die from a particular health problem, and who are most at risk, for example, men or women? which age groups? which ethnic group? which social class? which occupation? which geographical area? fat or thin people? smokers or non-smokers? sedentary or active people?

Detailed discussion of the sources and limitations of epidemiological data is outside the scope of this book, but see Recommended Reading at the end of this chapter. The important point to make here is that epidemiological data provide essential information on the health of the population, the causes and risk factors related to ill health and, consequently, the potential for prevention and health promotion.

Mortality and morbidity data are collected nationally, and some data are also available on a regional and local basis. (Mortality data are concerned with causes of death; morbidity data with types of illness and disability.) Mortality data are derived from death certificates; morbidity data from a wide range of sources, including general practice records, hospital records, sickness absence certificates, child health records, returns of notifiable diseases, disability registers and many others. In addition, surveys such as the government's General Household Survey and those carried out for research purposes provide a considerable amount of health information.[10]

Your local NHS organisation, such as a primary care trust, may have information about the local population including mortality and morbidity data (such as hospital admission rates for particular conditions). This may be broken down to the level of the population of smaller areas such as electoral wards. It might be helpful to compare data for the whole population and electoral ward data (for a neighbourhood) on, for example:

- the major causes of death
- the key causes of childhood admission to hospital
- the main conditions for which adults are admitted to hospital.

Exercise 6.2 is designed to help you to find out about local health information.[11]

Lifestyle Data

An increasing amount of information about people's health-related behaviour and lifestyle, such as physical activity, sexual behaviour, smoking and drinking is available

Exercise 6.2	Gathering Local Public Health Information

Ask your local NHS organisation, such as your local primary care trust (or equivalent in Scotland, Wales and Northern Ireland), for reports or data on the health status of your local population. They may have information available on the Internet. Some local data may also be available on national websites, such as www.statistics.gov.uk. Browse through the data and see if you can find out, for your local population:

- **What are the major causes of death?**
- **What are the major reasons for people to be admitted to hospital?**
- **What are the major risk factors for ill health? For example, is there information on what percentage of people smoke in your local population?**
- **How many people have had communicable diseases (diseases caught from other people) such as measles or sexually transmitted infections?**
- **Which neighbourhoods have the poorest health?**
- **What steps are being taken to prevent ill health and promote good health?**

Can you find information on anything else to help you in your health promotion work?

on a national basis from survey data.[12] You may also find that your local NHS organisation has done a lifestyle survey of your local population, and published the findings.

Socioeconomic Data

The planning or information departments of local councils should be able to help with information about housing, employment, social class and social/leisure/recreation/shopping facilities. Many produce summaries of census data. It might be helpful to compare district/borough/city and electoral ward data on social and economic factors, such as:

- unemployment
- household amenities
- income
- ethnicity.

It is advisable to ask for figures that are as full and recent as possible. Much information is obtained from the national census, which takes place every ten years. The last one was in 2001; information from the analysis of the data is available from 2003.

By setting illness data alongside social and economic data, you may be able to see patterns. In particular, you may see that areas where less well-off people live are also likely to be the areas of poorest health.

Professional Views

The views of fellow public health workers reflect experience and perceptions accumulated over the years, which it would be foolish to ignore. What do other workers in your area – teachers, youth workers, social workers, GPs, health visitors, district nurses, environmental health officers, police officers, community workers and religious leaders – consider to be the major health concerns?

Public Views

There is more about research methods for finding out people's views in Chapter 7, section Doing Your Own Small-scale Research.

Public sector organisations are now charged with the responsibility of seeking the views of the communities that they serve, but some organisations have developed good practice in this area over a number of years. Try contacting the local government in your area for information on this type of work, such as Citizens' Panels, which are representative samples of residents who give their views on local services, priorities and plans.

There are several methods of obtaining the views of the public at large, from informal discussions/interviews to large-scale surveys using questionnaires or in-depth interview techniques. Identifying priority groups and thinking clearly about them will influence the choice of methods used to contact and involve them.

It is best to start with the characteristics of the groups and then design the best approach. For instance, how large are the relevant groups? Do they have particular age, class or ethnic structures? What makes it a 'group' (geography, membership, current use of services and facilities)? Are the members of the group mobile? Do they have easy access to transport? What times of day are they likely to be available for meetings? Be absolutely clear about what sort of relationship you are proposing to have with local groups and individuals. For example, if you plan simply to establish consultation mechanisms, there may be hostility if local people have played a stronger role in other circumstances.

Public consultation and involvement are discussed in detail in Chapter 15.

The groups involved may include Patient Forums and Patient Advice and Liaison Services (PALS) (established from April 2002 to replace Community Health Councils in the NHS), local voluntary organisations and community groups such as self-help groups, black and minority ethnic groups, pensioners' clubs, tenants' associations, and a variety of local advisory groups or planning subcommittees, in addition to groups of key clients such as parents. Gathering views informally is useful but there are problems in ensuring accuracy and representativeness of subjective information. However, this subjective data can usefully feed into the wider picture.

There is more about research methods for finding out people's views in Chapter 7, section Doing Your Own Small-scale Research.

One of the most powerful ways of finding out what a service is really like is to experience it first-hand.[13] This can result in individual workers radically changing their working practices. However, it may not always be possible to translate this experience into general changes in the way services are delivered.

You might want to consider undertaking some first-hand research but first think about how much time and money it will take. Will the results justify the costs? If you still think it is worth doing, who could do it? If it is very small scale you could perhaps undertake it yourself, maybe in collaboration with some colleagues.

Local Media

The opinions and data collected will provide you with a picture at a particular point in time. Monitoring local radio, TV and newspapers will give a view of any major changes in the community. All this adds to the profile of local information you are building up, providing a basis for planning health promotion.

Exercise 6.3	Using Services That Promote Good Health or Prevent Ill Health: User Views

Find out about some services available locally, designed for the public, staff and/or health students (whichever is relevant to you) that aim to promote health or prevent ill health. (The public library, Human Resources Department of your employer, NHS Trust or college may be able to provide information about what services are available.) These could include swimming facilities, exercise classes, the Resources and Information service of your local Health Promotion Department or an NHS Walk-in Centre.

See also the section on Working for Quality in Chapter 8 for information on quality in health promotion services.

Select one of these, appropriate and acceptable to you, and visit it. Make notes about what happens. Look back at the section in this chapter on Adopting a Marketing Approach, if you need to remind yourself about how to make a service responsive to its users.

- **Is it easy to find out that the service exists?**
- **Is it easy to locate, with clear signposts where needed?**
- **Is transport easily available/is there easy access for parking your car?**
- **Are the opening times convenient to you?**
- **If there is a charge for the service, is it affordable and good value for money?**
- **How are you welcomed at reception? Are you given all the information you need? Do you feel at ease? Are the staff friendly?**
- **What do you think about the environment – is it safe, clean and comfortable?**
- **What do you think about the quality of the service you received? Do you have any ideas about how it could be improved? Will you use this service again?**
- **What have you learnt as a service user which you can now apply to health promotion practice?**

Assessing Health Promotion Needs

The assessment of health promotion needs can be approached systematically by asking a series of key questions. The answers will help you to decide whether to respond to a particular need, and if so, how.

1. What Sort of Need is It?

Is this a normative, felt, expressed or comparative need?

In a parent education class, for example, what kind of need is being met: the normative needs decided by the health professional, the felt or expressed needs of the parents or the comparative needs decided after looking at what was available elsewhere?

2. Who Decided That There is a Need?

Whose decision is it: the health promoter's, the client's or both?

Sometimes the answer to this question is not immediately obvious, because the need has emerged after discussion between the health promoter and client. People do not always know what they need or want, because their awareness and knowledge of the possibilities are limited. The health promoter may help by raising awareness and knowledge of health issues; in this way she may create a demand (an expressed need) for health promotion. For example, the public's demand for non-smoking in restaurants came only after health promoters had raised awareness of the hazards of passive smoking, which gave people the confidence to express their feelings about eating in a smoky atmosphere. The ideal situation is a joint decision by clients and health promoters.

3. What are the Grounds for Deciding That There is a Need?

Is there any evidence of need in the form of objective data, such as facts and figures? If local data are not available, has the information been collected in other localities and is it reasonable to assume that the same conditions will apply? Be aware that gathering data can be a delaying tactic to avoid doing something about an obvious problem. For example, surveys have shown that elderly people without cars find it difficult to get to hospitals if public transport is poor. It is reasonable to assume that this applies in most localities with poor public transport. So, collect information only if the answer to a question is really not known. Have the views of the clients been sought? Do they see this as a need?

4. What are the Aims and the Appropriate Response to the Need?

See the section on setting aims and objectives in Chapter 5 for a more detailed look at setting aims and objectives and identifying appropriate ways of achieving them.

Health promotion cannot solve all problems or meet all health needs. You need to be clear on what the need is, then what your aims are for meeting that need, then the appropriate way to meet it.

For example, there may be an identified need to increase the uptake of immunisation and aim to achieve an 80% uptake rate. You then need to decide the appropriate way to achieve your aim. It would be all too easy in this case to say that 'there is a need for a health education campaign to get parents to have their children immunised' because messages about attending immunisation clinics may be seen to be the answer. But this may make no difference because the appropriate response is to educate the health professionals who are withholding immunisation wrongly when a child has only a mild cold, and to move the time and place of the clinics so that working parents, and those without cars, are able to bring their children.

In Case Study 6.1 we assess an identified need for health promotion, applying the four assessment questions. Exercise 6.4 asks you to think about assessing a 'need' in your own work.

Setting Health Promotion Priorities

You may have a huge workload of health promotion needs that you feel should be met, but there are always constraints on time, resources and energy. Spreading efforts a mile

Assessing Health Promotion Needs

A Community Clinic[14]

The health visitors and primary care manager in a clinic wanted to make it into a focus for the local community. They felt that the clinic was an under-used local asset, and that the health visitors were failing to meet local needs and should extend their client group beyond mothers and babies to include more elderly and middle-aged people and schoolchildren. They also wanted to extend their role to become health advisers and counsellors.

The health visitors believed that offering an improved service would give them more satisfying jobs. They put considerable time and energy into planning how to achieve these goals. Yet much of the project never got off the ground and in the end the service remained virtually unchanged.

Although some reasons for this, such as staff changes, were outside the project's control, lack of clear ideas about how best to achieve the changes they wanted weakened the project from the start.

1. What sort of need is it?
Those involved in the project were anxious not to reinvent the wheel and made a number of contacts with other health visitors who had developed similar schemes.

This is a normative need based on a professional view. It is also a comparative need based on what other clinics provide.

2. Who decided that there is a need?
The professionals (the health visitors).

The views of existing and potential client groups were not sought. A letter was sent to existing users of the service, informing them of the proposed changes. No attempt was made to find out the needs and views of the additional client groups the health visitors wished to serve, although a plan was made to administer a questionnaire (see Question 3 for the outcome of this).

The other members of the primary health care team were not involved, and the receptionists were unsure about what was being proposed. Local community groups and other local health promoters had not been involved in drawing up the plans.

3. What are the grounds for deciding there is a need?
The grounds were the comparative under-use of the clinic, as perceived by the health visitors and primary care manager.

The proposed changes were not tied into the major priorities and objectives for the primary care trust, and the health visitor's manager was not involved in discussions. As a result a proposal to gather information from users about their need for services which the clinic could provide was the subject of cuts.

4. What are the aims and the appropriate response to the need?
The aims were not clear, and therefore the appropriate response to achieve the aims was not clearly thought through either.

One aim seemed to be to make the clinic accessible and attractive to a wider range of groups in the community. Who these potential users were, and what their specific needs were, remained unknown.

Another aim seemed to be for the health visitors to spend more time in face-to-face contacts with clients, acting as advisers and counsellors. Drop-in sessions were put on and advertised on a poster at the clinic. These sessions were found to be under-used and almost only existing users – mothers and babies – were attending them. This is not surprising when there was so little marketing of the new service. Attempts at proper counselling sessions were often frustrated by the receptionists continuing to put phone calls through.

Exercise 6.4   Assessing a Health Promotion Need

Use the following questions (discussed above in detail) to assess a health promotion need that you have identified in your own work, or one which you are likely to meet.

1. **What sort of need is it?**
2. **Who decided that there is a need?**
3. **What are the grounds for deciding that there is a need?**
4. **What are the aims and appropriate response to the need?**

wide and an inch deep is probably useless: concentrating effort on priority areas is more effective and rewarding.

Before attempting to set priorities it is helpful to analyse current 'real-life' practice and recognise the wide range of criteria that will affect such decisions (see Exercise 6.5).

The need to prioritise is vital, but one difficult issue to consider is how to approach work with people whose health experience is poor. It is automatic to consider that these people should be top priority, but it is important to stop and think whether focusing all health promotion effort on those most at risk will, in the end, be of greatest benefit.

We can consider two broad approaches to tackling a health issue such as reducing the incidence of coronary heart disease: the *high-risk* and the *whole population* approaches.[15]

The high-risk approach identifies people particularly at risk, such as smokers, people who are obese and those with high blood pressure, and work with these people to change lifestyle factors and treat their raised blood pressure, for example. But there may be poor return for effort, as these groups could include 'hard core' heavy smokers with poor diets who have no intention of changing, or people so overwhelmed with other issues in their lives that tackling smoking and eating habits is the last thing on their minds even if they would like to make changes.

The whole population approach works at community rather than individual level, with, for example, strategies to improve access to cheap healthy food, increase skills and confidence in producing healthy meals for families, and community development approaches to build up social support. At the same time, supporting changes at a wider population level, such as clamping down on under-age sales of cigarettes, and lobbying for increased income support, could result in better health gain across whole populations.

Generally, both approaches need to be taken (not necessarily by the same health promoters), as they complement each other. This is why developing partnership working is so important – it allows different aspects of the same issue to be addressed by whichever health promoters are best placed to tackle a particular aspect at a particular time, thus achieving greater impact.

There can be no watertight method for setting priorities because priorities ultimately depend upon the value judgements of the workers involved. But it may be helpful to work through the checklist in Exercise 6.6.

Exercise 6.5   Analysing the 'Real-life' Reasons for Health Promotion Priorities

Identify a health promotion activity which has a high priority in your work. This could be work that you undertake with a number of clients (e.g. antenatal education) or just one (e.g. a particular patient); it could be part of your usual work or a special event such as a campaign. (It will be especially helpful for the purposes of this exercise if you can identify an area of work that has recently become a priority.)

Now work through the following tasks.

1. Identify who it was who decided that this work should take priority (e.g. you? your seniors? your clients? all three?).

2. List all the possible reasons why this work has priority – include the reasons that you are sure about as well as any that are speculation.

   Your reasons could include any of the following and probably many more:

   ■ I feel that it's important.
   ■ It is the established policy of senior officers.
   ■ We've always done it and saw no reason to change.
   ■ There was pressure from the public.
   ■ It was in response to a crisis.
   ■ We had to be seen to be doing something.
   ■ There is new evidence of need.
   ■ There is evidence that the work has been effective in a similar area.
   ■ Someone has a personal enthusiasm for it (a bee in her bonnet).
   ■ It was the current national/local theme (e.g. World AIDS Day).
   ■ We had a new staff member with special expertise, which we wanted to use.
   ■ We had to economise and be more efficient.
   ■ It was politically expedient.
   ■ There was a change in national policy.

3. Identify what you think the most important reasons are. Do you think that they are sound reasons for setting priorities?

Exercise 6.6   **Setting Priorities for Health Promotion**

1. Health Promotion Issues, Approaches and Activities

Do you define your priorities in terms of:

- Issues that have an influence on health (e.g. poverty, unemployment, racism, ageism, inequalities)?
- Health promotion approaches (e.g. medical, behaviour change, educational, client-centred, societal/environmental change)?
- Health promotion activities (preventive health services, community-based work, organisational development, economic and regulatory activities, environmental measures, health education programmes, healthy public policies)?
- Health problems (e.g. heart disease, food poisoning, cancer, HIV/AIDS, overweight, mental health problems)?

Why?

2. Consumer Groups

Who are the people your health promotion is aimed at?

- Policy-makers and planners?
- Individual clients or service users?
- Families?
- Selected groups?
- The whole community? If so, how do you define your 'community'?

Why?

3. Age Groups

- Do you define your priority consumer groups further in terms of age: children, young people, parents, older people, etc.?

Why?

4. 'At-risk' Groups

- Do you define your priority consumer groups further in terms of high-risk categories such as smokers, people with high blood pressure, unemployed people or those living on low incomes?

  If so, why? Have you examined the evidence leading to the identification of these 'at-risk' groups?

- If your group includes people with highest health needs, for example people living in areas of social deprivation with many health and social needs, do you know whether there is evidence that work focusing on specific issues will be successful? Would you get more health gain for your effort if you focused on whole populations rather than those most in need?

5. Effectiveness

See Chapter 7 for information on how to collect evidence.

- Have you any evidence that health promotion in your priority areas is likely to be effective?
- Have you any evidence that it will provide good value for money?
- How could such evidence be collected?

6. Feasibility

- Is it feasible for you to spend time with your priority groups?
- Do you have access to these groups?
- Do you have credibility with these groups?
- Do you have the skills and resources to work with these groups?

7. Working With Other People

- Do you know what work is already being done with your priority groups, by other health promoters, community groups and voluntary organisations?
- Are you sure that your work will complement any other work that is going on – and not be seen as duplication or interference?
- Does your work fit in with existing local strategies and plans for health promotion?
- Are there any local partnership groups already set up to address the needs of your priority group?

8. Ethics

- Are there ethical aspects to your work which you need to consider?
- Is your work ethically acceptable to you?
- Will it be acceptable to your consumer groups?
- Will it be congruent with their values?
- How may the desired outcome affect their lives?

9. Add Anything Else You Feel it is Important to Consider

Now identify your top priority and add any other high priorities.

- You will have some scope for making choices about the range of health promotion activities you undertake. These choices must be based on a careful assessment of health promotion needs. The starting point is to gather various kinds of information.

- The views of users and receivers of services are paramount, therefore developing skills in gathering information directly from them is especially important.

- You can assess health promotion needs systematically by asking four key questions: What kind of need is it? Who decided that there was a need? What is the evidence for deciding that there is a need? What is the appropriate response to the need?

- Like all health promoters, you have a duty to reassess priorities regularly, through analysing whether your activities are targeted effectively, are feasible, complement the work of other practitioners and are acceptable to local people.

- Priorities depend ultimately on the value judgements of those involved. Best practice involves in-depth discussion on these matters with other health promotion workers and local people.

Recommended Reading

On Health Needs and Health Needs Assessment

➤ Bowling A 1997 Research methods in health – investigating health and health services. Buckinghamshire: Open University Press. (Chapter 3, Health Needs and Their Assessment, is an in-depth look at how health needs can be assessed, including demography, epidemiology and health economics.)

➤ Naidoo J, Wills J 2000 Health promotion: foundations for practice, 2nd edn. Chapter 17, Assessing Health Needs. London: Baillière Tindall

➤ NHS Executive Eastern Regional Office 1999 Public health practice resource pack. Cambridge: NHS Executive, Eastern Region. (This is a self-directed learning pack aimed at to enhancing public health skills. It includes health needs assessment and epidemiology. Available from: Communications Directorate, NHS Regional Office, Capital Park, Cambridge CB1 5XB. Also on the website: www.doh.gov.uk/ero/publications/ phealthpack.htm)

On the Experience of Ill Health and Health Services

➤ Davey B, Gray A, Seale C (eds) 2001 Health and disease – a reader, 3rd edn. Part 2, Experiencing Health, Disease and Health Care. Buckingham: Open University Press

On Targeting

➤ Naidoo J, Wills J 1998 Practising health promotion: dilemmas and challenges. London: Baillière Tindall. (Chapter 5, Targeting Health Promotion, critically examines the concepts of 'health risk behaviour' and targeting specific groups of people.)

On Marketing

➤ Irons K 1997 The marketing of services: a total approach to achieving competitive advantage. Maidenhead: McGraw-Hill. (Written for service-providing organisations.)

➤ Naidoo J, Wills J 1998 Practising health promotion: dilemmas and challenges. London: Baillière Tindall. (Chapter 6, Marketing Health, discusses and analyses social marketing and marketing health, including advertising and ethical aspects.)

On User Participation in the Development of Services

➤ Kemshall H, Littlechild R 2000 User involvement and participation in social care. London: Jessica Kingsley. (Explores strategies for effectively involving users in the planning, delivery and evaluation of services.)

Basic Epidemiology

➤ Barker D V P, Cooper C, Rose G 1998 Epidemiology in medical practice, 5th edn. London: Churchill Livingstone

Studying and Measuring the Health of Populations

➤ Bowling A 1997 Measuring health, 2nd edn. Buckinghan: Open University Press
➤ Katz J, Peberdy A, Douglas J (eds) 2001 Promoting health: knowledge and practice, Part 3, Investigating Health Information. Basingstoke: Open University and Palgrave
➤ McConway K, Davey B (eds) 2001 Studying health and disease, 2nd edn. Health and Disease series. Buckingham: Open University Press
➤ Naidoo J, Wills J 2000 Health promotion: foundations for practice. 2nd edition. Chapter 3 Measuring Health. London: Baillière Tindall

Notes and References

1   This is a classic analysis of the concept of 'need', based on:
Bradshaw J 1972 The concept of social need. New Society, 30 March

2   Cooper M 1975 Rationing health care. London: Croom Helm, p. 20

3   Buck D 1999 The distribution of health authority health promotion and education expenditure in England: a preliminary assessment. International Journal of Health Promotion and Education 37 (2), 52–56

4   All produced by Department of Health, London:
■ National Service Framework for Coronary Heart Disease (2000)
■ National Service Framework for Older People (2000)
■ National Service Framework for Mental Health (2001)
■ National Service Framework for Diabetes (2001)
Available on www.doh.gov.uk/nsf.

5   Some of this is adapted from:
Winn E, Quick A 1989 User friendly services – guidelines for managers of community health services. London: King's Fund Centre

6   Irons K 1997 The marketing of services: a total approach to achieving competitive advantage. Maidenhead: McGraw-Hill

7   For example, see:
Eadie D, Smith C 1995 The role of applied research in public health advertising: some comparisons with commercial advertising. Health Education Journal 54, 367–380. (On the relevance to public health advertising of methods and techniques from commercial advertising.)

Arnold-McColloch R, McKie L 1995 The potential application of social marketing techniques in health promotion. Journal of the Institute of Health Education 32(4), 120–124. (Draws out the advantages of employing social marketing techniques in health information campaigns.)

8   This is adapted from a definition of marketing in:
Willsmer R L 1976 The basic arts of marketing. London: Business Books, p. 7

9   This exercise is based on one in:
English National Board 1989 Health promotion in primary health care – an open learning package for practice nurses. London: English National Board with Learning Materials Design. Introduction, p. 8. (Reproduced by kind permission of the English National Board.)

10   The government website for statistics www.statistics.gov.uk has a wealth of information useful in public health work. It includes:
■ neighbourhood statistics, at local authority and ward level, including population, employment and indices of deprivation
■ health and personal social services statistics, including life expectancy, death rates, and health behaviour such as smoking rates

- results of the Health Survey for England, which includes self-reported health status, height, weight, smoking and alcohol consumption
- results of the General Household Survey, which includes smoking, alcohol consumption, health, use of health services
- social surveys, including some on health issues such as diet
- census data.

11   Until 2002, all directors of public health in health authorities and health boards in the UK were required to produce an annual report; this was a useful source of information on the health of the local population. In 2002, health authorities were abolished, and at the time of writing (2002) we do not know whether annual health reports will be required from, or produced by, new NHS organisations such as strategic health authorities and primary care trusts.

12   Lifestyle data on aspects of health such as nutrition, smoking and alcohol consumption, can be found on www.statistics.gov.uk – see Note 10.

13   See Recommended Reading and these further examples of accounts of personal experience of health care:

Berwick D 2001 Quality comes home. In: Heller T, Muston R, Sidell M, Lloyd C (eds) Working for health.

London: The Open University in association with Sage Publications. (The author uses the experience of observing the care of his father to make recommendations for health care organisations in the USA.)

Personal experiences of the health service from a user's point of view have been recounted in occasional articles in the Health Service Journal, for example:

Coker N 1997 Smoke and dust. Health Service Journal 107, 17 July, p. 29

Friend B 1997 Sickness benefit. Health Service Journal 107, 7 August, pp. 24–27

McQueen R 1997 Hip, hip hooray! Health Service Journal 107, 16 January, p. 27

14   This case study is based on a more detailed one in:

Winn E, Quick A 1989 User friendly services – guidelines for managers of community health services. London: King's Fund Centre, pp. 22–24

15   Whent H 1997 High risk v. whole population strategies. Healthlines, Issue 43, June, 14–16

Fowler G 1996 The population and individual strategies. In: Lawrence M, Neil A, Mant D, Fowler G (eds) Prevention of cardio-vascular disease: an evidence based approach. Oxford General Practice Series 33. Oxford: University Press, Chapter 21, pp 301–308

7 Skills of Effective Planning and Research

SUMMARY

In this chapter we look at particular aspects of knowledge and skill that help you to plan successful health promotion and use or undertake research to inform your work. These are: linking your work into broader national and local health promotion plans and strategies; basing your work on evidence of effectiveness; getting value for money; using published research; doing your own small-scale research; audit; health impact assessment.

Linking Your Work into Broader Health Promotion Plans and Strategies

The role of the NHS and local government in planning health strategies is outlined in Chapter 4. How local policy is made and implemented is discussed in Chapter 16.

The value of strategies at local and national level is in focusing efforts on agreed priorities, and providing a framework for setting objectives and monitoring progress towards their achievement.

The relevance of national and local strategy to the everyday work of a health promoter is that you can identify how your own work *contributes* to a broader strategy, and how it *complements* work that other people are doing. This can:

- increase your job satisfaction, as you see that you are not alone but are part of a broader movement
- help you and your colleagues focus your work on agreed national and local priorities
- increase the chance of successful funding and managerial support
- decrease the likelihood of unhelpful duplication of effort.

Figure 7.1 illustrates the many people in a range of agencies at local level who may contribute to the aim of increasing physical activity in the population, complementing each other's efforts. These, in turn, contribute to national goals about heart disease and stroke, accident prevention, mental health and cancer.

A key task is to become familiar with the national and local strategies relevant to your work. By 'strategy' we mean a broad plan of action that specifies what is to be achieved, how and by when; it provides a framework for more detailed planning. For health promoters there will usually be plans at a local primary care trust or local government level; these plans will themselves be informed by strategy at a higher level, such as national strategy.

First, we look at national strategies for health, then we consider what local plans there may be in your area.

Fig 7.1   **Contributing to Priorities in National Strategies. Local complementary contributions to promoting physical activity. (Heart disease and stroke, accidents, cancer and mental health feature as priorities in national strategies for health in England, Scotland, Wales and Northern Ireland)**

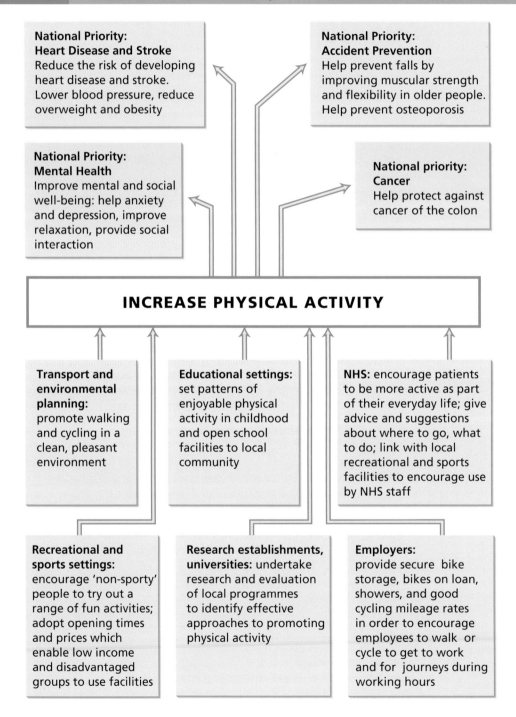

National Priority: Heart Disease and Stroke
Reduce the risk of developing heart disease and stroke. Lower blood pressure, reduce overweight and obesity

National Priority: Accident Prevention
Help prevent falls by improving muscular strength and flexibility in older people. Help prevent osteoporosis

National Priority: Mental Health
Improve mental and social well-being: help anxiety and depression, improve relaxation, provide social interaction

National priority: Cancer
Help protect against cancer of the colon

INCREASE PHYSICAL ACTIVITY

Transport and environmental planning: promote walking and cycling in a clean, pleasant environment

Educational settings: set patterns of enjoyable physical activity in childhood and open school facilities to local community

NHS: encourage patients to be more active as part of their everyday life; give advice and suggestions about where to go, what to do; link with local recreational and sports facilities to encourage use by NHS staff

Recreational and sports settings: encourage 'non-sporty' people to try out a range of fun activities; adopt opening times and prices which enable low income and disadvantaged groups to use facilities

Research establishments, universities: undertake research and evaluation of local programmes to identify effective approaches to promoting physical activity

Employers: provide secure bike storage, bikes on loan, showers, and good cycling mileage rates in order to encourage employees to walk or cycle to get to work and for journeys during working hours

National Public Health Strategies

We say more about the role of the WHO and other international bodies in Chapters 1, 4 and 16.

In health promotion, we have international planning led by the World Health Organization (WHO). The main focus in the UK is on national strategies and targets.

The First National Strategies in the UK

See also Chapter 1, section National Initiatives.

An important development for the UK in the early 1990s was the advent of national strategies for health: *The Health of the Nation* in England, and comparable strategies for Wales, Scotland, and Northern Ireland.[1]

For the first time we had national strategies for public health (as opposed to strategies for health *services*), with a clear emphasis on planning for improving, maintaining and restoring health. Health promotion had a key role in these strategies, although effective treatment and care also, of course, played a part. The aim of the NHS had been reoriented, to some extent, towards improving the health of the population rather than solely providing treatment and care.

How successful were these early national strategies? A report in 1996 from the National Audit Office on progress towards *The Health of the Nation* targets concluded that, while the initiative was making an impact, progress was uneven and slow.[2] Although good progress was being made to cut the number of deaths from heart disease, strokes and certain cancers, rising levels of obesity, alcohol consumption by women and smoking by children threatened to undermine health gains significantly.

In the areas where targets were being reached and trends in death, illness and health behaviour were going in the right direction, it was impossible to say how far this good news was due to efforts to implement the strategy.[3] For example, there was a decrease in the rate of accidental deaths (many due to road accidents) in children. But why? It could have been because of improved education about accident prevention or a safer environment, such as more traffic calming schemes. Or it could have been because more injured children were saved from dying with better or quicker treatment, or maybe even because more parents were afraid to risk letting their children out to play, walk to school or cycle on the roads, so that their exposure to life-threatening risks was reduced.

The government commissioned an assessment of the five years of *The Health of the Nation* 1992 to 1997.[4] The research found that, although the strategy was widely welcomed, it did not realise its full potential and was not seen to be as important as other health service priorities, for example waiting lists and balancing the books. Some key findings were that *The Health of the Nation* made little impact on local policy making, caused only a slight increase in health promotion spending (which peaked in 1994/95 and then tailed off), did not impact on primary care practitioners or hospital services, and was generally disliked by local authorities because of its disease-led, medically dominated approach. On the positive side, *The Health of the Nation* helped health promotion efforts to be coordinated, providing a focus on the key areas that encouraged organisations outside the NHS to be involved. It was a spur to multi-agency action where previous joint work had not existed, and the national targets were a useful rallying point.

The report makes recommendations for future public health strategy focused on:

■ the need for central government leadership, and committed local ownership and partnerships

■ developing a strong evidence base for setting targets and implementing activities

■ strong performance management so that public health workers at local level know how well they are doing in terms of both the process of implementing the strategy and the health outcomes.

These factors are important for the success of present and future health strategies.

1997 – New Directions in National Strategies

There were significant developments following the election of a Labour government in 1997, with new national strategies published in the late 1990s and early in the 21st century.

■ In Northern Ireland the Department of Health and Social Services published *Health and wellbeing: into the next millennium* in 1997.[5]
■ The Department of Health in England published *Saving lives: our healthier nation* in 1999.[6]
■ The Scottish Office published *Towards a healthier Scotland* in 1999.[7]
■ In 2001 The National Assembly for Wales published *Improving health in Wales: a summary plan for the NHS with its partners* and its action plan *Promoting health and wellbeing: implementing the national health promotion strategy.*[8]

There was a change in emphasis in these documents, with a move away from individual lifestyles towards people's conditions of living, tackling inequalities in health and the importance of partnership working.

England

See Chapter 1, section National Initiatives, for more about these inequalities targets.

Box 7.1 summarises the main features of England's *Saving lives: our healthier nation* strategy. A further significant development was that in 2001 the government published national targets to reduce inequalities in England.[9]

Northern Ireland

In Northern Ireland, the strategy for 1997–2002 (*Health and wellbeing: into the next millennium*) sets the overall direction for both health and personal social services, and identifies priorities and key areas for action: family and child health and welfare; physical and sensory disability; learning disability; mental health; circulatory diseases; cancers; and other non-communicable diseases of diabetes, respiratory diseases, and back pain. Specific aims and (in some cases) quantitative targets are set.

Scotland

Towards a healthier Scotland calls for a coherent attack on health inequalities, a special focus on improving children and young people's health, and major initiatives to reduce cancer and heart disease rates. It sets out action at three levels: life circumstances (social inclusion, jobs, income, housing, education, and environment), lifestyles (diet, exercise, tobacco, alcohol and drug misuse), and direct work to tackle what can be prevented – such as heart disease, cancer, and accidents – and to improve child, mental, oral, and sexual health. There is an emphasis on many agencies working together. Targets are set for coronary heart disease, cancer, smoking, alcohol, unwanted teenage pregnancies, and dental health.

Box 7.1	*Saving Lives: Our Healthier Nation.* **Summary of the National Strategy for Health in England, Published in 1999**

The goals of the White Paper *Saving lives: our healthier nation* are:

- to improve the health of the population as a whole by increasing the length of people's lives and the number of years people spend free from illness and
- to improve the health of the worst off in society and narrow the health gap.

Saving lives stresses that there is much that people can do to improve their own health, and emphasises the need to provide information, advice, support and opportunities to help them. It also puts great emphasis on tackling the social, economic and environmental factors in the community that affect people's health and mean that the health and well-being of people in the poorest communities have suffered most.

Saving lives identifies four major causes of illness and death – cancer, heart disease and stroke, accidents, and mental health – and sets targets and action plans for each one.

Cancer

Target: to reduce the death rate from cancer in people under 75 by at least one-fifth by 2010.

Action on: smoking; healthier eating; breast and cervical screening and the quality of screening services; evidence-based advice on introducing new screening programmes; more effective cancer treatment; a more strategic approach to research.

Coronary Heart Disease (CHD) and Stroke

Target: to reduce the death rate from CHD and stroke and related diseases in people under 75 by at least two-fifths by 2010.

Action on: smoking, healthier eating, obesity, physical activity, high blood pressure, sensible drinking, stress, more effective treatments.

Accidents

Target: to reduce the death rate from accidents by at least one-fifth and reduce the rate of serious injury from accidents by at least one-tenth by 2010.

Action on: road safety and traffic calming; safer design of motor vehicles, homes, playgrounds and leisure facilities; seat belts and cycle helmets; smoke alarms; more effective treatment.

Mental health

Target: to reduce the death rate from suicide and undetermined injury by at least one-fifth by 2010.

Action on: wide action to promote good mental health and reduce risk, including strengthening support systems for people with mental ill health and their relatives and carers; social networking and advice on parenting for young isolated parents; self-help support groups; early recognition and effective treatment for mental health problems.

Wider Action on Public Health

Saving lives identifies action on other key issues that affect health. These include sexual health, drugs, alcohol, food safety, fluoride in water, and communicable diseases such as tuberculosis, HIV, and AIDS. Work will also go forward with black and minority ethnic groups to tackle discrimination and poor access to services, issues of communication and recognition of different cultural practices, and diseases that particularly affect black and minority ethnic groups.

Making it Work

Saving lives sets out how the government expects local health workers to implement the strategy and monitor progress. There is strong emphasis on working in partnerships with other agencies, and developing local Health Improvement Programmes (now called Health Improvement and Modernisation Plans) with local targets and plans.

Wales

The action plan *Promoting health and wellbeing: implementing the national health promotion strategy* sets out key elements of helping communities through local health alliances, health-promoting schools, community health development, reaching young adults, and developing a healthy workforce. There are targeted programmes covering action on smoking, sexual health and teenage pregnancy, healthy eating, physical activ-

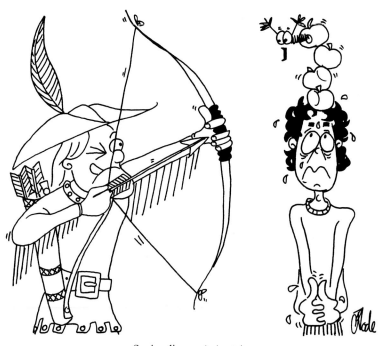

Saving lives *sets targets*

ity, substance misuse, older people, mental health, oral health, pregnant mothers and babies, people in prisons, and accident and injury prevention. Other elements of the plan cover improving the skills and knowledge of health promoters, better communication of health information, health impact assessment, and research and evaluation. Measures to monitor progress are specified for all action areas.

Local Health Strategies and Initiatives

See also Chapter 4 for the role of the health service and local government in promoting health.

The task of setting local strategies was given new impetus in 1997/98 with the publication of white papers outlining the Labour government's plans for the NHS in England, Scotland and Wales.[10] A key feature of these white papers was that health authorities or boards, in collaboration with local authorities and other partners, were required to develop health improvement programmes – later known as Health Improvement and Modernisation Plans (HIMPs) – for their populations.[11] This required more coordination between local agencies at both a strategic and operational level than had often previously been the case. HIMPs are programmes for action, based on local needs that cover prevention and health promotion as well as treatment and care services. They emphasise reducing inequalities and developing local partnerships to address locally identified needs and national health strategy priorities.

HIMPS are one vehicle for local planning for health improvement. Others are:

Local Strategic Partnerships[12]

At a local level the NHS is helping to develop Local Strategic Partnerships (LSPs), which will have the oversight of the Community Plan (see below), and be responsible, in areas of deprivation, for developing a local strategy for neighbourhood renewal. Health Action Zones (see below) have already made a valuable contribution towards the development of LSPs.

Community Strategies[13]

Part one of the Local Government Act 2000 gave local authorities new powers to promote or improve local economic, social and environmental well-being. It also requires them to prepare Community Strategies or Plans to coordinate these activities.

Neighbourhood Renewal Strategy[14]

The Neighbourhood Renewal Strategy and Fund was launched in 2001, and sets out a 'joined-up' approach to tackling the social and economic determinants of health in the most deprived local authority areas.[15]

It is also useful to be aware of the many government initiatives for different programmes and sources of funding, so that you can link into them. They include:

Healthy Living Centres[16]

The Healthy Living Centres (HLCs) initiative was launched in 1999, funded from the National Lottery to develop a network of HLCs across the UK. This funding is usually used for programmes of activity rather than a physical building. Local organisations, including those from the health service, local government, voluntary and private sectors, work together to bid for and run the kind of HLC that will meet the needs of local people. HLCs may include exercise facilities, parenting classes, complementary therapy, or support for people who are mentally ill, for example.

Health Action Zones[17]

Action zones for health, education and employment have been funded by the government in the most deprived areas throughout the country. The first wave of Health Action Zones (HAZs) was set up in 1998, with special government funding to develop and implement a programme of challenging targets. HAZs are pioneering new ways of tackling health inequalities through partnership working between the NHS, local authorities, community groups, the voluntary and private sectors; they link health, regeneration, education, housing, and anti-poverty initiatives. A central aim for HAZs is integrating the services and approaches they develop into mainstream activity.

There is a parallel development in education: Education Action Zones (EAZs) aim to raise standards and promote lifelong learning; many are also designated as HAZs with the links between education and health acknowledged. There are also Employment Action Zones.

The New Deal for Communities[18]

Funding has been allocated to 39 of the poorest neighbourhoods in the country for ten years. Funding supports plans that bring together local people, community and voluntary organisations, public agencies and local business in an attempt to make improvements that last in health, employment, education and the physical environment.

Sure Start[19]

This is a government scheme which aims to support parents and children under four in areas of high health need.

Exercise 7.1 aims to help you find out about national and local health strategies relevant to your work.

Evidence-based Health Promotion

The term *evidence-based* has now come into common use, especially in the phrase 'evidence-based medicine'.[20] It means that we should aim to do only those medical activities that we have evidence will work successfully. For example, someone believing that decisions about health care interventions should be based on evidence would argue that we should not undertake operations that research has shown do not benefit patients. This is the reason why, for example, it now uncommon to take out a child's tonsils, whereas years ago it was very common practice. Research over time has shown that it does not do the good that doctors had hoped that it would.

The same arguments can be applied to health promotion activities, and this is the subject of much discussion.[21] It is worth noting that health professionals, particularly

---

Exercise 7.1   **Finding out About National and Local**

1. Have a look at the national strategy for health in you
   National Health Strategies above to find out about y
   at educational institutions or at work, colleagues in h
   at your place of work, or contact the public health de
   organisation.

2. What do you think are the good and not-so-good poin
   strategy?

3. How does your own health promotion work contribute
   national strategy?

4. If you work in the NHS or local authority, have a look through your Local Health
   Improvement and Modernisation Plan or Health Action Zone plan and consider:

   ■ What are the good and not-so-good points about your local plan?

   ■ How does the local plan relate to your national strategy?

   ■ How does your own health promotion work contribute to the aims set out in your
     local plan?

---

doctors, often use the word 'evidence' in a specialised way, and only 'count' quantitative research studies. The results of both quantitative and qualitative studies are, however, essential to inform health promotion practice. An evidence-based approach to health promotion implies a rigorous approach to collecting and analysing data whether the study in question is qualitative or quantitative.

What is Evidence-based Health Promotion?

An evidence-based approach to health promotion means having an attitude of mind that constantly questions what you are doing, asking yourself: What do I know about what will be effective in this situation or with this client? How do I know? Who says so? It means that you do *not*:[22]

■ Say 'I know because I've worked here for 25 years'.

■ Use casual conversations and anecdotes to support major initiatives. ('Yes, we did a needs assessment – I talked to a couple of nurses and then we wrote a pack.')

■ Grow a bright idea with some colleagues and then carry it out without checking whether anyone else has done something similar and whether it worked.

■ Carry on doing things without question. ('But we've always given out toothbrushes.' Does it improve their dental health? 'But we've always done it ...')

■ Reinvent the wheel by researching work that is already well documented.

The evidence-based approach provides a defence against the indiscriminate use of practices in situations which have no research-based legitimacy, such as arousing fear to try to persuade people to change their behaviour.

Evidence-based health promotion also implies a willingness to write up and publish your work, which enables others to learn from your successes and failures. It is about building a culture where criticism is constructive and health promoters can penly share their experience. It uses the skills of reflective practice – thinking about what you do and questioning whether it is the right approach in your situation – and extends them by finding out what other people's experience might have to contribute.

It is important to recognise that there can be a gap between evidence and practice: if the research says that X works, practitioners do not, as rule, immediately change their work practices to implement X. There are many reasons, including the fact that it is not always easy for practitioners to keep up-to-date with new research findings, or to apply research findings in their own particular situation. Above all, change takes time, and health promotion practitioners can be set up to fail by being expected to achieve success within months when in reality it will take years. More attention needs to be focused on how research findings can best be put into practice – we need more studies of the processes of disseminating and implementing health promotion research.

According to those believing that health promotion work should be driven solely by evidence, we should aim to undertake only those health promotion activities that we know will work and will achieve the aims and objectives we have set. Arguably, however, as David Seedhouse demonstrates in his book on the philosophy of health promotion,[23] health promotion is driven by both values and evidence, which are often intertwined. So there are two key questions: *Do we think this ought to be done?* and *Will it work?*

See Chapter 3 for more about values and ethics in health promotion.

So, health promotion must be based on sound research. This is not to stifle innovative practice but is a requirement of the ethical principles of justice and beneficence (the duty to do good), as well as the political demand to be able to justify policies and practice on the basis of reliable evidence.

See Chapter 5 section on Stage 3 of the planning cycle.

How do we Know What Works?

We discuss how you can find and appraise research later in this chapter.

Another question is: How do we know what works? We looked at this briefly when discussing the basic planning cycle for health promotion (Stage 3, deciding the best way of achieving your aims).

One source of evidence is published research. There are many published research studies that help to show which health promotion interventions work best; these are easily accessible on the Internet.[24] Through the secure NHS 'Information Superhighway' NHSnet, health care professionals can access the National Electronic Library for Health, which aims to provide accredited reference material to develop evidence-based practice. Other electronic databases that can be accessed through the Internet include the Cochrane Library, CINAHL and Medline.[25]

Often it is not one single activity that produces results, but a combination of activities, of which you may be involved in just one. In the case study of physical activity (see Figure 7.1), we indicated a range of action that is likely to contribute to an increase in physical activity levels. Another example is child accident prevention work, where research indicates that we need a combination of educating people about safety and accident prevention, coupled with legislation and changes in the environment to make accidental injuries less likely.[26] For example, to reduce road accidents, we need a combination of road safety education for drivers and pedestrians, well-designed and maintained roads that include features such as traffic-calming schemes to slow motorists down, speed cameras to detect and deter speeding motorists, and legislation to enforce drink–driving laws. To reduce home accidents, we need education of parents and child carers on reducing risks around the home, provision of affordable (or free) home safety equipment such as fireguards and smoke alarms, and legislation on safety standards for buildings and items such as flame-retardant furniture. Research shows that for many health promotion issues a combination of complementary activities is the most effective.[27]

A major problem with the evidence-based approach is that evidence is not always to hand. The particular piece of work you plan to undertake may not have been done before, and indeed the particular set of circumstances in which you are working will be unique. So the best that can be done is to be aware of what the published research in *related* areas of work tells you, and to reflect on how what was learned might apply to your circumstances.

It also helps to think carefully about what constitutes *evidence*: evidence is not necessarily confined to formal research. The views of local people may be reliable evidence; your own experience may be evidence. Your job as a health promoter is to use your judgement to decide whether the evidence available applies to your clients and circumstances, and if so how. For example, GPs quote a number of factors which they believe provide evidence that health promotion is effective, including: 'I'm convinced because I have seen changes in the health of my patients over the last eight or nine years – patients don't keep coming back, they are more aware of their physical health, have better control of their sugar levels, blood pressure, diabetes, and so on'.[28]

In addition, you can plan carefully and evaluate or audit what you do. In this way you will be building up your own body of knowledge about what is effective.

We discuss audit later in this chapter.

Finally, it is also important to bear in mind that your decision about whether to do a particular piece of health promotion work is ultimately a moral and ethical one. You could decide that it is your responsibility to intervene, even though you have little or no information about what might work.

Using Published Research[29]

Health promoters need not only to be well informed about relevant research but also to *use* their knowledge of research findings to improve their practice. Familiarity with research findings can also give you ammunition to use in making a case for more, or different and better, health promotion. Scanning journals and digests (which highlight recent articles of interest to health promoters) should be part of your everyday working life.[30]

How to do a Literature Search

You may sometimes wish to find out about research on a particular topic, perhaps because you are proposing to introduce new health promotion work and want to know what has been shown to work best. For example, imagine you are a nurse working in cancer care and you are considering introducing a counselling service for women who are undergoing mastectomy (surgery to remove a breast, usually because of breast cancer). You want to know if research shows what the needs and concerns of these women are and how best to meet them. Where do you start?

First you need to clarify exactly what your research question is. It pays to take time to discuss this with colleagues. For the mastectomy counselling service, you could also discuss it with someone who has recently had a mastectomy. What did she find helpful, and what was unhelpful?

Once you are clear about what you want to find out, list no more than six key words that feature in your question. The cancer care nurse might include the words mastectomy, needs, and counselling in her list. Then write words that mean the same thing (these are referred to as 'synonyms'), or are similar in meaning, by each key word. For example, you might put breast cancer as an alternative to mastectomy, and advice as an alternative to counselling. These key words and their synonyms/alternatives will be helpful when you go to the library or search on the Internet.[31] In addition, many journal articles include a list of key words after the title, which will help you to know whether the article is likely to be of interest to you. When you have found a few references, you can start by reading the most recent one. This will provide you with more references. Once you are under way, the next problem is to avoid being swamped by information. Here again, your key words should be useful in stopping you from being side-tracked and in keeping your research question in mind.

It is important to keep records of what you read. Doing this may seem a chore, but it will save you time in the long run. There is computer software designed to help you store and retrieve references, but if you are using a paper system you can write up a separate index card for each article or book. For a book, you need to record:

- author's (or editor's) surname and initials
- year published
- title and subtitle
- edition if not the first
- chapter, or numbers of pages, if you are only going to refer to part of the book
- place of publication
- publisher.

For articles in journals you need to record:

- author's surname and initials
- year of publication
- title and subtitles of article
- journal title
- volume and part numbers
- the inclusive page numbers of the article
- date of publication.

If you are gathering research evidence that will be used to inform a health promotion decision or action, then the first thing you need to know when reading an article is whether it is a report of actual research or just a knowledgeable account of facts and opinions. The first thing that may help you to know about this is the *abstract*. This is a summary of why a study was done and the main findings. Abstracts usually take the form of a paragraph at the start of an article. Research reports also usually follow the following format:

- introduction – background to the study
- literature review – summary of previous and related research
- method – a description of how the study was carried out
- results – the findings of the study
- discussion – a discussion of the findings
- conclusions – the implications of the findings
- references – all the studies and books referred to in the article.

Having identified an article as a report of research that was actually carried out, you now need to read it critically, bearing a few crucial questions in mind:

When was the research carried out? Although the article is recent, it could be reporting on research that was carried out some years previously and has been superseded by more up-to-date research.

Why was the research done? Do you see the need for this research? Will it contribute new knowledge on the subject? Will this knowledge be useful in practice?

How was the research carried out? Did it use methods and tools that were likely to provide answers to the questions posed by the researchers? What type of research was carried out? For example, if the researchers wanted to find out what works in changing the behaviour of sedentary people with angina to cause them to take more exercise, then *experimental research* would be required. (This is research that establishes a relationship between cause and effect, often through studying subgroups of people, where the *experimental* subgroup experiences the intervention under consideration, and the *control* subgroup does not.) Another type of research is *action research*. This is used to find out exactly how to implement changes, or solve problems, in a specific situation through watching and documenting in a systematic manner how the changes are introduced.

Does the researcher draw reasonable conclusions from the results? This can be the most difficult question to answer, especially if you are blinded by statistics. If you are not sure that you understand, get help! This is of crucial importance if you are thinking of implementing the findings.

How could or should this research affect health promotion practice or policy? Even if the research was not carried out in your specialty or particular area of work, it could have implications for them. For example, findings about how best to communicate with patients who are very anxious after a heart attack could be used to help to improve communication with patients who have cancer.

Through asking these, and other, questions you should be able to come to a judgement about whether a piece of research is sound. It should have:

- been carried out by competent researchers
- used sound research design
- contained sound baseline data
- used a research instrument (such as a questionnaire) that has been piloted (which means tried and tested first to iron out any problems) and validated (which means that it has been tested to show that it really does measure what it was supposed to measure).

So, you do not need to do research yourself – you can improve your effectiveness through examining research findings and considering whether and how they apply to your work. However, in certain situations you may wish to carry out a modest piece of research yourself. We discuss this in the next section.

Doing Your Own Small-scale Research

We have included suggestions for further study on research skills in the Notes and References throughout this section, and in the Recommended Reading at the end of this chapter.

There may be times when you might want to undertake some research yourself. For example, you may be studying for a qualification in a particular aspect of health or health promotion and the course may include a research project, or you and a group of colleagues may have uncovered an unmet health promotion need and your manager has agreed to fund a study to look in more detail at the need and how it could best be met.

By *research* we mean a planned, systematic gathering of information for the purpose of increasing the total body of knowledge. Research involves gathering information that is not readily available. If you are inexperienced, it is important for you to get some help from an experienced researcher, right from the start. The following information should also help, but it should not be used as a guide to doing research on its own.

The research process involves carrying out some specific tasks, which are set out in Box 7.2.

Although the tasks will tend to be carried out in the sequence set out in the box, this is not necessarily so. For example, you may write parts of the research report as you go through each task, so that all the relevant information is set down as you go along. And you may have a much clearer idea about the purpose of the research *after* you have read the literature on other investigations in your area of interest.

The most important task in this list is the first one – the kind of question you want to answer will form the basis of the whole project. For example, suppose that you want to find out the best way to encourage a particular group of patients with angina to take more physical activity. This question is concerned with ways of motivating a specific group of patients. The experts in this field are psychologists, so it is to the body of psychological research literature that you will turn for soundly based principles. However, you may instead be concerned to know which of a number of alternative effective ways to motivate patients to take more physical exercise is best value for money. If so, you will want to look at cost-effectiveness studies and make use of the work of health economists. It is vital that you are clear about the practical reasons for engaging in this research. If you are very sure about why you are doing it, who will use the findings and for what purposes, then you are likely to come up with some useful answers. If you are distracted by interesting but irrelevant information, your research could be confused and therefore flawed.

Time spent on task 3, planning, always proves to be a good investment. If you are going to apply for funding, your planning must include investigating sources of funding and the particular interests of different potential funders. Most tasks take longer than you think they will, and you will need to allow plenty of time for consulting people; for example, to arrange interviews with people. Ethical issues and the need to apply for permission from ethical committees must also not be forgotten:[32] They will want to see the research proposal and may require additional information about issues such as confidentiality.[33]

You will also need to consider ways of collecting the information you need. Any information collected needs to be *valid* and *reliable*. By *validity* we simply mean actu-

Box 7.2	**Research Tasks**

1. Define the purpose of the research.
2. Review the literature.
3. Plan the study and the method(s) of investigation.
4. Test the method by carrying out a pilot study.
5. Collect the information.
6. Analyse the information.
7. Draw conclusions based on the findings of the analysis.
8. Compile the research report.

ally measuring what you purport to measure. For example, if you are attempting to measure the success of health education in encouraging a group of people to take more physical exercise, a valid measure would be directly to observe whether or not they spend more time on physical activities. Asking them to complete a written questionnaire may not give valid responses because research shows that people often respond to questions and questionnaires in ways they think the experts want them to. By *reliability* we mean that if the research is repeated, it will give the same results.

Basic Tools of Research

There are a number of basic tools used in health promotion research.

Questionnaires[34]

These are useful when you want to collect information from relatively large numbers of people. Questionnaires should be kept as simple as possible, but this does not mean that they are easy to design. A great deal of care is needed in the formulation of questions to ensure that valid conclusions can be drawn from the answers. Questionnaires are most useful for collecting information that is quantifiable, such as factual knowledge. Advantages of questionnaires include: they can be answered anonymously, and respondents may therefore be more truthful; they can be given to a whole group of people at the same time, so using respondents' and researcher's time effectively.

Your questionnaire should always first be tried out (piloted) on a small sample of people from the group it is intended for. You will then be able to identify any questions that have been misinterpreted, and can redesign them.

The response rate to questionnaires can be low, and you may need to think about the implications of this; for example, will the results really reflect the views of the target population? Also, some people hate filling in forms and even if they fill one in they may do so casually, without giving it careful thought.

You need to consider right from the start how the information collected will be analysed. Decisions about whether a computer will be needed to analyse the information may affect the design of the questionnaire. Consultation with a statistician and/or an experienced researcher may be helpful at this point.[35]

See Chapter 10, section Asking Questions and Getting Feedback, for more about open and closed questions.

You have to put a lot of effort into the design of quantitative questionnaires by clarifying closed questions with defined ways of responding (such as tick boxes), so that they will give accurate results. On the other hand, qualitative questionnaires (those with open questions, which can be responded to in a variety of ways) are easier to design, but it can be very complicated to analyse the responses. There is no 'right' way to solve these problems: it is a matter of trading off the advantages and the disadvantages of one approach.

Personal Interviews[36]

With face-to-face interviews you can develop rapport and encourage people to talk more openly. You may find out things that you did not think to ask about, but which are very relevant. The main advantage of personal interviews is that there is more scope for initiative by the interviewee. For example, the interviewee can seek clarification, and may be able to express views and opinions more easily verbally than in writing. The disadvantage is that, unless you are very skilled, you may bias the

The basic skills of asking questions and helping people to talk are discussed in Chapter 10.

response – that is, you may get the responses you want to get or expect to get. For example, asking 'you do feel better, don't you?' biases the answer towards 'yes', whereas 'do you feel better?' removes this bias.

Interviews can be one-to-one or with groups. They can be organised through using pre-prepared questions (this is often described as a *structured interview*) or allowed to flow more freely. At one extreme, you could design an interview schedule that looks like a questionnaire; at the other extreme, you might simply have three or four broad headings which you wish to discuss (a *semi-structured interview*). Special interview groups, such as focus groups, have also been developed. Focus groups concentrate on a particular issue through 'focusing' on pre-determined questions.

Participant and Non-participant Observation

Observation can include observing behaviour, such as how well a person performs an exercise routine, and physiological observations, such as monitoring weight. *Participant observation* happens when the researcher is also actively involved in what is being observed, such as actively contributing to discussions in a meeting. *Non-participant observation* means that the researcher takes no part in what is being observed.

Advantages of participant observation are that the researcher may be more aware of what is going on, including less tangible things such as the mood of a group of people. However, the researcher could have difficulty in making objective observations and may find it difficult to record what is happening, so that information could be lost. The non-participant researcher may find it easier to make objective observations, and may be able to plan and record observations more easily. On the other hand, having an observer who does not participate can seem threatening; people might not open up or may not behave as they normally do. This could have a big effect on what is observed, and invalidate the research.

Sampling

If it is too expensive or time consuming to collect information from the whole population or group you are interested in, then you need to select individuals so that you avoid getting a biased response. The techniques of random sampling or quota sampling can be used to ensure that the sample is representative of the whole population.

Random sampling This involves identifying people at random from the whole group. For example, imagine you are a practice nurse. Using the practice age–sex register you could decide at random on a number between 1 and 10 (say 5) and send out questionnaires to the 5th, 15th, 25th, 35th (and so on) persons on the list.

Quota sampling This uses your knowledge of a particular group to help set criteria about who to include in the sample. Criteria you might use include age, sex, and ethnicity. Once the group has been divided into segments, using your criteria, you can use a proportion from each segment for your sample. This ensures that people with certain characteristics are not over- or under-represented.

Convenience sampling This means that researchers question the people they can get hold of at the time. This is biased but, accepting that it is very difficult to avoid bias altogether, it is important to decide whether the particular bias that has been introduced is acceptable. It will also be important to discuss this aspect of the research in the report, in order to avoid misleading readers.

The Research Report

See also the section Report Writing in Chapter 8, and the section Written Communication in Chapter 10.

The final stage of your research will be to produce a written report, which will make your findings available to all those with an interest. People who read the report may be interested in assessing the validity of the findings for themselves, in repeating the research in similar circumstances and avoiding any pitfalls, or in applying the research findings in the context of commissioning or providing health promotion work. So the report should be written with the objective of helping readers to use it in these ways. You may need to consider producing more than one version of the report for different groups of readers; for example, a two-page summary for community groups, and a full report for your health service colleagues and managers.

The contents of your research report may include the information set out in Box 7.3, although not every point will be applicable to a particular report, which should be written with the needs of the readers in mind.

Finally, a warning: in a field like health promotion, interpretation of research data is a complex matter, often because of underlying differences of opinion on what is health and what constitutes success. It is therefore all too easy for the sceptical to dismiss research findings. So it is extremely important that any health promotion research is of good quality. Poor research is worse than no research because it wastes resources and misleads.

Box 7.3	**Checklist of Research Report Content**[37]

- An abstract or summary of the report.
- A statement about the purpose of the research, the background circumstances and the questions to be answered.
- The reasons for carrying out the research.
- A review of the literature to assess the current state of knowledge.
- The information the research was designed to collect.
- A description of the population sample studied, the sampling methods and response rates.
- A description of the methods used for collecting the information and the reasons for selecting these methods.
- A discussion of the ethical implications.
- Descriptions of the methods used for analysing the information and the reasons for selecting these methods.
- A description of the pilot study and any changes that were made as a result.
- The findings and all statistical data (where appropriate) on which the conclusions were based.
- A discussion of the findings, stating clearly the limitations of the study and providing recommendations for further research.
- An account of the difficulties encountered, how they were dealt with and whether they affected the results.
- A reference list providing information about all source material.

Value for Money[38]

When planning, you need to think not only about what resources you need but also the wider question of whether you are getting value for money. Health economics is a discipline that provides a way of thinking about value for money and making efficient use of scarce resources. It is not about doing things more cheaply, but about choosing priorities and making the best choices with the resources available. To help with this, the economist focuses on costs and outcomes. *Costs* involve much more than money: they may include people, equipment, buildings and intangible costs, such as distress. *Outcomes* include length of life and things that are difficult to measure, such as relief of stress.

Opportunity Cost

This is an important concept. If resources are scarce, doing one thing means giving up the potential benefits of doing another thing. So, for example, money devoted to drugs mass media campaigns cannot be used on drug education in schools. All health promotion activities involve the use of resources that are expected to produce benefits, but at the same time incur opportunity costs – benefits that will be forgone. It is often a matter, in practice, of getting the right *balance* between alternative activities; for example, in health education about smoking getting a balance between national advertising and local facilities to help people stop smoking.

Cost–Benefit Analysis

This is the process of comparing benefits with costs. Failing the cost–benefit test does not mean that an activity is not worth investing in, but it does mean that the cost of pursuing these benefits, in terms of other benefits that will have to be forgone, cannot be justified. Formal cost–benefit analysis is a complex process, not least because it is difficult to decide how different benefits should be measured and valued. Nevertheless, it can be useful to apply the basic concepts of analysing the costs and the benefits when you are allocating resources.

Cost-effectiveness Analysis

This means comparing the costs and outcomes of alternative activities to achieve the same goal.[39] It can be used when it is possible to measure the outcomes of alternative activities in the same unit of measurement, such as measuring blood pressure. For example, supposing that research had shown that exercise, drugs and diet (or a combination of these) were effective in lowering high blood pressure, these interventions could then be costed to see which ones were the most cost effective. This approach is used in considering alternative health interventions.

At a national level the National Institute for Clinical Excellence (NICE), funded by the Department of Health, undertakes this kind of cost-effectiveness analysis.[40] Established in 1999, its role is to provide patients, health professionals and the public with authoritative, robust and reliable guidance on 'best practice' in relation to drugs, treatments and services across the NHS. NICE reviews current research evidence and issues recommendations in the form of clinical guidelines for health professionals. An example of its work is the review of the cost effectiveness of using beta-interferon for people with multiple sclerosis.

Audit

What is 'Audit'?

See Chapter 5 for the basic planning and evaluation cycle.

Audit is the systematic examination of the operations of a service, followed by the implementation of recommendations to improve quality. Basically, an audit will scrutinise how the service carries out each stage of the planning/evaluation cycle, which we described in Chapter 5.

Strengths and weaknesses will be revealed, and ways of overcoming weaknesses will be identified. Audit can involve either an internal review by the people responsible for delivering a service or scrutiny by an independent external auditor. For example, all NHS trusts now have clinical auditors who audit the clinical activities of the trust.[41]

At national level, the Audit Commission is responsible for auditing NHS activities.[42] The audit cycle normally starts with the specification of standards or criteria, followed by the collection of data, the assessment of performance, the identification of the need for change and implementing the improvements (see Figure 7.2).

It is in the nature of cycles that you can, in practice, start anywhere. So you might start with collecting data on performance, assess performance, and recommend the need to specify standards. The difficulty with auditing health promotion practice is that it is often embedded in other work. For example, audit of health promotion in clinical settings may involve scrutinising issues about relationships, communication, and staff training and supervision, all of which are vital to the quality of health promotion work, but non-clinical. In addition, the most serious problems are often between professions and departments and agencies, in the areas of communication and coordination, while

Fig 7.2   **An Audit Cycle**

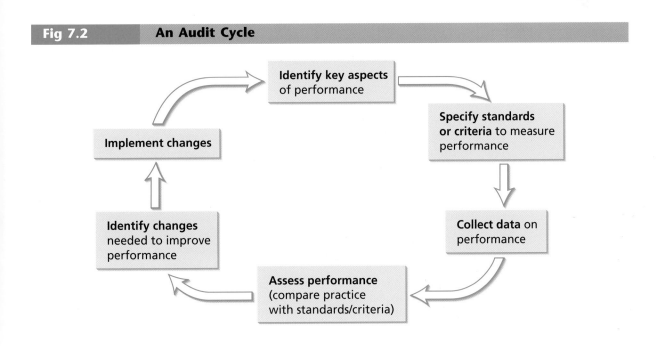

audit is usually conducted on a uniprofessional basis (confined to a single profession such as doctors or nurses), for example medical audit.

However, there are a number of good reasons why it may be wise to make a start on auditing health promotion on a uniprofessional basis:[43]

- Many services are structured by profession.
- Audit may be unfamiliar and may seem threatening to health promoters.
- Most existing experience of audit, and proof of its value, is within each profession (for example, within nursing audit and medical audit). This experience can help.
- Problems that involve other professions, departments or agencies can be noted and later tackled through establishing interprofessional or inter-agency health promotion quality groups.

For further reading on quality standards see Chapter 8, section Working for Quality.

Many of the tools described in the section above on 'Doing your own research' can also be used in audit. So, for example, you could use a telephone survey after discharge to study the satisfaction of patients with information and education they received as inpatients. When telephoning patients, you would need to reassure them that participation in the survey is voluntary, and that their comments would be completely confidential. The sort of questions you might like to ask are set out in Box 7.4.

Box 7.4	**Patient Satisfaction with Health Education and Information: Telephone Survey Schedule**

- When you were in hospital what information were you given about your illness?
- Do you now feel you have sufficient information about what was wrong with you?
- Were you able to discuss your anxieties with anyone while you were in hospital?
- Who did you prefer to discuss things with? *Prompt: Was it a nurse, a doctor, another professional or a domestic helper?*
- Did you have sufficient privacy to feel able to open up? *Prompt: Did you have access to a comfortable, private room for private conversations?*

Audit, Research and Evaluation

Audit, research and evaluation are complementary activities. Research is concerned with generating new knowledge and new approaches, which can be applied beyond the specific context of the study. Evaluation involves making a judgement about one specific intervention or project, which is the focus of its concern. Audit seeks to improve the performance of a continuing service, such as an environmental health service or a midwifery service, through reviewing its practice. All three are crucial to the pursuit of evidence-based health promotion.

You should not need to do a detailed evaluation of everything you do, because you will be basing what you do on techniques and materials that have already been evaluated by others and form part of the published evidence. What you *should* do is to audit your health promotion practices regularly to check whether what you have planned and the techniques you have chosen are working properly. Health promoters are inhibited from doing this by a lack of audit skills.[44] If you need further training in how to carry out an audit of your health promotion practice, it would be worth finding out about local opportunities for training in clinical audit – the basic concepts can be applied to health promotion. Another area to pursue could be training related to measuring and improving quality or quality assurance. Quality cycles and audit cycles are very closely related and the purpose of audit is to improve quality. You could also discuss, with your manager, local arrangements for performance appraisal (mechanisms for checking on and improving the performance of staff), professional development plans, and supervision, since these are all related to audit.

See the section Working for Quality in Chapter 8.

From the viewpoint of the individual client or patient, we need to audit their total experience of a service, including non-clinical or non-technical aspects such as health education and health promotion practice.

Health Impact Assessment

It is appropriate here to mention *health impact assessment* (sometimes abbreviated to HIA).[45] This has been defined as the estimation of the effects of a specified action on the health of a defined population.[46]

HIA is a relatively new approach, which accepts that social, economic and environmental factors, as well as genetic make-up and health care, make a difference to people's health. It is a systematic way of assessing what difference a policy, programme or project (often about social, economic, or environmental factors) makes to people's health. For example, it has been used when public-sector organisations and partnerships have wanted to understand the effect on people's health of policies on transport, air quality, economic development, regeneration, or housing.

The assessment can be carried out before, during or after a policy is implemented, but ideally it is done before, so that the findings can inform decisions about whether and how to implement the policy. Key steps are to:

- select and analyse policies, programmes or projects for assessment
- profile the affected population – who is likely to be affected and their characteristics
- identify the potential health impacts by getting information from the range of people who have an interest in the policy, or who are likely to be affected by it
- evaluate the importance, scale and likelihood of the potential impacts
- report on the impacts and make recommendations for managing the impacts.

HIA is a tool for bringing public health issues into the foreground when organisations and partnerships are making policies and decisions. Public health workers may find HIA useful if they are considering new policies on, for example, transport or regenerating areas of social deprivation.

PRACTICE POINTS

- It is important to identify how your health promotion work contributes to local and national strategies. Your effectiveness depends not only on what you do but also on how well your work complements, and avoids conflict with, that of other health promoters.

- All health promoters have a duty to appraise relevant research regularly, and to base their work on evidence of effectiveness when such evidence exists.

- Doing research involves specialised skills, and you should not attempt it unless you have developed the appropriate competencies that the particular type of research requires.

PRACTICE POINTS

- When planning, you need to think about whether you are getting value for money, through using the ways of thinking developed in health economics.

- Any service should regularly undertake audit: take stock of how it operates and identify how things can be improved.

- If your work involves making or implementing policies that affect people's health, Health Impact Assessment may be a useful tool.

Recommended Reading

National Strategies for Health

➤ Find the most up-to-date national strategy for health in your country. You should be able to find it on the Internet or borrow a copy from:

- your local NHS health promotion department
- national health education/promotion libraries (Health Development Agency, Health Education Board for Scotland, Health Promotion Division of the National Assembly for Wales, Health Promotion Agency for Northern Ireland)
- your local primary care trust, care trust, strategic health authority or board
- libraries in colleges and universities running health courses.

In 2002, the most recent strategies were:
England: Department of Health (1999) Saving lives: our healthier nation. London: The Stationery Office. Cm 4386. Website: www.official-documents.co.uk and www.ohn.gov.uk
Scotland: The Scottish Office (1999) Towards a healthier Scotland. London: The Stationery Office. Cm 4269. Website: www.scotland.gov.uk/library
Wales: The National Assembly for Wales (2001) Improving health in Wales: a summary plan for the NHS with its partners. Cardiff: National Assembly for Wales. The National Assembly for Wales, Health Promotion Division (2001) Promoting health and wellbeing: implementing the National Health Promotion Strategy. Cardiff: National Assembly for Wales. Website: www.wales.nhs.uk/pubs.cfm
Northern Ireland: Department of Health and Social Services (1997) Health and wellbeing: into the next millennium. Belfast: DHSS. Full and summary version available from: Department of Health and Social Services, Belfast. Website: www.dhsspsni.gov.uk

National Service Frameworks

➤ All published by the Department of Health, London. The purpose of these frameworks is to have national standards of care and treatment and a national approach to addressing health promotion and disease prevention.

- National service framework for coronary heart disease (2000)
- National service framework for older people (2000)
- National service framework for mental health (2001)
- National service framework for diabetes (2001)

Available on www.doh.gov.uk/nsf
For Scotland:
Scottish diabetes framework. Consultation paper issued by the Scottish Executive September 2001. See www.scotland.gov.uk

On Evidence-based Health Care and Health Promotion

➤ Fletcher A, Breeze E, Walters R 2000 The evidence of health promotion effectiveness: shaping public health in a new Europe. Brussels: International Union for Health Promotion and Education, European Commission. (International perspective.)

➤ Katz J, Peberdy A, Douglas J (eds) 2001 Promoting health: knowledge and practice, 2nd edn. Basingstoke: The Open University in association with Palgrave. Chapter 12, What counts as evidence in health promotion?

➤ Muir Gray J A 2001 Evidence-based health care – how to make health policy and management decisions, 2nd edn. London: Churchill Livingstone. (Explains how evidence can be applied to health policy and management decisions which affect the health and health care of populations. Accessible to non-clinicians and clinicians alike, and recommended for any professional working in, or training for, the health service.)

➤ NHS Executive Eastern Regional Office 1999 Public health practice resource pack. Cambridge, NHS Executive Eastern Regional Office. (A self-directed learning pack which aims to enhance public health skills, including taking an evidence-based approach to public health work. Available from: Communications Directorate, NHS Regional Office, Capital Park, Cambridge CB1 5XB. Also on the website: www.doh.gov.uk/ero/publications/pubhealth)

➤ Perkins E R, Simnett I, Wright L 1999 (eds) Evidence-based health promotion. Chichester: Wiley

➤ Sidell M, Jones L, Katz J, Peberdy A (eds) 1997 Debates and dilemmas in promoting health. Basingstoke: Macmillan/Open University Press. (Section 2, Questioning the evidence base of health promotion, looks in depth at what counts as evidence in health promotion and includes chapters about epidemiological, economic and social work approaches to collecting and assessing evidence.)

On Health Economics

➤ Naidoo J, Wills J (eds) 2001 Health studies: an introduction. Basingstoke: Palgrave. (Chapter 8, Health economics, is a good basic overview of health economics)

On Finding and Using Published Research

➤ Boulton M, Fitzpatrick R, Swinburn C 1996 Qualitative research in health care: 2. A structure review and evaluation of studies. Journal of Evaluation in Clinical Practice 2, 171–179

➤ Ogier M 1998 Reading research: or how to make research more approachable, 2nd edn. London: Baillière Tindall/Royal College of Nursing

On Doing Your Own Research

➤ Bell J (ed.) 1999 Doing your research project: a guide for first time researchers in education and social science, 3rd edn. Buckingham: Open University Press. (Basic guidance on how to do small-scale research projects)

➤ Denscombe M 1998 The good research guide for small-scale social research projects. Buckingham: Open University Press. (Covers strategies and methods; includes analysis of qualitative and quantitative data, surveys, case studies, action research, questionnaires, interviews, observation, writing up)

➤ Katz J, Peberdy A, Douglas J (eds) 2001 Promoting health: knowledge and practice, 2nd edn. Basingstoke: The Open University in association with Palgrave. Chapter 13, Studying populations; Chapter 14, Analysing numerical data; Chapter 18, Enquiring and reporting

➤ McConway K, Davey B (eds) 2001 Studying health and disease, 2nd edn. Health and Disease series. Buckingham: Open University Press. (Broad introduction to main methods of research and investigation used in the area of health and disease)

➤ Maslin-Prothero S (ed.) 1997 Baillière's study skills for nurses. London: Baillière Tindall. (Includes study skills, reading skills, using libraries and information technology, how to do literature searches, and writing skills – including writing reflectively for academic publications)

➤ Swetham D 2000 Writing your dissertation – how to plan, prepare and present successful work, 3rd edn. Oxford: How To Books. (Basics of research, research techniques and writing up)

On Audit of Health Promotion Practice

▲ Simnett I 1996 Auditing quality in health promotion work. British Journal of Health Care Management 2 (4), 205–207

Notes and References

1   Secretary of State for Health 1992 The health of the nation: a strategy for health in England. London: HMSO

Welsh Office 1989 Strategic intent and direction for the NHS in Wales. Welsh Office NHS Directorate: The Welsh Health Planning Forum

Scottish Office 1992 Scotland's health: a challenge to us all. Edinburgh: HMSO

Department of Health and Social Services 1991 A regional strategy for the Northern Ireland health and personal social services 1992–1997. London: HMSO

2   National Audit Office 1996 Health of the nation: a progress report. London: HMSO

For a summary of the National Audit Office report on The Health of the Nation, see:

News focus 'Variations on a theme.' Health Service Journal 1996 22 August, 12–13.

3   For a review of Health of the Nation, its choice of targets, how well it has performed, and whether some of the successes have anything to do with the strategy, see:

Appleby J 1997 Feelgood factors. Health Service Journal 3 July, 24–27

4   Department of Health 1998 The health of the nation: a policy assessed. London: The Stationery Office. www.doh.gov.uk/pub/docs/doh

5   Department of Health and Social Services 1997 Health and wellbeing: into the next millennium. Belfast: DHSS. www.dhsspsni.gov.uk

6   Department of Health 1999 Saving lives: our healthier nation. London: The Stationery Office. www.ohn.gov.uk

7   The Scottish Office 1999 Towards a healthier Scotland. London: The Stationery Office. www.scotland.gov.uk/library

8   The National Assembly for Wales 2001 Improving health in Wales: a summary plan for the NHS with its partners. Cardiff: National Assembly for Wales

    The National Assembly for Wales, Health Promotion Division 2001 Promoting health and wellbeing: implementing the national health promotion strategy. Cardiff: National Assembly for Wales. www.wales.nhs.uk/pubs.cfm

9   See Department of Health website: www.doh.gov.uk/healthinequalities/targets.pdf

10 Secretary of State for Health 1997 The new NHS: modern, dependable. London: The Stationery Office

    Department of Health Scottish Executive 2000 Working together to build a healthy caring Scotland. London: The Stationery Office

    Secretary of State for Wales 1998 NHS Wales: putting patients first. London: The Stationery Office

11 For further information on Health Improvement and Modernisation Plans, see www.doh.gov.uk/hrforhimps/

12 Department for the Environment, Transport and the Regions 2000 Local strategic partnerships: consultation document. London: DETR

    For further information see: www.local-regions.dtlr.gov.uk/index.htm

13 Department of the Environment, Transport and the Regions 2000 Preparing community strategies. Government guidance to local authorities. London: DETR

    For further information see: www.local-regions.dtlr.gov.uk/index.htm

14 Social Exclusion Unit 2001 A new commitment to neighbourhood renewal. National strategy action plan. London: Cabinet Office. www.cabinet-office.gov.uk/seu/2001/Action_Plan/default.htm

15 Social Exclusion Unit 2001 A new commitment to neighbourhood renewal: national strategy action plan.

    For further information on regeneration, see: www.regeneration.dtlr.gov.uk

16 For further information on Healthy Living Centres, see www.doh.gov.uk/hlc.htm or contact the New Opportunities Fund enquiry line. For England:

0845 0000 121; for Scotland: 0845 0000 123; for Wales: 0845 0000 122; for Northern Ireland: 0845 0000 124. Website: www.nof.org.uk

17 For further information on Action Zones, see: www.haznet.org.uk/; www.dfes.gov.uk/index.htm; www.dfee.gov.uk/employmentzones/map/map.htm

18 For further information on New Deal, see: www.regeneration.dtlr.gov.uk/ndc.htm

19 For further information on Sure Start, see: www.surestart.gov.uk

20 See Recommended Reading and:

    Holloway P J, Worthington H 1997 What does 'evidence-based medicine' mean? International Journal of Health Education 35(2), 40–43

21 For discussion on evidence-based health promotion, see Recommended Reading and:

    Learmonth A, Mackie P 2000 Evaluating effectiveness in health promotion: a case of re-inventing the millstone? Health Education Journal 59, 267–280

    Macdonald G 2000 A new evidence framework for health promotion practice. Health Education Journal 59, 3–11

    Nutbeam D 1999 The challenge to provide 'evidence' in health promotion. Health Promotion International 14, 99–101

    Raphael D 2000 The question of evidence in health promotion. Health Promotion International 15 (4), 355–366

    Speller V, Learmonth A, Harrison D 1997 The search for evidence of effective health promotion. British Medical Journal 315, 361–363

22 Adapted from Perkins E R, Simnett I, Wright L (eds) 1999 Evidence-based health promotion. Chichester: Wiley, pp. 5–6

23 Seedhouse D 1997 Health promotion: philosophy, prejudice and practice. Chichester: Wiley, Chapter 4 (Seedhouse argues that health promoters have a responsibility to arrive at their opinions through reflecting on both values and evidence, and should be continually prepared to question, and if necessary to revise, their judgements)

24 The Health Development Agency has a website called HealthPromis (http://healthpromis.hda-online.org.uk). It is a national bibliographic database of health promotion materials, and includes books, resources and journal articles of use to health professionals. It has a current awareness facility where you can find the latest journal publications on health promotion. Searching the database is free, and it is updated on a daily basis. It provides easy access to the best available information on what works

to improve health and reduce inequalities and includes effectiveness reviews, which can be downloaded.

25 Medline can be accessed on www.ncbi.nlm.nih.gov/PubMed

More information about access to the CINAHL database can be found on www.cinahl.com

The Cochrane Library can be accessed through the National Electronic Library for Health website (www.nelh.nhs.uk).

26 Health Education Authority 1996 Health promotion effectiveness reviews: health promotion in childhood and young adolescence for the prevention of unintentional injuries. London: HEA

Hogg C 1996 Preventing children's accidents: a guide for health authorities and boards. London: Child Accident Prevention Trust

NHS Centre for Review and Dissemination, University of Leeds 1996 Preventing unintentional injuries in children and young adolescents

27 Other examples are:

Teenage smoking prevention work:

Staed M, Hastings G, Tudor-Smith C 1996 Preventing adolescent smoking: a review of options. Health Education Journal 55(1), 31–54

Preventing teenage pregnancy:

NHS Centre for Reviews and Dissemination, University of York 1997 Preventing and reducing the adverse effects of unintended teenage pregnancies

28 Office for Public Management 1997 Achieving health gain through health promotion in a primary care-led NHS. London: Health Education Authority, p. 42

29 This section is partly based on:

Ogier M 1996 Reading research: or how to make research more approachable. London: Baillière Tindall/Royal College of Nursing

30 One helpful way to keep in touch is through the Health Development Agency's HealthPromis website – see Note 24 (http://healthpromis.hda-online.org.uk)

31 A useful place to start researching any health promotion topic is the Health Development Agency's HealthPromis website – see Note 24 (http://healthpromis.hda-online.org.uk)

If you need help with using the Internet, try:

Kennedy A 1999 The Internet: the rough guide. London: Rough Guides

32 For further reading on ethical issues in research, see:

Ayer S 1994 Submitting a research proposal for ethical approval. Professional Nurse September, 805–806

Behi R, Nolan M 1995 Ethical issues in research. British Journal of Nursing 4(12), 712–716

33 For more on writing a research proposal, see:

Parahoo K, Reid N 1998 Research skills no. 3: writing a research proposal. Nursing Times 84(41), 49–52

34 For guidance on designing questionnaires see Recommended Reading.

35 For basic concepts of statistics and their application in the design of research, see:

Bowers D 1996 Statistics from scratch: an introduction for health care professionals. Chichester: Wiley

36 For more on interviewing see Recommended Reading above

37 Adapted from: Partridge C S, Barnitt R E 1987 Research guidelines: a handbook for therapists. London: Heinemann

38 On performance indicators, targets and value for money as applied to health promotion:

Buck D, Godfrey C, Morgan A 1996 Performance indicators and health promotion targets. University of York: Centre for Health Economics

39 For more on cost-effectiveness and prevention see:

Tengs T O 1996 Enormous variation in the cost-effectiveness of prevention: implications for public policy. Current Issues in Public Health 2 (1), 13–17

Examples of studies on the cost-effectiveness of health promotion include:

On smoking:
Buck D 1997 The cost-effectiveness of smoking cessation interventions: what do we know? International Journal of Health Education 35(2), 44–52

Lennox A S et al 2001 Cost effectiveness of computer tailored and non-tailored smoking cessation letters in general practice: randomised controlled trial. British Medical Journal 322, 1396–1400

On health promotion in primary care:

Langham S, Thorogood M, Normand C, Muir J 1996 Costs and effectiveness of health checks conducted by nurses in primary care: the Oxcheck study. British Medical Journal 312, 1265–1268

On heart disease screening and primary care programmes:

Wonderling D, McDermott C, Buxton M, Kinmouth A 1996 Costs and the cost effectiveness of cardiovascular screening and intervention: the British Family Heart Study. British Medical Journal 312, 1269–1273

Wonderling D, Langham S, Buxton M, Normand C 1996 What can be concluded from the Oxcheck and British family heart studies: commentary on cost effectiveness analyses. British Medical Journal 312, 1274–1278

On whether mass media health education is cost effective:

Reid D 1996 How effective is health education via mass communications? Health Education Journal 55 (3), 332–344

On skin cancer prevention:
Carter R, Marks R, Hill D 1999 Could a national skin cancer primary prevention campaign in Australia be worthwhile? An economic perspective. Health Promotion International 14 (1), 73–82

40   For more about the National Institute for Clinical Excellence see www.nice.org.uk

41   For an example of clinical audit of health promotion, see:

Learmonth A, Jackson M, English C 1997 Calling in the auditors. Healthlines March, 8–9

42   See, for example:
Audit Commission 1995 Dear to our hearts? Commissioning services for the treatment and prevention of coronary heart disease. London: HMSO

43   These reasons are adapted from those set out in:

Ovretveit J 1992 Health service quality: an introduction to quality methods for health services. Oxford: Blackwell Science, p. 65

44   Fox J 1997 Clinical audit and the practice nurse. Practice Nursing 8(6), 18–20

45   For a useful introduction to health impact assessment see:

A short guide to health impact assessment – informing healthy decisions. Commissioned in 2000 by the NHS Executive, London. Available at: www.londonshealth.gov.uk, including fuller details and some practical tools for use in different situations.

See also:
Scott-Samuel A 2001 Health impact assessment. In Heller T, Muston R, Sidell M, Lloyd C (eds) Working for health, Chapter 14. London: The Open University in association with Sage Publications

46   Scott-Samuel A 1998 Health impact assessment – theory into practice. Journal of Epidemiology and Community Health 52, 704–5

8 Skills of Personal Effectiveness

SUMMARY

This chapter is about developing skills to manage your health promotion work effectively. We cover: managing information; writing reports; using time effectively; managing project work; managing change; and finally, working for quality. We include case studies and practical exercises.

Management Skills in Health Promotion

See also Chapters 5, 6 and 7. Working well in health promotion means not only having a clear view of your aims and plans but also having management skills to implement your plans.

It is not easy to define what management is, but in general terms we can say it is about being effective and efficient in your work. *Effectiveness* is the extent to which the results you set out to achieve are actually achieved. *Efficiency* is about how you achieve those results compared with other ways of achieving them.

We have already discussed some important aspects of management, such as setting aims and objectives, setting priorities, planning and evaluating work. A comprehensive introduction to management is beyond the scope of this book, but interested readers are provided with some suggestions for further study[1] and recommended reading at the end of this chapter.

In this chapter we identify and discuss a number of managerial skills you will need to be effective and efficient as a health promoter. However, it is important to emphasise that possessing these skills will not automatically make you effective and efficient. Other factors also influence this, including:

For further reading on ethics and values in health promotion, see Chapter 3.
■ How well you integrate ethical principles into your basic everyday work; how you exercise your *responsibility* as a health promoter. ('Response-ability' is your ability to choose your response and is a product of your conscious choice, based on values, rather than a reaction to your circumstances.) A fundamental aspect of health promotion is that it involves empowering ourselves, and others, to have more control over our health and our lives, and this in turn empowers us each to fulfil our unique potential.

■ The people you work with. Your effectiveness and efficiency are limited or enhanced by the competencies and motivation of those you work with – receptionists, secretaries and colleagues within and outside your organisation, for example.

- Your organisation. Both the structure and culture of your organisation will influence what you are able to achieve.
- The wider world. The state of the economy, government legislation, the organisation of local government and the impact of social trends are just a few examples of factors in the world outside your organisation that influence how effective you can be.

This book is designed to increase your awareness of these wider influences on your work, as well as to develop your own skills; both will help you to improve your competencies.

We now discuss some key aspects of personal effectiveness which will help you to manage health promotion.

Managing Information

Whether you keep information on computer or have a manual filing system it is easy to be swamped by documents and papers, so keep only what is essential for your job and cannot be kept by someone else or in another existing system.

Think about who else collects information in your workplace and how they store it. Is there a central filing system? Does it work? Which things could you keep in it?

Principles of Effective Information Systems

When reviewing or setting up your information system, it is useful to keep reminding yourself of three basic principles:

1. Keep it simple! Systems are only as effective as the people who put in and take out the information. The simpler the system the more likely it is that busy people will use it correctly.
2. Do not devise any more systems than are absolutely necessary.
3. Organise systems so that anyone who might want to use them can easily understand them.

Exercise 8.1	What Information do You Need to Store?

Make a list of all the types of information you collect at present and analyse it by asking yourself the following questions about each one.

1. **Do I need to keep this information?**
2. **How easy is it for me to find the information when I need it?**
3. **Could someone else, or another information system, keep the information for me?**
4. **Who else might need access to this information? How easy would it be for them to find it?**
5. **How could this information best be stored?**

Writing Reports

Important information is often conveyed through written reports. For example, you are likely to need to write a report on plans for health promotion, or an evaluation report on a specific project. You may need to write reports for your manager, or formal reports for committees. With written reports like these, they are likely to be read when you are not there, so there is no immediate feedback about whether your key points have been understood. To reduce the danger of being misunderstood, good skills in preparing and writing reports are essential.

See Chapter 10, section on written communication skills.

Work through the following stages each time you prepare and write a report.

Stage 1. Define the Purpose

To help to clarify the purpose, complete the following sentence: 'As a result of reading this report, the reader will...' What?

The purpose could be to inform, to influence decision-making, to initiate a course of action, or to persuade. Whatever it is, keep it clearly in mind throughout all the later stages.

Stage 2. Define the Readers

Identify the readers and consider them at all stages. Direct the report to the needs and interests of the readers. What do they already know about the subject? How much time do they have for reading? What kind of style is appropriate, for example, formal or chatty?

Stage 3. Prepare the Structure

Decide on the structure of the report. The usual parts of a report are:

- **Title** – this should accurately describe what the report is about.
- **Origins** – for example the author's name, occupation, work base and date.
- **Distribution list** – it is a great help to readers if they know who else has seen the report. They may detect that someone vital has not received a copy.
- **Contents list** – a long report will need a contents list, showing the main sections of the report and the pages on which the reader can find them. This is not necessary for short reports.
- **Summary** – this is vital for all except the very shortest of reports (less than a page or two). It helps the reader if the summary is easy to find at the beginning of the report. Remember that busy people will often read only the summary (and perhaps the conclusions and recommendations), or at least read the summary first in order to decide whether it is worth spending time reading any more. So the summary needs to set out the essence of the report clearly and concisely.
- **Introduction** – this sets the context for the report, for example why the work was done.
- **The 'body' of the report** – this will be the bulk of the report. You need to break up the content into sections and subsections, all with clear headings. Headings should be signposts to help the reader to see a route through the document and have an overview just by skimming through the headings. Sections need to be ordered in a way which will be logical for the reader. It may help to organise material into

sections by writing headings on index cards or sticky notes, then grouping them into a logical sequence. This can also be done on a computer: write all the possible headings down, then move them around until you are satisfied that they are in the most logical order.

- **Conclusions** – summarises the conclusions which can be clearly drawn from the information in the report.
- **Recommendations** – these relate to the future, and summarise any changes the author thinks are needed.
- **References** – putting any references at the end makes the report easier to read.
- **Appendices** – a much-misused feature of many reports, to be avoided unless really necessary. Ask yourself 'What information will most of my readers need the first time they read this report?' If they need this information straight away, put it in the main body of the report.

Stage 4. Write the Report

Tackle the various sections in the order that makes it easiest. For example, it may be easiest to write the detailed body of the report first, then summarise the information, then discuss the information, then draw your conclusions, then set out your recommendations, then write the summary of the report and lastly finish it off with the title, contents list, origin, distribution list and other essential details.

Stage 5. Review and Revision

After the draft report has been produced, review it and revise as necessary. Make sure pages are numbered and check that sections and subsections are correctly numbered. It is a good idea to show the report to one or two colleagues, preferably those who have good report writing skills and who will give constructive comments.

Stage 6. Final Check

Always do a final check for writing and typing errors, spelling mistakes, etc. It can be helpful to ask someone who has not seen the report before to check it for typing and layout errors.

Using Time Effectively

How well organised and effective are you at your work? The following paragraphs should give you some ideas about how to improve your effectiveness by looking at how you use your time. Time is an expensive resource, and the one that many health promoters find hardest to manage. First of all, you need to know where your time goes, so we look at ways of analysing and improving the use of your time. Then we outline an approach to scheduling your work.

Time Logs and Time Diaries

A time log involves keeping a record of how you spend your time at regular intervals, which may be as often as every five or ten minutes. It is useful if you wish to know exactly how you are using your time on an activity that seems to be taking longer than you think it should, and can help you to pinpoint the source of the problem. But keeping a log is time consuming itself, so is really worthwhile only if a particular activity is causing you problems.

If you want to know more about how you generally use your time you can keep a time diary. This records how you have spent your time day by day and should take only a few minutes to fill it in at the end of each day. If you have a short memory you might find it better to fill in your diary more frequently, say at the end of the morning and at the end of the afternoon, or at any other convenient break between blocks of work.

Exercise 8.2	Analysing and Improving Your Use of Time

1.   Devise a Recording Format That Suits You, Based on the Example Below

Then photocopy a supply of the sheets. Use as many sheets as necessary each day. Remember to include any work you do away from your base, for example at home.

If you discover that a particular activity, for example telephone interruptions, is causing you a problem, then make a detailed log of what happens each time. *Do this immediately* – do not leave it till the end of the day. Keep the diary for at least a week. If none of your weeks is 'typical' you will need to keep it for several weeks.

Using codes will save you time. For example, you could use M for meetings, I for interruptions, P for phone calls, IP for phone interruptions.

Time diary

Day _____   Date _____   Page no. _____

Activity	Time spent	Comments
_____	_____	_____
_____	_____	_____
_____	_____	_____

2.   Now Analyse How You Used Your Time

Each week, analyse your use of time by answering the following questions:

- How did you actually use your time compared with how you planned to use it?
- How much of your time do you spend on different activities? Does this reflect the importance of the different activities? Important activities are those that help you to achieve your objectives.
- Which jobs did not get done? Does it matter? Did you finish all the *important and urgent* jobs?
- How much time do you lose through interruptions? What sort of interruptions?
- How much of your time is spent on other people's work?
- Do you do the right job at the right time? Most people have a time of day when they work best. Do you use this time for your most important work?

3.   Now Plan How to Improve Your Time Management

Some of the changes you could make will be obvious. For example:

- You discover that jobs started early in the morning tend to get completed quickly. So you decide in future to do your most important work at this time.
- You discover that you spend about eight hours each week handling interruptions. You decide to experiment with techniques to cut down this time.
- You discover that urgent jobs are generally done but important long-term projects tend to be neglected. You decide to make realistic plans to ensure that these jobs will be done.
- What else can you do?

Scheduling Your Work

See Chapter 6, section Setting Health Promotion Priorities.

Health promoters generally find that they want to do far more than their time permits, and that they are faced daily with an almost bottomless pit of requests and demands. This means that, first and foremost, they must be very clear about their priorities. Secondly, they must be assertive about saying 'no' to requests to take on non-priority tasks. Thirdly, they need to develop skills of organising time to ensure that work which should get done actually does get done – scheduling work.

Scheduling work into the time available involves three steps:

1.   Identify how long you need to spend on a job. This depends on:

- The nature of the activity; for example, whether it is possible to cut corners without endangering people or the outcomes.
- How important the job is. If it is unimportant it does not merit a large investment of your time. Ask yourself 'What am I employed for? Will doing this job contribute to my main aims and objectives?' If not, it is unimportant. If the job is important it merits a large investment.

2.   Identify how soon you need to have the job completed. This depends on how urgent it is. Urgent jobs are ones that have imminent deadlines. If an urgent job can be completed quickly, deal with it right away. That means it will not interfere with you getting on with the most important jobs.

3.   Plan when the work will be done. This involves the following steps:

- Break the job down into manageable parts. If the job is big or difficult, or parts of it are boring, try setting aside regular, but small, amounts of time to complete specific bits. Using this 'salami' method (dividing it into thin segments) will help you to see that you are progressing.
- Estimate how long each part will take to complete. It can be difficult to estimate how long it will take you to complete a particular task, but an informed guess will at least help you to be more realistic in future. Here are some suggestions that may help:
  – ask someone you know who has experience in doing the job
  – use your experience from similar jobs
  – consult colleagues
  – build in some contingency time

– keep a note of how long the task actually takes, so that you can make a better estimate next time.

■ Schedule in your diary or organiser when the work will be done. You may find that you need to re-schedule daily, to take account of changing priorities. The important thing is to ensure that the key tasks you need to undertake are scheduled to allow enough time for their completion.

Managing Project Work

First, we need to know what a 'project' is, and why planning and managing it is different from other managerial activities you undertake. When you are first given responsibility for a project, it can seem rather daunting. You must turn something that does not yet exist into reality, and control its progress so that it delivers effectively and efficiently.

The most obvious thing about a project is that it has a particular (unique) purpose, which may be encapsulated in its name, such as 'Bromley Active Lifestyles Project' or 'Portsmouth Needle Exchange Project'. It is probably most useful to think of a project as an instrument of change, which, when it is successfully completed, will have made an impact as defined in its aims and objectives.

Another key aspect of projects is that they are time-limited: they have clearly identifiable start and finish times. Projects vary enormously in their scope. Small projects can last only a few days and involve activities by a single person; large projects can involve many people (and indeed many agencies) and last for several years.

All projects, however, have the same basic underlying structure and go through a number of stages, as set out in Box 8.1.

Box 8.1	The Stages of a Project

1. The **start** is the most important stage of any project and covers areas such as setting the overall aims, gaining approval, and the allocation of a budget. It will set the foundations for the lifetime of the project.

2. **Specification** involves defining the detailed objectives of the project, i.e. what the outcomes will be and the targets for delivering these outcomes in terms of quantity, quality and timing.

3. The **design** stage is when the 'what' is translated into 'how'. It may take the form of detailed plans.

4. In the **implementation** stage the plans are put into operation. It is important to note that the end of implementation is *not* the end of the project.

5. The **evaluation, review and final completion** stage will be marked by delivery of the final report, which includes evaluation of the findings and the details of a post-implementation review. This review should take place some time after the end of the implementation stage, so that it is possible to include data on the long-term outcomes of the project.

See Chapter 5,
The Basic Planning and
Evaluation Process.
These stages are, of course, very similar to the basic planning and evaluation cycle that was described in Chapter 5, and you should read the present section in conjunction with Chapter 5. The difference is that when you are delivering an on-going service, rather than a one-off project, the cycle repeats itself over and over again.

See Chapter 7, section
Linking Your Work into
Broader Health Promotion
Plans and Strategies.
Because projects vary so much in terms of their scale and length of life it is particularly important that they are planned systematically. It is also vital to understand how the project contributes to the wider strategic plans of the organisation concerned.

Starting a Project

A project will start with a proposal or written document, which can take a number of guises, such as 'terms of reference' or 'report of a feasibility study'. The key elements that must be described in this document include the following:

- Who is proposing to carry out the project, for example, a primary care trust or voluntary organisation.
- Who is the purchaser or commissioner of the project, for example the local authority.
- The aims and outcomes of the project.
- The scope of the project, for example who will use or receive it, the setting in which it will be delivered, which departments, agencies and people will be affected.
- The costs of the project, in terms of staffing, buildings, equipment and other resources.
- The project stages and timescales.
- Methods and standards: the use of any particular techniques or methods and the adoption of any recognised quality standards.
- Roles and responsibilities of participants in the project (especially important when the project is commissioned by a partnership of a number of agencies).

Detailed Planning

For anything but the very smallest of projects, you will need to develop a detailed plan of each stage immediately before you enter it. Typically, one of the last tasks in the planning of a stage will be planning the next stage. The bar chart (also known as the Gantt chart after the man credited with inventing it) is the primary tool to use for scheduling project tasks and controlling progress.

The Gantt or bar chart is made up of a task information side (on the left) and a task bar side (on the right). The task information side sets out the nature of each task and the person or people responsible for it. The task bar is a line that represents the period during which the task will be carried out. The precise content of a Gantt chart should be determined by what you intend to use it for. Such a chart is easy to draw and presents the plan in a visual form, which is easily understood by most people.

The chart can be used at every level in the planning process, from initial outline planning down to the detailed planning of individual tasks. For complex projects any single bar on the master chart for the whole project might have to be represented by a more detailed bar for that particular task or stage.

One major benefit of Gantt charts is that they highlight critical points, for example where progress in X is dependent on Y already being completed.

It pays to remember that planning tools such as Gantt charts are only aids to help you to achieve your purpose. Sticking slavishly to your plan will not necessarily bring success; you may have to alter your plan because of unforeseen circumstances. However, without systematic planning you are unlikely to be able to keep your project on course at all. An example of a Gantt chart is set out and described in Case Study 8.1 and Figure 8.1.

| Case study 8.1 | **Using a Gantt Chart in Project Planning** |

This small pilot 8-month project aimed to explore the feasibility of using community pharmacists (retail chemists) to promote physical activity with customers. Its objectives included identifying barriers and opportunities, and seeing whether training helped.

The plan was to recruit ten volunteer pharmacists, interview them to ascertain their attitudes towards promoting physical activity with customers and their current practice, and then work with them in a training session. After the training, the pharmacists had a 6-week period to implement the training, followed by another interview to see if their attitude and actions had changed.

A project manager had responsibility for planning and managing the project; a researcher was employed to design and carry out the interviews and help with the final report.

Figure 8.1 shows the Gantt chart drawn up by the project manager. It was useful for clarifying what needed to be done when, and for seeing when possible timing difficulties could arise. For example, would pharmacists' or researcher's holidays interfere with the schedule? Were there too many tasks to be completed at one time (for example, recruiting pharmacists and appointing the research worker in February and March)? The Gantt chart also showed which stages required the research worker, so that the project manager could negotiate the appropriate numbers of hours worked at appropriate stages.

Controlling Implementation

For more about quality, see section on p. 161 Working for Quality.

In addition to detailed plans any project needs to have built-in control procedures: controlling projects is about identifying problems as soon as they arise, working out what needs to be done to ameliorate them, and then doing it. Things that need to be controlled include time, the budget (costs) and quality. Methods for control include progress reports and one-to-one and group progress meetings. Large projects will need to use all of these methods. Progress reports can sometimes be best presented in a standardised form, which compares progress with the project plan.

Some problems will be outside the immediate control of the project. For example, a project could be influenced by the training policies of an organisation or other factors deeply embedded in the structure and culture of an organisation. In these cases project managers should do what they can to reduce the impact of these issues on the project, but should also remember that they have a duty to highlight these issues in reports, and not cover them up.

Managing Change

Health promoters may experience change in two ways. One is being a part of an organisation that is undergoing change itself – in other words, finding yourself being

Fig 8.1   A Gantt Chart

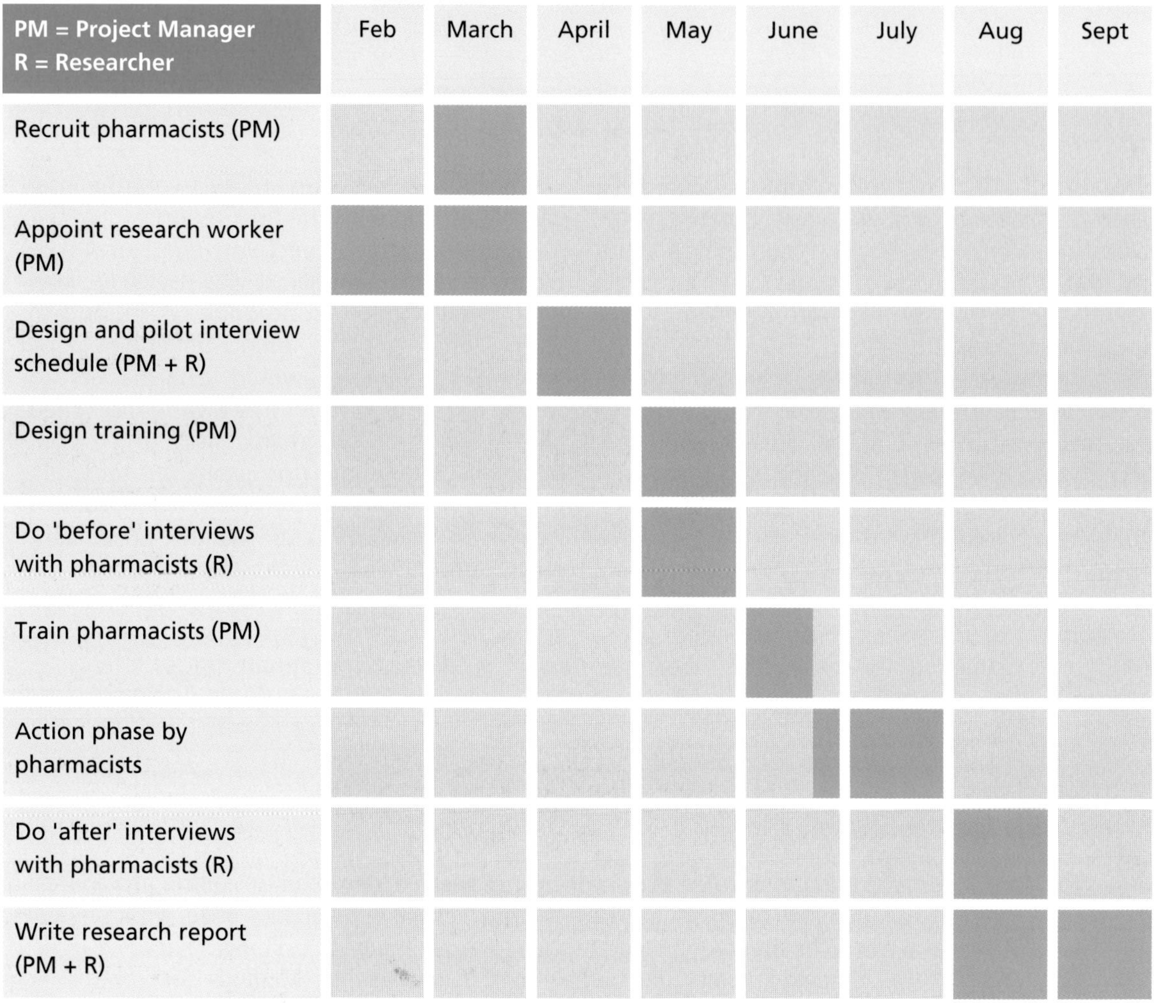

PM = Project Manager R = Researcher	Feb	March	April	May	June	July	Aug	Sept
Recruit pharmacists (PM)		■						
Appoint research worker (PM)	■	■						
Design and pilot interview schedule (PM + R)			■					
Design training (PM)				■				
Do 'before' interviews with pharmacists (R)				■				
Train pharmacists (PM)					■			
Action phase by pharmacists					■	■		
Do 'after' interviews with pharmacists (R)							■	
Write research report (PM + R)							■	■

reorganised, with your job and your location within your organisational structure changed. The second way is by being a change agent yourself, by implementing changes in public health policy or practice.

The first way, experiencing organisational change, has been particularly common in statutory agencies since the 1990s as modernisation and reorganisation have affected the NHS and local authorities in particular. The topic of understanding and surviving organisational change, and feeling positive about it, is outside the scope of this book. However, thinking about the second way – how to implement change successfully – may help you to understand and cope better with being part of an organisational change.

Implementing Change

You may want to introduce a change in your public health practice, such as a different way of running health promotion programmes, introducing a health-related policy at your place of work, or starting off new health promotion activities. Implementing change can be very challenging, and it will help to spend some time thinking through your strategy. The following sections on key factors for successful change, identifying reasons for resistance, and overcoming resistance, may help.

Key Factors for Successful Change

The key to gaining commitment to change, and overcoming resistance to change, lies in understanding the motivation of all the people who could be affected by the change and how they feel about it. Overall, do they feel positive or negative about the proposed change? The balance between positive and negative factors can be expressed in a 'change equation' developed as a tool to help analyse the key factors involved (Box 8.2).[2]

Box 8.2	The Change Equation

A = the individual's or group's level of dissatisfaction with things as they are now.
B = the individual's or group's shared vision of a better future.
C = the existence of an acceptable, safe first step.
D = the costs to the individual or group.
Change is likely to be viewed positively, and be implemented successfully, if:
A + B + C is greater than D

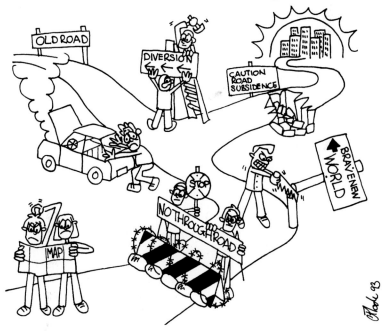

Implementing change can be very challenging

The basis of the equation is the simple assumption that people are rarely interested in change unless the factors supporting change outweigh the costs. As a change agent your job is either to reduce D (the perceived costs) or to increase the sum of A, B, and C. We shall now examine each of the elements in the equation briefly in turn.

A: Dissatisfaction with the way things are If we are dissatisfied, we may wrongly assume that others are too. If people are comfortable with the way things are they are unlikely to support change.

B: A shared vision of a better future If a vision of a better future does not exist, or is unclear, people will not strive to achieve it. If there are several competing visions, energy will be dissipated in arguments. Few people would buy into a vision that threatens their livelihood or other cherished aspects of their lives. A vision that threatens important aspects of an individual's or a group's life is almost bound to fail.

C: An acceptable, safe first step The size of the change and the risks involved can seem overwhelming. Many of us could share a common view of what better health for all would mean. But where do we begin? First steps are acceptable if they are small, are likely to be successful or, if they fail, do not cause too much damage and the situation is retrievable.

D: The costs to the individual or group What is important here is how people *perceive* the costs, not how they actually are. There will always be costs; change is often painful and unfair. Costs can be tangible things like time, money, resources, or more intangible costs like stress or loss of status.

Reasons for Resistance

We now look more closely at some of the main reasons why people resist change. Different people react differently to change for a variety of reasons. While one person passively resists a change, another may actively try to sabotage it, whereas a third may not be resistant and may actually bring change about.

Whether you are campaigning for a change, or implementing a change in policy or practice in your work, you will need to deal with the fact that many people resist change for a number of reasons, including the following.

Self interest While a change may be in the interest of most people, it may not be in everyone's best interest. For example, while most people, including some smokers, may support a smoking policy, others may see it as an infringement of personal liberty.

Misunderstanding People can easily misunderstand what is being proposed. For example, people may think that an alcohol policy is letting people with drinking problems 'off the hook', so that they do not have to meet the same standards of work performance and behaviour as everyone else. Misunderstandings are particularly frequent in organisations where there is a lack of trust between the managers and the workforce.

Belief that a change is not in the interest of the people it is intended to benefit People may believe that the costs of a change will outweigh the benefits, not only to themselves but also to other people or a whole organisation. For example, people may feel that the introduction of ethnic monitoring as part of an equal oppor-

Case study 8.2 — Change in a District General Hospital[3]

An example of significant change originating from a few people started in the physiotherapy outpatients' department of a district general hospital. One of the physiotherapists found that, in addition to giving instructions verbally, it was useful to write down instructions for patients who needed to do exercises at home. She enlisted the help of the Medical Illustration Department in designing and printing some leaflets based on these instructions. A second physiotherapist had begun to collect a small library of books, such as those produced by the Arthritis and Rheumatism Council. Meanwhile, the receptionist had taken another initiative. A friend had told her about a local support group for arthritis sufferers, and she pinned up a poster, giving information about it, in the waiting area.

The superintendent physiotherapist in charge encouraged the staff to share their ideas. As a result a departmental strategy to improve the provision of information to patients was launched, and patients were asked about their needs and preferences.

Other outpatients' departments in the hospital heard about the venture and expressed interest. As a result, a number of other initiatives took place across the hospital to improve patient information. Plans are now under way for a Patient Education Centre to be located in the foyer of the main hospital entrance, and this has the support of the Community Health Council and the Friends of the Hospital.

This case study illustrates the factors in the 'change equation':

A. The individual's or group's level of dissatisfaction with things as they are now: two of the physiotherapists and the receptionist, and through them their supervisor and the rest of the department, saw that there was room for improvement.

B. The individual's or group's shared vision of a better future: the idea of improved help for patients was shared and spread through an increasing number of people in the hospital.

C. The existence of an acceptable, safe first step: this change was built on a number of small successes, and did not present any major hurdles which could have induced resistance. If the *first step* had been to propose a Patient Education Centre, people may well have perceived major difficulties.

D. The costs to the individual or group were small in the first instance, just a little time and effort. By the time major investment was required for the Patient Education Centre, everybody was committed.

tunities policy could actually increase discrimination against black and minority ethnic groups.

Awareness of these opinions is important for the policy maker, because they may be based on knowledge of what goes on in parts of the organisation with which the policy maker has little contact. Policy formation must be based on an accurate analysis of the situation; this is particularly relevant in large organisations, like the health service and local councils.

Low tolerance for change People may resist change because they are anxious about new demands that will be made of them. For example, there may be demands to provide separate rest rooms for smokers, or to provide health counselling for people with alcohol problems. Organisational change can require people to change too much, or fail to provide them with the time and support they need.

Methods for Overcoming Resistance to Change

In order to overcome resistance to change it is vital to select the best approach, or combination of approaches, for the situation and the people involved. Five possible options are given below.

1. **Education and communication** This involves educating people about a change before it happens and communicating with them in a variety of ways, including one-to-one, group discussion and written documents. An educational and communication approach is indicated when resistance to change is based on inadequate or inaccurate information. The limitation is that it can be time consuming, especially if a lot of people are involved.

2. **Participation and involvement** Resistance to change may be forestalled if those initiating the change identify the people that they think will be resistant, and actively involve them in the process of designing and implementing the change. The initiators of the change must genuinely be prepared to listen and learn. A token effort is liable to provoke more resistance, because people will feel tricked if their advice is not heeded.

Participation and involvement are indicated when people need to be committed to a policy change in order to make it work; policies work when people feel ownership for them because they have been involved in their development. This approach is also useful when the initiators do not have full information about the implications of the change for certain groups of people or certain departments. It could also be the preferred option where the initiators of change have little power, because it harnesses the power of others as a force for change.

Nevertheless, this approach does have limitations. It is very time consuming and demands a high degree of coordination. It can lead to a poor outcome if it tries to please everybody.

3. **Facilitation and support** This involves helping people to identify what changes are required and providing them with support to plan and manage the change themselves. This could be done, for example, by providing 'time out' for people to reflect on the situation, and to identify their own objectives and how to meet them. Support could include emotional support to cope with stress and 'burn out', and the development of 'mentoring' or 'facilitator' schemes, where more experienced people help others with their managerial or professional development. This approach works best where anxiety and fear lie at the heart of resistance. The limitation of this approach is that it, too, can be time consuming and expensive (for example, if it is necessary to employ counsellors for a large workforce).

4. **Negotiation and agreement** This involves offering incentives to actual or potential resisters, for example, through negotiating with trade unions about the effects of the change on their members' pay. This is particularly appropriate when it is obvious that some people will lose out as a consequence of the changes. It can be effective if there are specific pockets of resistance, but could be expensive if everyone leaps on the bandwagon and tries to argue that they are also losing out.

5. **Political influencing** This approach can be useful where one, or a few, powerful individuals are the source of resistance. It can be relatively quick, but has the drawback that it can lead to problems in the future if people feel that they have been manipulated.

See also Chapter 16, section The Politics of Influence.

Working for Quality

There is now a lot of emphasis on the *quality* of services, that is, looking at the nature of the service, and assessing how 'good' it is when judged against a number of criteria.

Criteria for Quality

What are the criteria for quality in health promotion work? The checklist in Box 8.3 may be helpful in identifying aspects of quality in your health promotion work. The checklist can be applied to your work overall, or to a particular health promotion programme.

Box 8.3	Checklist: Criteria for Quality in Health Promotion[4]

1. **Appropriateness:** is it relevant and acceptable to clients – the individual, group or community concerned?
2. **Effectiveness:** does it achieve the aims and objectives you set?
3. **Social justice:** does it produce health improvement for all concerned, not for some people at the expense of others? In other words, is it 'fair'?
4. **Equity and access:** is it provided to all people whatever their racial, cultural or social background on the basis of equal access for equal need? (This may mean, for example, unconventional clinic times, wheelchair access, leaflets in Braille and ethnic minority languages, information on audio and video cassettes, etc.)
5. **Dignity and choice:** does it treat all groups of people with dignity and recognise the rights of people to choose for themselves how they live their lives? Is it non-judgmental, accepting that people have the right to withdraw from, or reject, health promotion if they so wish?
6. **Environment:** does it ensure an environment conducive to people's health, safety and well-being? Does it recognise that people feel at home in different environments, and may feel uncomfortable or intimidated in some settings? Is the social environment friendly and welcoming?
7. **Participant satisfaction:** does it satisfy all those with an interest in the outcomes of the health promotion work, such as commissioners, managers, clients and other interest groups, acknowledging that the views of clients should be paramount?
8. **Involvement:** does it involve all those with an interest, including clients, in planning, design and implementation? Does it avoid 'tokenism', with clients' views genuinely sought and incorporated in a non-patronising way?
9. **Efficiency:** does it achieve the best possible use of the resources available, and provide value for money?

Improving Quality

Initiatives to improve quality are usually successful if people work together to pool ideas. This could be a group of people authorised by management to examine a particular issue or problem, such as improving the quality of patient information literature, the way in which antenatal advice is being given to prospective parents, or the way a GP practice is helping patients to stop smoking.

Sometimes such groups are called *quality circles*. These are 'natural work groups' of between about three and twelve employees who do the same (or similar) work, who meet regularly to address work-related problems. The issues to tackle are selected by the group itself and the outcomes are presented to management. In many cases the group is also involved in implementing the solutions. Management commitment to taking account of the outcomes and implementing recommended changes is crucial to success.

Typically, a quality circle will:

- begin by drawing up a list of issues for consideration, using techniques such as brainstorming
- select the issue to be addressed
- gather information about the nature of the problem, and analyse the causes
- generate a range of solutions, and establish the best options or combination of options
- prepare a report on their findings for management decision.

An example of a quality circle might be a group of nurses working in a coronary care unit looking at how to improve the quality of the patient education programmes which are run for discharged patients. The activities of such a group are described in Case Study 8.3.

Case study 8.3 **Bloggsville Royal Hospital: Coronary Care Unit**

Improving the Quality of Patient Education

A group of four nurses in the Coronary Care Unit have been meeting regularly as a quality circle, and have decided to investigate how to improve the quality of education for discharged patients. At present a course of six group sessions is provided for patients after discharge, and nurses take turns to organise and run the courses.

The group first looked at the data for attendance at the group sessions. They discovered that, over the last year, 60% of discharged patients attended at least one session, but of these, only 20% attended three or more sessions.

They conducted a series of interviews with discharged patients to investigate the reasons for attendance or non-attendance, and to find out patients' preferences about how they would like the education to be provided. They discovered that some patients do not like attending a group under any circumstances, and some strongly dislike coming back into the hospital environment. But some of these would like one-to-one opportunities for guidance from specialists such as a dietitian (on healthy eating), a physiotherapist (on exercise and fitness) and a psychologist (on how to stop smoking, stress management and relaxation).

Other patients would prefer to have written information, audiotapes (for relaxation and self-hypnosis) and videotapes (of appropriate exercise routines), rather than come back to the hospital. Others would like more information about community groups and facilities for exercise tailored to their needs; for example, free trials of fitness classes, swimming sessions for elderly people. Others are interested in knowing if there are self-help or voluntary groups they could join, such as clubs for people who are being rehabilitated following heart disease. Some patients, especially those who are socially isolated, have particularly valued the opportunity to meet as a group and to exchange experiences.

After analysing these findings, the group of nurses produced a report for their manager recommending that a range of educational opportunities is provided for the education of discharged patients including:

- putting patients in touch with local self-help and cardiac rehabilitation schemes
- setting up a video- and audiotape library providing appropriate material for discharged patients on free loan
- offering opportunities for counselling by specialists (dietitian, physiotherapist, psychologist) before discharge
- selecting or producing appropriate written material, and making it available to patients before discharge
- inviting all patients to return for an open evening, with information and demonstrations about facilities and activities available locally. This would include local authority exercise and leisure facilities, alternative medicine practitioners, community and self-help groups and commercial leisure organisations.

The report includes a financial breakdown, which demonstrates that the recommendations will have additional costs, primarily related to the proposed services to be provided by the professions allied to medicine. However, savings will be made on the nursing staff time currently devoted to running the courses and through financial sponsorship of written material by approved 'ethical' commercial sponsors.

This case study shows how the quality of the patient education programme could be improved on a number of criteria:

- **Appropriateness**: clients would find the new approach more acceptable and relevant.
- **Effectiveness**: more clients would gain from the programme.
- **Equity and access**: clients could access advice and help in different ways, and those who disliked group meetings, or found attendance difficult, would have their needs met in other ways.
- **Environment**: it was recognised that some people disliked the hospital environment.
- **Participant satisfaction**: clients and nurses would be more satisfied with the results.
- **Involvement**: clients were involved in redesigning the programme, with their views taken into account.
- **Efficiency**: it would be a better use of resources because it would reach the people intended, and avoid wasting resources on a programme that reached very few.

Developing Quality Standards

It may be helpful to look at improving quality by setting specific quality standards to aim for. A quality standard can be defined as:

an agreed level of performance negotiated within available resources.[5]

Examples of standards are those used by the ambulance service. A quality issue for an ambulance service is that it reaches the scene of an accident quickly. A quality standard is the specified maximum length of time this takes.

Quality standards in health promotion work have been developed.[6] For example, quality standards can be set for health promotion materials, and the criteria listed in Chapter 11 could be developed as a list of quality standards for health education leaflets:

See section Health Promotion Resources: Criteria for Choice in Chapter 11.

- appropriate for achieving your health promotion aims
- content consistent with your values and approach
- relevant for the people you are working with
- not racist or sexist
- easily understood by the people for whom the leaflets are intended
- accurate, up-to-date information
- free of inappropriate advertising.

A further challenge is to develop standards that are *quantifiable* in some way. This is a difficult task, but you could, for example, develop a five-point scale for assessing the quality of your leaflets, so that you score them out of five for the extent to which they fulfil each quality standard. Another example could be that you decide that a quality management issue is to respond quickly to requests from your clients. You could develop this by setting a standard such as returning telephone calls within 24 hours, and written requests within 3 days.

Setting, monitoring and reviewing quality standards can involve a great deal of time and effort. The benefit comes from seeing clearly identified improvements in service. There is considerable literature on developing quality in services, and we make suggestions for further study in the Recommended Reading below.

PRACTICE POINTS

- To implement health promotion work successfully you need to develop management skills, including information management, report writing, time management, project management, managing change, and developing quality.

- Managing information: keep only paperwork that is essential and cannot be kept by someone else or in another information-retrieval system (for example, on a computer). Store information in the simplest possible way, so that it is easily understood by everyone who might need access to it.

- Writing a report: be clear about the report's purpose and who will read it; decide the structure and outline content; write the sections in the order you find easiest; allow time for what you have written to 'sink in' and then review, edit and change as necessary. Always get your report checked at the final stage by someone else.

- Managing time: know more about how you spend your time through using time logs and diaries. Schedule your time by thinking about how long a job is likely to take (usually longer than you think), when it must be completed by, and when you can devote time to it.

- Planning your project work: even the smallest project is unlikely to succeed without detailed and systematic planning. A Gantt chart is a useful tool. Planning tools are aids to success, but good management means that plans may be subject to change.

- Managing change: change is more likely to be successful if people believe that the factors in favour of the change outweigh the costs. A shared vision

PRACTICE POINTS

of a desirable future and a small, safe, first step forward help to make change acceptable. It is important to identify reasons why people resist change and design an effective change strategy.

■ Working for quality: working to improve quality is best achieved through groups of people working together and pooling ideas. Management support and involvement are essential for success, but the staff who do the job are in the best position to know what is practical and feasible.

Recommended Reading

On Personal Effectiveness

➤ Covey S R 1992 The seven habits of highly effective people: powerful lessons in personal change. London: Simon and Schuster. (A highly acclaimed book on a principle-centred approach to personal effectiveness, which argues that highly effective people integrate ethical principles into their basic character. Also available as an audio cassette.)

On Management

➤ Archer M 2001 Call yourself a manager! Chalford: Management Books 2000. (Packed with techniques to improve management performance.)
➤ Johnson H T, Broms A 2001 Profit beyond measure: extraordinary results through attention to work and people. New York: Free Press. (Describes an approach to management based on self-organisation, interdependence and diversity: i.e. the characteristics of living systems.)

On the Management of Health Services

➤ Clark J E, Copcutt L (eds) 1997 Management for nurses and health care professionals. London: Churchill Livingstone
➤ Iles V 1997 Really managing health care. Buckingham: Open University Press
➤ Joyce P 2000 Strategy in the public sector: a guide to effective change management. London: Wiley

On the Management of Voluntary Organisations and Other Not-For-Profit Organisations, Such as NHS Trusts

➤ Wolf T 1999 Managing a non-profit organization in the twenty-first century. New York: Simon and Schuster. (The 'bible' for non-profit organisations.)

On Writing Reports and Proposals

➤ Burnard P 1996 Writing for health professionals: a manual for writers, 2nd edn. London: Chapman & Hall
➤ Heritage K 1998 Successful report writing in a week. London: Hodder & Stoughton/Institute of Management Foundation
➤ Jay R 1999 How to write proposals and reports that get results. Harlow: Pearson Professional Education
➤ Mort S 2000 Professional report writing. Aldershot: Gower

On Time Management

➤ Yager J 1999 Creative time management for the new millennium. Stanford: Hannacroix Creek Books

On Project Management

➤ Billows R 2001 Essentials of project management. Denver: The Hampton Group. (Includes instructions for using Microsoft Project software.)

On Organisational Change

➤ Hopkins R 2001 How to survive the information age at work: peak performance amid never-ending change. Chalford: Management Books 2000
➤ Wille E, Hodgson P 2001 Making change work. Chalford: Management Books 2000. (A practical manual providing for active participation by readers.)
➤ See also the website of the Change Management Resource Library (a reference site for publications on change management): www.change-management.com

On Developing Quality

➤ Marsh J 1998 The continuous improvement toolkit. London: B T Batsford

➤   Scherkenbach W 2001 The Deming route to quality and productivity. Chalford: Management Books 2000. (A practical guide to the philosophy and teachings of W. Edwards Deming, the founder of the Total Quality Management (TQM) movement.)

On Quality Assurance in Health Promotion, With Examples of Quality Standards

➤   Evans D, Head M J, Speller V 1994 Assuring quality in health promotion: developing standards of good practice. London: Health Education Authority

Notes and References

1   The Open University Business School provides a comprehensive distance learning course in management – The Effective Manager. For further details contact The Open University, Open Business School, Walton Hall, Milton Keynes MK7 6AG. Tel: 01908 274066.

    The Directory of Social Change organises masterclasses on management for the voluntary sector. For further details contact the Directory of Social Change, 24 Stephenson Way, London NW1 2DP. Tel: 020 7209 4422.

2   The change equation was developed by David Gleicher as a pseudomathematical tool. For further information see:

    Open Business School/Institute of Health Services Management/NHS Training Authority 1990 Managing Health Services. Milton Keynes: The Open University Book 9, pp 36–37, Managing Change

3   This case study is based on case material described in:

    Spurgeon P, Barwell F 1991 Implementing change in the NHS. London: Chapman & Hall/Health Services Management Centre

4   This checklist draws on the main principles of the WHO Health For All Movement (see Chapter 1, International Initiatives for Improving Health) and the White Paper Working for Patients:

    WHO Regional Office for Europe 1985 Targets for Health For All. Geneva: WHO

    Secretary of State for Health 1989 Working for patients. London: HMSO

5   Wessex Regional Health Authority 1991 Using information in managing the nursing resource – quality. Macclesfield: Greenhalgh

6   A useful quality assurance framework for health promotion, and examples of quality standards, is:

    Evans D, Head M J, Speller V 1994 Assuring quality in health promotion: developing standards of good practice. Wessex Institute of Public Health Medicine/London: Health Education Authority

9 Working Effectively with Other People

SUMMARY

In this chapter we focus on developing skills of working effectively with other people and organisations in order to plan and implement health promotion. We discuss the following key aspects: communicating with colleagues; coordination and teamwork; participating in meetings; effective committee work; working in local partnerships for health with other organisations. We include practical exercises and a case study.

You may plan and undertake your health promotion work entirely on your own, but you are more likely to be working with other people, including those from the wide range of professional backgrounds that make up the public health workforce:

- colleagues, who may be your peers, your managers, or people you manage
- colleagues in other parts of your own organisation
- people drawn from the community and/or from different organisations who are working with you on a health promotion activity of mutual interest and importance.

A key aspect of success will be how well you work with other people, and in this chapter we discuss the knowledge and skills needed. First, we look at the basics of your communication with your own colleagues.

Communicating with Colleagues

See Chapter 10.

Some fundamentals of good face-to-face and written communication are dealt with in Chapter 10. Whilst these are presented primarily with health promoter: client contact in mind, they are also applicable to contact between health promotion colleagues. We suggest that the following factors are particularly important to ensure effective working relationships:

- working in a partnership with colleagues which recognises and builds on their strengths, developing their self-confidence and mutual trust
- actively listening to colleagues, so that you understand clearly their opinions, thoughts and feelings.

A considerable proportion of your time may be taken up by communications with working colleagues, including telephone conversations, face-to-face discussions and written communications on paper and via computer (e-mail). Try Exercise 9.1 to help increase your awareness of how you communicate with colleagues, and how your communication might be improved.

Coordination and Teamwork

Health promotion often involves different professions and disciplines working together; it will include working with colleagues from other departments and from different agencies. Therefore good coordination and teamwork are required.

Poor coordination can result in dramatic losses in efficiency and even the total breakdown of programmes; it is especially difficult when big bureaucracies like the

---

Exercise 9.1   How You Communicate with Colleagues

Record all the types of communication with colleagues that you carry out over one working day, by making a tally of all the occasions in four categories, as set out below. Then add up your total for each category, and your grand total for the day.

You might like to compare your results with those of your colleagues.

	Face-to-face verbal	Telephone	Paper: letters and memos	Electronic: e-mail, web cam/ computer conferencing
	___	___	___	___
	___	___	___	___
	___	___	___	___
	___	___	___	___
	___	___	___	___
	___	___	___	___
TOTALS	___	___	___	___

Think about whether there is anything you would like to change or improve; for example:

■ If you spend a lot of time on the telephone, could you improve your telephone skills?
■ Could you use your time more efficiently if you used less time-consuming methods of communications (for example, phone or e-mail) instead of writing letters or having meetings?
■ Are there ways that you can use technology to communicate more effectively and efficiently with colleagues?
■ Do you need to selectively spend more time face-to-face in order to understand colleagues and establish a closer working relationship?

NHS and local authorities are working together. There are several ways of coordinating, and it is important to use the one best suited to the situation.

Appointing a Coordinator

The problem for coordinators is that they do not directly manage the people they are trying to coordinate and therefore cannot control them in the same way as a manager can; they must convince people that any requests they make are legitimate. Often coordinators are at a modest level in a hierarchical organisation. A diabetic nurse trying to coordinate the production of a patient information leaflet, for example, might find it difficult to obtain the commitment of a consultant. The very word *coordinator* may provoke resistance in some people because they think they will be 'organised' by someone else.

Although resistance to coordination cannot be magically spirited away, there are several tactics that can help.

Using Your Reputation

People will find it difficult to turn down any reasonable requests if your work is well known and well thought of locally and you are respected by those who work with you. So you need to publicise your work and seek to establish a good reputation.

Establishing Good Relationships

There is no substitute for building and maintaining good relationships, and there is no denying that this requires a lot of continuing effort. It may be tempting to think that this is not 'getting on with the job' but it is an essential investment for every coordinator.

Bargaining

It may be possible to bargain with individual people or departments – could you offer them something in return for their cooperation?

Out-ranking

This should be used only in extreme circumstances. It means getting a senior manager from your hierarchy to request cooperation through the other person's manager. While the other tactics build trust and goodwill, this one endangers it and may give you even more headaches in the future.

Discussion and Negotiation

Talking to all involved could result in clarification of responsibilities and improved mutual understanding, leading to the group giving you more legitimate authority. This could mean first discussing the issue with individuals, and later convening a meeting when you have got sufficient commitment to solving the problem.

Policies, Rules and Procedures, Protocols

Making and implementing policies is discussed in Chapter 16.

Policies are increasingly important in coordinating health promotion work. Using *rules* and *set procedures* are ways of coordinating routine tasks. *Protocols* are agreed written procedures that everyone follows, ensuring that everyone carries out a particular task in the same way. For example, there may be a protocol in a GP surgery about how to help a patient to stop smoking. The protocol ensures that whoever is dealing with the patient (the doctor, the practice nurse, the district nurse, or the health visitor) will offer the same range of help and follow the same follow-up procedures.

Joint Planning

In this approach the parties involved not only agree objectives but also meet regularly to develop and implement a joint plan. This may minimise the need for one individual to be given the job of coordinator and prevent the problem of one agency or department being perceived as telling another what to do. However, it can be very difficult to get all the people involved together on a regular basis, and to make sure that communications are always clear to all those involved.

Joint Working Through Creating Teams

A particular team is given the authority, training, money, staff, premises and equipment to carry out the programme. The team is autonomous and gets the satisfaction of 'running their own show'. There is no need for a coordinator, since the whole team is working together from the same base. Joint working of this kind is not suitable for short-term programmes, but can be excellent for long-term projects, such as a community development project.

Creation of Lateral Relations

This type of coordination depends on strengthening relationships between individuals in broadly equivalent jobs in different departments or agencies. Setting up project teams, which are dissolved once the particular project is completed, can do this. It could also be done by forming interdepartmental or multidisciplinary teams, who are given more authority for making decisions 'at the sharp end', without having to refer them up the different hierarchies. However, this can lead to conflict with the existing vertical lines of command, and works best where there are good links between the various managers.

Characteristics of Successful Teams

There are different sorts of teams. Some are competitive, like sports teams; others are associations of people with a common work purpose, for example a primary health care team. Successful teams have the characteristics set out in Box 9.1. If you experience a team that does not seem to be working well, it can be helpful for the team to consider this list together, to identify the roots of the difficulties.

Participating in Meetings

The detailed planning and organisation of meetings are beyond the scope of this book, but we offer you some guidance below on how to be an effective participant at meetings. As a participant there are a number of constructive things you can do:

- Encourage the Chair into good practices, for example, ask for clarification on the purpose of the meeting, and ask for a summary of what has been agreed at the end.
- Come prepared and arrive on time. Insist on ending on time too!
- Acknowledge the authority of the Chair.
- Agree what to do about taking notes: does each person take their own, or does one person take them and circulate a copy to everyone else? Do you want detailed notes of everything you discussed, or just action points?
- Do not speak for more than a minute or two at a time.
- Actively contribute to the meeting – express your views, keep an open mind and listen to other people's opinions.
- Encourage everyone to participate – draw in quieter people by referring to their relevant experience or expertise.

Exercise 9.2   Improving Coordination and Teamworking

In the health promotion work you do that involves working with other people, can you think of any ways by which you could improve coordination and teamworking?

- **What steps could you take to enhance the reputation of your health promotion work?**
- **With whom could you build a better relationship to improve coordination or teamwork?**
- **What have you got to offer if you are bargaining?**
- **Can you think of any health promotion activities that you undertake routinely together with other people, which could be more efficient with a set procedure?**
- **Are there any ways by which you could develop stronger links with other staff at your level in different departments or agencies, to facilitate joint working in health promotion?**
- **Have you any opportunities for joint objective-setting or joint planning that could help to coordinate health promotion in your situation?**
- **Can you think of anything else? Discuss this with colleagues who are also involved in health promotion.**

Box 9.1   Characteristics of Successful Teams

- A team consists of a group of identified people.
- The team has a common purpose and shared objectives, which are known and agreed by all members.
- Members are selected because they have relevant expertise.
- Members know and agree their own role and know the roles of the other members.
- Members support each other in achieving the common purpose.
- Members trust each other, and communicate with each other in an open, honest way.
- The team has a leader, whose authority is accepted by all members.

- Only make commitments that you are genuinely able to fulfil, and make sure you fulfil them on time. Say 'no' clearly and non-defensively if you are unable or unwilling to do something.
- Remember that discussion and argument about ideas will help decision-making but personal rivalries will not.

Effective Committee Work

A committee is a group of people appointed for a specific purpose accountable to a larger group or organisation; examples are the management committee of a voluntary organisation or the health committee of a local authority. There are many common routines and procedures that help to oil the wheels of committees, and it is useful to be familiar with them. The details will vary from committee to committee, although the principles remain the same. Some committees start their life with recommendations from a steering group, which include proposals for the interim committee rules. These are then approved at the first committee meeting. After review and modification, a set of rules will be agreed which become the accepted rules for the committee.

Officers

The officers are servants of the committee and carry out its instructions. In practice, these are powerful positions that can be abused and a good Chair will work for the active involvement of all committee members. Many committees have three key officers – the Chair, the Secretary and the Treasurer. As committees grow the officers often need help with their work and additional appointments may be necessary, for example, a Minutes Secretary.

Chair

Much of the work of the Chair may be done between meetings, but it is at the meetings when the Chair is most visible, and has responsibility for ensuring that the committee successfully completes its tasks. It is vital for the Chair to be heard clearly during meetings, so that all the committee can be involved. Good Chairs delegate as much as possible, to ensure active involvement of all members. The Chair also has the responsibility of preparing or 'grooming' the next Chair and must ensure that opportunities are provided for the Vice-Chair to develop.

Secretary

The Secretary is responsible for all the non-financial papers and reports, for general planning and organisation (often in collaboration with the other officers), and for seeing that the committee's work is coordinated and nothing is forgotten. Ability to use word-processing software on a computer and skill in the use of words are extremely helpful. Good organisation and coordination skills are needed.

The Secretary is responsible for compiling the agenda for the committee meetings. This is the list of things to be done or agreed during the meeting. It will often include standard items such as 'apologies for absence', 'minutes of the previous meeting', 'matters arising from the previous meeting' and 'any other business'. The important point is that the agenda acts as an advance organiser for everyone attending the meeting, so that they are able to prepare. The committee members need to receive the agenda in good time before the meeting.

The Secretary is also responsible for the final version of the minutes, and for agreeing these with the Chair, even if a Minutes Secretary takes the notes at the meetings. Minutes are accurate records of the meeting, and should always precisely identify who has responsibility for what action by what date, and when a report back will be made to the committee.

Treasurer

A Treasurer will be necessary if the committee is responsible for any financial matters. Treasurers are expected to report on the financial position quickly and precisely at any time by recording and summarising every transaction as it happens, so that it is easy to see the current situation. At the end of the financial year all financial transactions are summarised in an annual statement – a clear one-page summary.

Quorum

In the real world it is unlikely that all committee members will be able to attend all meetings. The rules usually state the minimum number of members who must be present for the meeting to be considered representative of members' views and to have the authority to make decisions. This is called a quorum and is usually one-third or one-half of the total voting membership.

Committee Behaviour

Committees tend to be more informal than they were in the past. Nevertheless, it is good to bear in mind the reasons for various formal behaviours. For example, the rule that only one person speaks at a time, and is not interrupted, is meant to ensure a fair hearing for everyone. The Chair should not allow a vociferous few to dominate the meeting.

The rule of everyone speaking by addressing the meeting through the Chair helps to prevent a number of sub-discussions developing at the same time. On the other hand, it may seem more natural and helpful to address another committee member directly. Ultimately it is the job of the Chair to set a tone that encourages all members to participate whilst keeping the meeting under control.

For further information, including conduct of elections of officers and annual general meetings, see the suggestions at the end of this chapter.

Understanding Conflict

In itself, conflict is not bad. Conflict is inevitable at times in any group because of differences in needs, objectives or values. The results of conflict will be positive or negative depending on how the group handles it. Handled well, conflict can be a creative source of new ideas and can help a group to change and develop. It can also strengthen the ability of group members to work together. Conflict is badly handled when it is either ignored ('burying your head in the sand') so that negative feelings are left to fester, or approached on a win/lose basis (one person only can win, the rest of the group lose).

Exercise 9.3	**Your Conflict Resolution Style**

When confronted with conflict in a group you work in, which of these styles do you use?

Style	Characteristic behaviour
Avoidance	Ignores the problem; avoids raising the issue; denies that there is a problem
Accommodating	Attempts to cooperate with everyone, even at the expense of not meeting personal or team objectives
Win/lose	Fights to win at any cost, even if it means alienating colleagues or causing the rest of the team to fail in meeting their objectives
Compromising	Suggests a compromise that would meet everyone's basic needs and maintain good relationships
Problem-solving	Openly confronts the problem and encourages everyone to face the disagreements and to express fully their opinions and ideas. Searches for a new solution which meets everyone's needs as fully as possible

Review this chart with other members of groups you work in. Can you think of situations in which these different approaches to conflict resolution were used? Discuss what worked and what did not. What could have been done differently to improve the outcome?

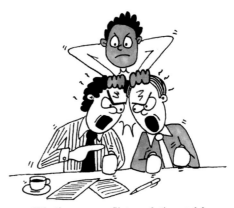

What's your conflict resolution style?

Working in Partnership with Other Organisations

Health promotion programmes and projects often require people from different organisations to work together; it is a way of working that has been recognised in health promotion for many decades. In the 1990s the term 'health alliance' came into prominent use because it featured in the first national strategy for health in England, *The Health of the Nation*.[1] The term 'health alliance' (sometimes shortened to 'alliance') is still in use by many health promoters to refer to formally recognised working partnerships between two or more organisations drawn from the NHS, local authorities, voluntary and/or community groups.

The most recent national strategy for England, *Saving Lives: Our Healthier Nation*, however, replaces the term 'alliances' with 'partnerships'.[2] NHS primary care trusts are

See Chapter 4, section on Primary Care Trusts for more on local strategic partnerships.

charged with forging powerful local partnerships to deliver shared health goals. Like the alliances that preceded them, local partnerships may be formally structured, with 'partners' or 'members' at different levels from chief executives to field workers. There may be a written constitution and terms of reference, or arrangements may be fairly informal. They may be long term, or set up for a time-limited period to work on a specific project.

The main reasons for setting up local partnerships are:

- to harness a range of complementary skills and resources to work towards common goals
- to avoid duplication and fragmentation of effort
- to avoid gaps in services or programmes.

See Chapter 4, Figure 4.1 for an overview of the organisations working for public health.

Recent government health reforms have created the opportunity for new styles of partnerships that the government wants to promote.[3] There is a broad approach to public health work and new financial flexibility, including giving health services and local authorities the power to pool their budgets for work they are both undertaking. This will help people working in the NHS and local authorities to form partnerships for planning, commissioning and delivering services. Local Health Improvement and Modernisation Plans (HIMPs) reflect these new-style partnerships, which are genuine joint enterprises with local authorities and others (Case Study 9.1 [p177] is a good example of this). Integrating HIMPs and local authority community plans will further enhance partnership working. Health Action Zones (HAZs) and neighbourhood renewal strategies are also leading the way in breaking down organisational barriers and engaging members of communities in partnership arrangements.

See Chapter 4, sections on primary care trusts and local authorities, for information on HIMPs, HAZs and neighbourhood renewal strategies. Also see Chapter 6, section Local Strategies and Initiatives.

In general, partnerships can take different forms, and vary in terms of how closely members work together. It is useful to think of three main ways of working, spanning a range of degrees of involvement between partners:[4]

Networking – Cooperating – Joint working

Networking

Networking means coming together with other people from different agencies, and exchanging information and ideas on activities and plans.[5] This is useful for coordinating activities, avoiding duplication and sharing knowledge of mutual interest. Members meet and talk, but they do not actually work together. Networking has the lowest degree of involvement between organisations.

Cooperating

Cooperating means that member agencies help each other in ways that are compatible with their own goals. They meet, talk, and agree to participate in each other's work when this is helpful for their own work plans. For example, in an accident prevention partnership (or alliance), people who work in the accident and emergency (A&E) department of a hospital may cooperate with a local alcohol advisory service (a voluntary organisation) to ensure that patients brought in with a drink problem know that they can go to the alcohol agency for help. This cooperation helps the alcohol agency to reach needy potential clients, and helps the A&E department to fulfil its role of helping patients with their health problems, possibly even preventing patients from coming back in a similar state. This way of working in partnership means a moderate degree of involvement between partners.

Joint Working

Joint working means coming together to agree a mutually acceptable plan, and working together to carry it out. This necessitates a high degree of involvement between partners. For example, the police, the probation service, road safety officers from the local authority, and a local alcohol advisory service may all work together to plan, implement, and evaluate a joint programme of work on drink/driving.

Partnerships can operate in one, two or all of these ways. Sometimes joint working is thought to be the 'gold standard', but networking and cooperating can be useful in themselves. It is not always feasible or worthwhile to aim for full joint working.

Factors for Successful Partnership Working[6]

See also earlier sections in this chapter on coordination and teamwork.

Successful partnerships do not 'just happen': they are usually the result of investing a considerable amount of resources, skill and time to enable members to work well together. The Verona Benchmark, a partnership benchmarking tool that has undergone a two-stage pilot, is useful in informing and assessing partnership processes and outputs.[7] Key factors for success are:

- All partners need to be working towards the same thing: a shared vision of what the partnership should achieve, with an agenda and goals which all partners agree to.
- There must be an agreed approach to partnership; all partners need to feel a sense of ownership of the partnership/alliance, and not that one partner dominates, with others as 'second class' fringe members.
- Commitment from the highest level of member organisations is vital to ensure that belonging to the partnership fits in with the organisation's strategic aims and that there will be management support for input of time and other resources.
- There must be commitment of sufficient time and resources and realistic expectations. Partnership working is time consuming, and it may take months or years to develop a shared understanding and joint plans, let alone achieve results from joint health promotion activities. On the other hand, there must be demonstrable achievements, otherwise the partnership/alliance will be regarded as a mere 'talking shop'.

See section on coordination earlier in this chapter.

- Someone acceptable to all partners needs to take responsibility for running the partnership/alliance (for example, setting up, chairing and servicing meetings) and coordinating action. A full-time coordinator can be extremely helpful.
- There must be mutual respect between partners; all partners need to feel that others value their input.
- Working relationships need to be characterised by openness and trust. Partners need to recognise and resolve potential areas of conflict.
- There must be an agreed framework for reviewing the partnership, changing the way of working if necessary, and even bringing it to an end if it has outlived its usefulness or is unproductive.
- Awareness and understanding of partner organisations should be promoted through joint training programmes and incentives to work across organisational boundaries.
- Partnership arrangements need to be regularly reviewed and adapted to reflect the lessons learned from experience.

Potential Difficulties

Partnership working can result in many difficulties. Major problems are:

- organisational change, which blights long-term commitment and planning
- competition between member agencies for funding, for example between different voluntary organisations who are seeking funding from the same source
- lack of resources, both money and person-power
- lack of top-level commitment from members of the partnership
- individual personalities who dominate partnership working (for good or bad)
- an imbalance of input from different agencies, which can lead to resentment and issues about ownership of joint activities and who takes the credit for success
- professional jealousy and unwillingness to share expertise and information
- differences between agencies and individuals in terms of different goals and values; different organisational cultures and ways of working; different levels of expertise and experience.

It is worth bearing in mind that not all partnerships are successful. Many fade out or are wound up. Partnership working is not an end in itself; it is a means to an end, and there are circumstances where the end is better achieved by an organisation working alone.

Case study 9.1	HEAL: a Case Study on Community Development and Partnership Working[8]

Health and Empowerment through Active Learning (HEAL) was set up in the London Borough of Hillingdon to enable minority ethnic communities to be involved in assessing their health needs and developing health initiatives with a range of partners. The aim was to use community development approaches to develop confidence and ability in Asian communities. A key influence was the Local Government Act 2000, which requires local authorities to work with communities to produce a community plan addressing economic, social and environmental well-being.

HEAL was initiated by Healthy Hillingdon with support from the statutory and voluntary partners involved in the Hillingdon HIMP. Healthy Hillingdon is a strategic health promotion partnership involving the London Borough of Hillingdon and the local NHS organisations. The overall strategy used by Healthy Hillingdon is based on a 'Healthy Cities' partnership approach to health promotion.

For more about 'Healthy Cities' see Chapter 16, section Developing and Implementing Policies.

HEAL was informed by the experience of community development work with ethnic minority groups throughout the UK, especially the following points.

- Although communities want to address health needs, they often perceive issues within holistic concepts of health and not in terms of government targets. But health service staff often see health needs in terms defined by government targets, and sometimes find it difficult to engage with the holistic health concepts embraced by community groups.
- Staff in the NHS with remits for community education are often unaware of the potential for working in partnership with ethnic minority community groups and unnecessarily assume that there will be insurmountable language barriers.

Recognition of the relevance of these factors in Hillingdon led to emphasis on developing working partnerships between Asian women's groups and health service staff. Consequently the objectives for the HEAL project were defined as:

- in Hillingdon NHS services, to develop ways of working with ethnic minority communities in order to assess their needs and promote health
- to overcome the communication barriers faced by ethnic minority communities in participatory and partnership work with the people providing services
- to develop the ability to tackle inequalities in *Saving lives – our healthier nation* topic areas (cancer, heart disease and strokes, accidents, mental health) and ethnic minority communities.

Process

HEAL contacted established community groups to explain the initiative. Negotiations with community groups and health service staff were held to arrange discussions about participatory and partnership health promotion and assessing health needs. Key steps were:

- discussions with community groups on health subjects they were concerned about
- identification of NHS staff who had remits to work with ethnic minority communities
- agreement of a work plan for a series of participatory workshops on health themes.

Meetings facilitated understanding between the professionals and the community and helped to form effective partnerships. The meetings focused on agreed health topics, explored concerns, and developed awareness of related issues.

Outcomes

In the first year five sessions were held, covering diabetes, food, activity, mental health, sexual health and general health. The holistic approach used enabled people to explore a broad range of issues, typically covering access to services, individual and community attitudes to health, and lifestyle.

Follow-up requests included expansion of discussion groups in other communities, joint working on a community-run drugs awareness project, and organisation of community-led workshops with service providers to look at access to services.

For professionals involved in the programme the key learning outcome was the openness of the women's groups to discussion and learning, and their desire to communicate without using translators. Although translation was occasionally needed, the group emphasised that they wanted to develop skills for direct communication and to access information without depending on intermediaries.

Community Work and Partnership: Practice Points Learnt From the HEAL Experience

- Recognise that the approach used to define health promotion needs may influence outcome as much as the method chosen to promote health.
- Before attempting to assess need, aim to develop sound working relationships between community groups and the partnership agencies that support them.
- Accept that expressed need is what is important and relevant to the community. It might not coincide with needs identified by partnership agencies.
- Plan for the long term. Building trust and relationships takes time in partnership initiatives.
- Start with small practical community-based initiatives. In work with communities it is essential to work together on achievable partnership projects.
- To be effective there is a need to 'legitimise' work and investment of time and resources. Providing a nationally defined strategic context is important for getting partners on board. Equally, community groups need to see that their involvement is relevant to their needs.
- The agencies and communities involved in partnerships need to see that joint work is

relevant to their own need to meet personal, community, operational and strategic objectives.

■ Partnership approaches require a commitment to facilitating shared learning, empowering people to take initiatives and a clear focus on enabling the translation of ideas into action.

PRACTICE POINTS

■ A key aspect of successfully implemented health promotion programmes is how well you and other health promoters work together.

■ You need to think about how you communicate with colleagues: the channels you use, how well you use them, and the quality of your relationships.

■ Health promotion often involves different professionals and disciplines working together; there is a range of ways in which you can encourage good teamwork and coordination.

■ For effective meetings and committee work, you require knowledge of how people behave in meetings, the roles and responsibilities of committee members, and skills of making the most use of meetings and committees.

■ Health partnerships between two or more organisations work at varying levels of involvement with each other, from networking at a local or national level to full joint working and from local partnerships to strategic partnership. Think about the many factors that contribute to success, and the potential pitfalls to avoid.

Recommended Reading

On Teamwork

➤ Barham K 1999 The teams audit: a complete self-assessment of company team working skills and performance. Cambridge: Cambridge Strategy Publications (CSP). (On measuring the effectiveness of your organisation in relation to teamwork.) Also included in CSP publications are High Performance Teams Portfolio and The Partnership and Alliance Audit. For further details of these and other publications see their website: http://www.cambridgestrategy.com/page_c.htm

➤ Gorman P 1998 Managing multi-disciplinary teams in the NHS. Basingstoke: Open University Press

➤ Lipnack J, Stamps J 2000 Virtual teams: people working across boundaries with technology, 2nd edn. Chichester: Wiley. (Information on web cams, video conferencing and the use of technology in teamwork.)

➤ Payne M 2000 Teamwork in multi professional care. Basingstoke: Palgrave. (Practical ideas on teamwork and teambuilding.)

On Running and Taking Part in Meetings

➤ Stanton N 1996 Mastering communication, 3rd edn. Chapter 9. Basingstoke: Macmillan

➤ Willcocks G, Morris S 2000 Making meetings work. London: Hodder and Stoughton

On Partnerships for Health

➤ Markwell S, Speller V 2001 Partnership working and interprofessional collaboration: policy and practice. In: Scriven A, Orme J (eds) Health promotion: professional perspectives, 2nd edn. Basingstoke: Palgrave, pp 19–31. (A succinct overview of partnership working.)

➤ Naidoo J, Wills J 1998 Practising health promotion: dilemmas and challenges. Chapter 8, Collaboration for health promotion. London: Baillière Tindall. (Explores collaboration between sectors and tensions in practice.)

➤ Naidoo J, Wills J 2000 Health promotion: foundations for practice, 2nd edn. Chapter 8, Partnerships for health – working together. London: Baillière Tindall. (Outlines and discusses partnerships and stakeholders in health promotion.)

Examples of Partnerships in Action, and Detailed Aspects of Partnership Working

➤ Evans N 2001 Tackling smoking through partnerships: lessons learned from the National Alliance Scheme. London: Health Development Agency

➤ Scriven A (ed.) 1998 Alliances in health promotion: theory and practice. Basingstoke: Macmillan

➤ Tones K, Tilford S 2001 Health education: effectiveness, efficiency and equity, 3rd edn. Chapter 10, Community-wide coalitions and inter-sectoral working. Cheltenham: Nelson Thornes

A Practical Framework for Planning, Evaluating or Developing Partnerships

➤ Funnell R, Oldfield K, Speller V 1995 Towards healthier alliances: a tool for planning, evaluating and developing alliances. London: Health Education Authority/Wessex Institute of Public Health Medicine

Notes and References

1 Department of Health 1993 Working together for better health. London: HMSO

Secretary of State for Health 1992 The health of the nation: a strategy for health in England. London: HMSO

2 Department of Health 1999 Saving lives: our healthier nation. London: HMSO

3 Department of Health 1997 The new NHS: modern, dependable. London: Department of Health

Department of Health 1997 Action for health – the ultimate partnership scheme. Press Office, DoH 97/309

Department of Health 1998 Partnerships in action (new opportunities for joint working between health and social services). London: HMSO

Department for Health 2001 Government response to the House of Commons Select Committee of Health's second report on public health. London: The Stationery Office

4 Based on:

Powell M 1992 Healthy alliances: a report to the HealthGain Standing Conference. London: Office for Public Management, pp. 31–32

5 Although in this chapter we focus on local networks of people, there are many wider networks in health promotion. They may be organised on a regional or national basis. For example, the Young People's Health Network is coordinated by the Health Development Agency and funded by the Department of Health. It publishes a regu-

lar newsletter on issues affecting young people's health and provides a means of exchanging information on research, news, projects, events and useful contacts (the database holds over 7000 contacts across a wide range of sectors and settings). For further details contact: Young People's Health Network, Health Development Agency, Holborn Gate, 330 High Holborn, London WC1V 7BA and/or their website: http://www.hda-online.org.uk/yphn/

6 These factors are drawn from the authors' experience, and from:

Department of Health 1993 Working together for better health. London: HMSO

Naidoo J, Wills J 2000 Health Promotion: foundations for practice, 2nd edn. Chapter 8, Partnerships for health – working together. London: Baillière Tindall

Powell M 1992 Healthy alliances: a report to the HealthGain Standing Conference. London: Office for Public Management

7 For further details on the Verona Benchmark see:

Watson J, Speller V, Markwell S, Platt S 2000 The Verona Benchmark – applying evidence to improve the quality of partnerships. Promotion and Education V11 (2), 16–23

8 Thanks to Terry Kelly and Andrew Knight of Healthy Hillingdon for providing this case study, which is a real-life example of a health promotion local partnership based on an HIMP.

3 DEVELOPING COMPETENCE IN HEALTH PROMOTION

Part 3 aims to provide you with guidance in how to assess, develop and improve your competencies in health promotion.

Competencies are the combinations of knowledge, attitudes and skills needed to perform work of a satisfactory standard in health promotion. As a health promoter, you need competencies to plan, evaluate, and implement health promotion activities, in different settings and with different goals, which we discussed in Part 2. You will also need to develop other core competencies of health promotion: communicating and educating, marketing and publicising, facilitating and networking, and influencing policy and practice. We address these in Part 3.

Some chapters of Part 3 will be more important to some professions or disciplines than others. So you may wish to start by studying the chapters most relevant to you, rather than going through them in sequence. We have provided cross-referencing to help you to identify which sections of other chapters may also be relevant to your particular needs.

In Chapter 10 we address the fundamentals of communication, including establishing relationships, and the links with promoting self-esteem and assertiveness. We identify four basic communication skills and provide guidance on how to improve them. We discuss communication and language barriers, non-verbal communication and written communication.

In Chapter 11 we start by suggesting some principles governing the choice of communication tools in health promotion. We look at the advantages and limitations of a variety of teaching and learning resources and provide guidance on how to produce and use displays, written materials and statistical information. We discuss how mass media can be used effectively in health promotion, including practical help about working with the local press, radio and television. We include a section on using information technology in health promotion.

In Chapter 12 we outline the principles of adult learning. We describe how you can help people to learn and evaluate the learning outcomes. We include guidelines on giving talks, and on patient education.

Chapter 13 is about working with clients in groups. We consider when it is appropriate to work with groups, how to lead groups, and how to understand group behaviour. We focus on the competencies required to work effectively with groups.

Chapter 14 is about how to help people to change their behaviour towards healthier living. We include information on models of the process of changing health-related behaviour. We describe strategies that can be used, such as working with a client's own motivation. We outline skills of counselling to help people to make decisions. We discuss principles that help with using strategies effectively.

In Chapter 15 we focus on community-based work in health promotion, including community participation, community development, and community health projects.

Chapter 16 is about how local and national policies, programmes, plans and strategies are made and how they can be influenced. We look at how health promoters can challenge health-damaging policies and develop, implement and evaluate health promotion policies. We include a section on the principles of campaigning and how to plan campaigns.

10 Fundamentals of Communication

SUMMARY

We start this chapter by exploring relationships with clients and discussing the links between self-esteem, self-confidence and communication, followed with a case study on relationship skills. Discussion on four basic communication skills follows: listening, helping people to talk, asking questions, and getting feedback. We continue by considering communication and language barriers, and non-verbal communication. We end with a section on written communication. Exercises are provided on overcoming communication barriers and on each basic communication skill.

Good communication between people is fundamental to successful health promotion, whether it happens in the context of a consultation with a patient, a conversation with a colleague, or a request to a manager. By 'good communication' we mean clear, unambiguous two-way constructive exchanges, without distortion of the message between when it is given and when it is received.

This chapter discusses some fundamentals of relationships with clients, communication barriers and basic communication skills. These skills will often be applied in one-to-one situations, though they may apply when working in groups or teaching as well as in more formal situations. These skills will help to develop better communication, but they should not be expected to provide a blueprint for every situation, or a quick and easy route to being a good communicator. They are a start, but improving communication is a life-long developmental process.[1]

See also Chapter 12, which discusses communication and education between health promoters and patients.

Exploring Relationships with Clients[2]

We start by asking health promoters to look at some fundamental (and possibly uncomfortable) questions. For example, what is your basic attitude towards the people you work with? Do you accept them on their own terms or do you judge them by your own standards? Do you aim to encourage people to be independent, make their own decisions, take charge of their health, and solve their own problems? Or are you actually encouraging dependency, solving their problems for them and thereby decreasing their own ability and confidence to take responsibility for themselves? We suggest that you work through the following questions, thinking about how you relate to the people you work with.

Accepting or Judging?

Accepting people means:

- recognising that people's knowledge and beliefs emerge from their life experience, whereas your own have been modified and extended by professional education and experience
- understanding your own knowledge, beliefs, values and standards
- understanding your clients' knowledge, beliefs, values and standards from their point of view
- recognising that you and the people you work with may differ in your knowledge, beliefs, values and standards
- recognising that these differences do not imply that you, the professional health promoter, are a person of greater worth than your clients.

Judging people means:

- Equating people's intrinsic worth with their knowledge, beliefs, values, standards and behaviour. For example, saying of someone who drinks 'people who get drunk are stupid' judges (and condemns) that person, and takes no account of life experience and cultural background. 'Drunkenness can result in people getting hurt' does not judge the person.
- Ranking knowledge and behaviour. For example, 'I'm the expert so I know better than you' is judgmental; 'I know more than you about this particular thing' is not – it is a statement of fact. 'My standards are higher than yours' is judgmental; 'My standards are different from yours' is not.

Autonomy or Dependency?

There are a number of ways in which you can help clients to take more control over their health.

Autonomy can be helped by:

- encouraging people to make their own decisions, and resisting the urge to 'take over' the decision-making
- encouraging people to think things out for themselves, even if this takes much longer than simply telling them
- respecting any unusual ideas they may have.

Autonomy can be hindered if:

- you impose your own solution on your clients' problems
- you tell them what to do because they are taking too long to think it out for themselves
- you tell them that their ideas are no good and won't work, without giving an adequate explanation or opportunity to try them out.

We suggest that the appropriate aim is to work towards as much autonomy as possible. By doing this, you are helping people to increase control over their own health, which is a basic aim of health promotion. Obviously, there are times when people are dependent on a health promoter, and rightly so; for example, they may be ill, confused, or likely to put themselves or other people in danger. There is also the very real problem that working towards autonomy is time-consuming. However, in the long run, it is time well spent.

A Partnership or a One-way Process?

Do you think of yourself as working in partnership with people in pursuit of health promotion aims, or do you see health promotion as your sole responsibility, with yourself as the 'expert'?

A partnership means:

- there is an atmosphere of trust and openness between yourself and your clients, so that they are not intimidated
- you ask people for their views and opinions, which you accept and respect even if you disagree with them
- you tell people when you learn something from them (e.g. 'I never thought of it that way before')
- you use informal, participative methods when you are involved in health education, drawing on the experience and knowledge that clients bring with them
- you encourage clients to share their knowledge and experience with each other. People do this all the time, of course (for example, knowledge and experience are discussed between patients in a hospital ward and parents in a baby clinic) but do you deliberately foster and encourage this?

A one-way process means:

- you do not encourage clients to ask questions and discuss problems
- you imply that you do not expect to learn anything from your clients (and if you do learn, you don't say so)
- you do not find out what people already know and have experienced
- you do not encourage people to learn from each other, only from you
- you use formal methods when you are undertaking health education, such as lectures, rather than participative methods.

Clients' Feelings – Positive or Negative?

A change in people's health knowledge, attitudes and actions will be helped if they feel good about themselves. It will rarely be helped if they are full of self-doubt, anxiety or guilt.

Clients will feel better about themselves if:

- you praise their progress, achievements, strengths and efforts, however small
- the consequences of 'unhealthy' behaviour (e.g. smoking) are discussed without implying that the behaviour is morally bad
- time is spent exploring how to overcome difficulties (e.g. practical strategies to help a client stop smoking). This will help to minimise feelings of helplessness.

Clients will feel bad about themselves if:

- you ignore their strengths and concentrate on their weaknesses
- you ignore or belittle their efforts
- you attempt to motivate them by raising guilt and anxiety (e.g. 'if you don't stop smoking you'll damage your baby' or 'you're killing yourself with what you eat').

To sum up, we suggest that the health promotion aim of enabling people to take control over, and improve, their health is best achieved by working in a non-judgmental partnership. This should seek to build on people's existing knowledge and experience, move them towards autonomy, empower them to take responsibility for their own health and help them to feel positive about themselves.[3]

Self-esteem, Self-confidence and Communication

The ability to communicate is closely linked to how people feel about themselves. People with a low sense of self-esteem tend to be over-critical of themselves and to underestimate their abilities. This lack of self-confidence is reflected in their ability to communicate. For example, they may lack assertiveness and thus may either fail to speak up for themselves or react with inappropriate anger and even violence.

By 'assertiveness' we mean saying what you think and asking for what you want openly, clearly and honestly. It does not mean being aggressive or bullying, but it is in contrast with hiding what you really feel, saying what you don't really mean or trying to manipulate people into doing what you want.

Assertiveness helps people to create win–win situations (situations where everyone involved feels that they have done all right) through direct and open communication and through avoiding aggressive behaviour (win–lose situations, where one party feels that they have won and the other party feels they have lost) or manipulation (lose–lose situations, where, for example, one party in a negotiation walks out). It builds the self-esteem of all concerned. Successful negotiation is a good example of how assertiveness can work. In a successful negotiation both parties come away with the following thoughts:[4]

- This is an agreement which, whilst not ideal, is good enough for both of us to support.
- Both of us made some compromises and sacrifices.
- We will be able to have successful negotiations with each other in future.

Many clients with low self-esteem will need to learn how to feel better about themselves before they can communicate better with professionals and others. This requires opportunities for 'life skills education', by which we mean education in the key skills necessary for living. These skills include how to improve self-esteem, and how to communicate and relate to others in a morally responsible manner, with respect for oneself and others, and with sensitivity towards the needs and views of others. Unfortunately, we are often expected to 'catch' these skills automatically, without any proper learning process to help us. Furthermore, the time allotted to personal and social education in schools may be insufficient.

For further reading on how to develop life skills and assertiveness and improve self-esteem, see the suggestions at the end of the chapter.

One way to develop these life skills is through relationships with people who are 'healthy' role models, and there is a body of research on the characteristics of the psychologically healthiest people.[5] However, we cannot choose our parents and many people have little choice of workmates or employers, so health promoters need to find opportunities for 'life skills education'.

Case study 10.1 illustrates how parents can learn to develop the self-esteem of their children and ensure that their children understand the rights of other people. While the case study refers to parents and children, and we have used this example because it is supported by research evidence, the same principles can be used by health promoters with their clients.

So, when working with clients with low self-esteem, you may find it helpful to:

| Case study 10.1 | **Relating Skills – Lorraine and Jack** |

Lorraine is late for work and tries to coax her three-year-old son, Jack, into his coat so that she can take him to nursery school. Jack starts to cry. Lorraine hugs him but tells him that he's got to go to school. She is at a loss about what else to do, and when she reaches nursery school Jack is still crying. One of the nursery nurses notices his distress and manages to calm him. When Jack has recovered, the nurse talks to Lorraine about what she's learnt from a book about good parenting which is based on up-to-date research.[6]

A week later in a similar situation Lorraine tries out what the nurse suggested. She starts in the same way as before, by empathising with Jack, but this time she goes further and provides him with guidance on what to do with his uncomfortable feelings. The conversation goes something like this:

Jack: 'It's not fair. I don't want to go to school'. (Starts to cry.)
Lorraine: 'Come here Jack'. (Takes him on her knee.) 'I'm sorry but we can't stay at home. I have lots to do at work. Does that make you feel sad?'
Jack: (nodding) 'Yes'.
Lorraine: 'I feel a bit sad too. It's OK for you to cry.' (Hugs him while he cries.) 'I know what. Let's think about what to do on Saturday when I don't have to go to work and you don't have

to go to school. Can you think of anything special you would like to do on Saturday?'
Jack: 'Can we go to the park and feed the ducks?'
Lorraine: 'Yes. That would be great.'
Jack: 'Can Nick come too?'
Lorraine: 'Perhaps. We'll have to ask his Mum. But right now it's time to get going.'
Jack: 'OK.'

Lorraine has gone through five steps:

1. She becomes aware of Jack's feelings.
2. She recognises the opportunity for helping Jack to learn about how to handle emotions.
3. She listens to Jack, tries to understand his feelings, and lets him know it is OK to feel bad and upset sometimes, and that she has these feelings too.
4. She helps Jack to find the words to label the emotion he is having.
5. She sets limits while exploring strategies to solve the problem.

Studies show[6] that children whose parents consistently practise these five steps have better physical health and score higher academically than children whose parents do not. They also get along better with friends, have fewer behaviour problems and are less prone to acts of violence.

- be aware of the client's feelings
- recognise the opportunity to help the client to learn about how to handle difficult feelings
- listen and acknowledge that you have these feelings too
- label the feelings
- set limits for the interaction while exploring strategies to solve the problem.

Listening

As a health promoter, you need to develop skills of effective listening so that you can help people to talk and identify their needs and feelings.

Listening is an active process. It is not the same as merely hearing words. It involves a conscious effort to listen to words, to the way they are said, to be aware of the feelings shown and of attempts to hide feelings. It means taking note of the non-verbal communication as well as the spoken words. The listener needs to concentrate on giving the speaker full attention, being on the same level as the speaker and adopting a non-threatening posture.

Figure 10.1 shows that active listening involves searching for an understanding of the underlying meaning behind the words used by the client. It shows how the meaning conveyed by the client can become distorted if the client cannot express exactly what he or she means. At the second step it shows that the health promoter may not hear what is being said. Thirdly, the health promoter may hear the words accurately, but interpret them in a different way from that which the client intended.

Fig 10.1	The Listening Process[7]

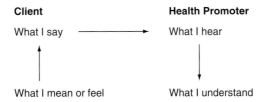

Client	Health Promoter
What I say ⟶	What I hear
↑	↓
What I mean or feel	What I understand

When listening, it is easy to allow attention to wander. Some of the things you may find yourself doing instead of listening are planning what to say next, thinking about a similar experience, interrupting, agreeing or disagreeing, judging, blaming or criticising, interpreting what the speaker says, thinking about the next job to be done or just plain day-dreaming.

The task of a listener is to help people to talk about their situation unhurriedly and without interruption, helping them to express their feelings, views and opinions, and to explore their knowledge, values and attitudes. This reinforces the speakers' responsibility for themselves and is essential for helping them towards greater responsibility for their own health choices.

Helping People to Talk

See also Chapter 14, section Strategies for Decision Making, which discusses counselling skills.

The main task of the listener is to help someone to talk. There are several useful techniques, as follows.

Giving an Invitation to Talk

To get someone started it may be helpful to give out a specific invitation to talk. Examples are:

'You don't seem to be your usual self today. Is something on your mind?'

'Can we talk some more about that matter you raised briefly at yesterday's meeting?'

'You look worried – are you?'

Exercise 10.1	Learning to Listen

Work in groups of three to six people. Appoint someone as a timekeeper.

1. Person A speaks for two minutes, without interruption, on a subject of her choice to do with work or other interests (e.g. sensible drinking guidelines, keeping fit and active, pets, holidays). Everyone else in the group listens, without interrupting or taking notes.
2. Person B repeats as much as she can remember, without anyone else interrupting. B may not:
    - add anything extra to what A said;
    - give interpretations (e.g. 'It's obvious from what she said that . . . ');
    - give comments (e.g. 'She's just like me . . . ').
3. A, and the rest of the group, identify what was inaccurate, forgotten or added.
4. Repeat, with a different topic, until everyone has had a turn at being A and B.
5. Discuss the following questions:
    - **What helped me to listen?**
    - **What helped me to remember?**
    - **What hindered my listening?**
    - **What hindered my remembering?**
    - **What did I learn about myself as a listener?**

Giving Attention

This means listening closely to what is being said, and being fully aware of all the channels of communication, including non-verbal behaviour. It requires effort and concentration to listen hard and give full, undivided attention.

Encouraging

This means making the occasional intervention to encourage someone to carry on talking. It tells the speaker that you really are listening, and want to hear more. Such interventions include noises like 'mm mm', words such as 'yes . . . ' and short phrases such as 'I see . . . ' or 'And then . . . ?' or 'Go on . . . '.

Another useful intervention is the repetition of a key word which the speaker has just used. For example, if the speaker says 'My work's getting on top of me' you could repeat the word 'work . . . ?'

Paraphrasing

This means responding to the speaker using your own words to state the essence of what the speaker has been saying. Use key words and phrases, for example, 'So you're not sure whether to have the baby vaccinated or not?' or 'So you think some people will be very angry if you ban smoking in the office?'

Reflecting Feelings

This involves mirroring back to the speaker, in verbal statements, the feeling he is communicating. To do this it helps to listen for words about feelings, and to observe body language. Examples are 'You seem pleased' or 'You are obviously upset about this'.

Reflecting Meanings

This means joining feelings and content in one succinct response, to get a reflection of meaning:

'You feel ... because ...'

'You are ... because ...'

'You're ... about ...'

For example:

'You feel pleased about your progress.'

'You're depressed because your children have grown up and left home.'

'You're angry about all the rubbish and dumped cars left lying in this neighbourhood.'

Summing Up

This is a brief re-statement of the main content and feelings which have been expressed throughout a conversation. Check back with the speaker to ensure that the statement is accurate. For example, say 'It seems to me that the main things you've been saying are ... Does that cover it?'

Exercise 10.2	Helping People to Talk

Work in pairs.
Each person chooses a topic she feels strongly about (which might be a personal experience or topic of general concern such as sex education, traffic jams, cuts in the health service or violence on television). Stay with the same topic for all three stages of the exercise.
(The whole exercise takes about 45 minutes.)

Stage 1. Giving Attention

One person speaks for two minutes, and the other listens, giving only non-verbal feedback. Then swap roles. After both of you have had your turn, spend 10 minutes discussing these questions:

When you were listening:

■ **What did you find difficult about listening?**
■ **Did your mind wander?**
■ **Did you maintain eye contact?**
■ **What did you notice about the speaker's non-verbal communication?**

When you were speaking:

- **What did the listener do which helped you to talk?**
- **Did the listener do anything that made it difficult for you to talk?**

Stage 2. Encouraging

One person speaks for two minutes. The other listens and gives encouraging interventions (such as 'mm mm'), words ('yes . . . ') and non-directive comments ('I see . . . ') or repeats key words. Swap roles. Then spend five minutes discussing these questions:

When you were listening:

- **What sort of interventions did you make?**
- **How did you feel about making them?**

When you were speaking:

- **What interventions did you notice?**
- **Did you find them helpful?**

Stage 3. Paraphrasing, Reflecting Back and Summing Up

One person speaks for five minutes and the other listens. The listener makes encouraging interventions as in Stage 2, but *also* paraphrases, reflects feelings and reflects meaning when she feels it is appropriate. At the end, she makes a brief statement summing up the main content and feelings of the speaker, checking with the speaker that her summing up is accurate. Exchange roles. Then spend ten minutes discussing these questions:

When you were listening:

- **What sort of interventions did you make?**
- **How did you feel about making them?**

When you were speaking:

- **What interventions did you notice?**
- **Did you find them helpful?**

Asking Questions and Getting Feedback

Skilful questioning will help people to give clear, full and honest replies. It is useful to distinguish different types of questions.

Types of Questions

Closed questions are questions that require short, factual answers, often only one word.
Examples are:

'What is your name?'

'Is this address correct?'

'Are you able to see me again next Tuesday?'

Closed questions are appropriate when brief, factual information is required. They are not appropriate when the aim is to encourage talking at more length. So 'did you get on OK with your healthy eating plan last week?', which could be answered by 'yes' or 'no', is not the best way to encourage people to express their experiences of trying to change what they eat. A better question would be 'How did you get on with your healthy eating plan last week?' This is an open question.

Open questions give an opportunity for full answers. Examples are:

'How did you get on at the meeting yesterday?'

'How do you feel about introducing a non-smoking area in the pub?'

'What do you think about trying to take a short brisk walk every day?'

Note that words like 'how', 'what', 'feel' and 'think' are useful for encouraging a full response.

Biased questions indicate the answer the questioner wants to hear, or expects to hear. In other words, biased questions (sometimes called 'leading questions') are likely to bias the response by leading the person who answers in a particular direction. Examples are:

'You're feeling better today, aren't you?' (This is biased because it would be easier to answer 'yes' than 'no'.)

'You have been doing what we discussed last time, haven't you?'

'Surely you aren't going to do that, are you?'

Multiple questions contain more than one question. Multiple questions are likely to confuse, because the listener will not know which question to answer, and probably will not remember all of them. Examples are:

'Is this a serious problem for you – when did it start?'

'Does your store have a policy on promoting healthy foods – do you stock low-alcohol drinks and did you promote displays of low-fat products during the special campaign last September?'

'What are you going to do to get the Council to take all this rubbish away and are you going to get more bottle banks and newspaper recycling bins?'

'Are you sure you know what to do or would you like me to explain it again?'

Getting Feedback

After people have been given some information, or have been taught a skill, it is very important to check to make sure that they really have understood what was said, and remembered it, or mastered the skill. This is especially important when there is any doubt about how much has been understood, perhaps because, for example, someone is in a state of anxiety or has a limited command of English. There are two key points to note about getting feedback.

Exercise 10.3   Asking Questions

Work in groups of about ten people.

Decide on a topic on which it is easy to think of questions – such as pets, holidays, my job, my family.

- Person A volunteers to answer questions.
- Person B observes the length of A's response to questions.
- Person C observes A's non-verbal behaviour (body language).
- Everyone else has the task of asking questions.

Firstly, everyone in turn asks a *closed* question on the topic.
Secondly, everyone in turn asks an *open* question on the topic.
Thirdly, everyone asks *biased* questions on the topic.
After these three rounds of questions:

- Person A says how she felt about having to answer the three different kinds of questions (e.g. clear? muddled? irritated? angry? confused?).
- Person B says what she observed about the length of A's responses to the three kinds of questions.
- Person C says what she observed about A's non-verbal behaviour when answering the three different kinds of questions.

Discuss the application of what you found out to your work.

It is *your* responsibility to ensure that the communication has been received and understood. It is not the fault of the listener if he tried but did not understand, and he should not be blamed or made to feel small or stupid.

It can be helpful to ask questions in a way which shows that it is your responsibility as a health promoter to 'get it across'. For example, say 'I'd like to make sure I've explained this properly, so could you please tell me what you're going to do about it tomorrow?' or 'May I check to make sure I've covered everything – could you just recap what you understand so far?' Avoid questions such as 'Let's see if you've learnt it yet – could you show me?' or 'I don't think you've totally understood – tell me what you think the main points are'.

Ask open questions. Closed questions such as 'do you understand?' are not an adequate way of getting feedback. People may answer 'yes' because they are embarrassed, intimidated or afraid of making a fool of themselves by admitting that they do not understand. Or they might just want to draw the conversation to a quick conclusion. Ask open questions, such as 'Could you please tell me what you're going to do . . .'

Communication Barriers

As a health promoter you may encounter numerous difficulties in communicating. Recognising that communication barriers exist is the necessary first stage before work can begin on tackling the problems. There are no easy solutions, but increased awareness and skill can go a long way towards improvement.

Common communication barriers may be categorised into six groups.

1.   Social and Cultural Gaps

A number of factors can cause gaps, among which are:

- different ethnic background
- different social group, which may be apparent in dress, language or accent
- different cultural or religious beliefs, for example about hygiene, nutrition or contraception
- different values, reflected in a different emphasis on the importance of health issues
- different gender or sexual orientation, reflected in different approaches, interests or values.

2.   Limited Receptiveness

You might want to communicate, but the reverse is not always true: people might not want to be communicated with. They may be unreceptive for many reasons, including:

- learning difficulty or confusion
- illness, tiredness or pain
- emotional distress
- being too busy, distracted or preoccupied
- not valuing themselves, or not believing that their health is important.

3.   Negative Attitude to the Health Promoter

Some people may be 'anti' you, even before you have met. This may be caused by:

- previous 'bad' experiences
- lack of trust in 'them' – that is, anyone seen as an authority figure or part of 'the establishment'
- lack of credibility of the health promoter (perhaps you set a poor example of good health yourself?)
- perceiving you as a threat, coming to criticise or pass judgment
- believing that 'I know it all anyway', and that you will be 'teaching your grandmother to suck eggs'
- believing that advice will be given which they cannot comply with because of financial or social constraints, or being asked to give up the 'few pleasures in life'
- not wishing to confront unpleasant issues such as results of medical tests, or the need to change policies and practices.

4.   Limited Understanding and Memory

There may be difficulties because people:

- understand and/or speak little or no English
- have limited education or learning difficulties, and may be unable to read and write

■ are being confronted with technical words, jargon or medical terminology that they do not understand

■ have poor or failing memories and cannot remember what was discussed previously.

5.   Insufficient Emphasis by the Health Promoter

Communication may fail because you do not give it sufficient time and attention. The reasons may be:

■ communication was given a low priority in basic training, so it is given low priority in practice

■ lack of confidence, skills and knowledge, which may be the result of inadequate training

■ being too busy with other things, and unable to find the time

■ managers not being supportive about time spent on health promotion

■ reluctance to 'demystify' and share professionally acquired health knowledge.

6.   Contradictory Messages

Communication barriers are erected when people receive different messages from different people. For example:

■ different health professionals give different advice

■ family, friends or neighbours contradict health promoters

■ 'the experts keep changing their minds' as information is updated.

Exercise 10.4   Identifying Communication Barriers

This exercise can be done alone, but it is best carried out in pairs or small groups so that ideas can be shared.

Consider the six kinds of communication barriers discussed.

1.   How many of them can you identify in your own experience?
2.   What other communication barriers can you add to this list?
3.   What communication barriers cause you the most problems?
4.   What suggestions can you make for helping to break down communication barriers? (Share examples from your own experience and make additional suggestions.)

Overcoming Language Barriers

See suggestions for further reading at the end of this chapter.

Language is only one facet of the gulf that may exist between people of different ethnic backgrounds. The root of many communication problems is racism; this is a huge topic, largely outside the scope of this book, but we recommend that all health promoters take time out for racism awareness training when working with people from different ethnic groups.

However, when we focus solely on the question of language barriers, learning a few key words and phrases in the other person's language may help. Words such as hello, goodbye, hot, cold, food and money may be useful. Help with learning the language may be available from multi-cultural education centres run by local education authorities.

When faced with a language barrier, there are some useful guidelines which you can follow to help someone with limited English to understand what is being said.[8] See Box 10.1 and Exercise 10.5.

| Box 10.1 | **Guidelines for Communicating with Someone who Speaks Little English** |

If a client who speaks little English has an appointment with you, you should attempt to find out whether a translator could be present. If you are able to find a translator, allocate more time for the meeting. Give information concisely and in stages; this will allow time for the translator to explain to the client and for the translator to translate back information that the client wants to say to you. Using children or relatives to translate information to clients is less reliable than using trained translators.

If you do not have a translator, the following points may be helpful:

1. Speak clearly and slowly, and resist the temptation to raise your voice in an effort to get through.
2. Repeat a sentence if you have not been understood; repeat it using the same words. This gives the listener more time to 'tune in' and understand; if you use different words you are likely to cause more confusion by introducing even more words which are not understood.
3. Keep it simple. Use simple words and sentences. Use active forms of verbs rather than passive forms, so say 'The nurse will see you' rather than 'You will be seen by the nurse'. Do not try to cover too much, and stick to one topic at a time.
4. Say things in a logical sequence: the sequence in which they are going to happen. So say 'Eat first, then take the tablet' rather than 'Take the tablet after you eat'. If the listener does not pick up the word 'after' correctly, he will take the tablet first, because that is the order in which he heard the instruction.
5. Be careful of idioms. Being 'fed up', 'popping out' and 'spending a penny' may be totally incomprehensible.
6. Do not attempt to speak pidgin English. It does not help people to learn correct English, and sounds patronising.
7. Use pictures, mime and simple written instructions, which may be read by relatives or friends who understand written English. Be careful of symbols on written material; ticks and crosses, for example, might not convey what you intend.

See section on asking questions and getting feedback earlier in this chapter.

8. Check to ensure that you have been understood, but avoid asking closed questions that require a one-word answer such as 'Do you understand?' A reply of 'Yes' is no guarantee that your client really has understood.

| Exercise 10.5 | Overcoming Language Barriers |

The following five extracts come from the district nurse's side of a conversation with a patient whose English is very limited.

'Hello – Oh, we are looking brighter today!'
'Have you been visited by the doctor today yet – did he give you a new prescription?'
'I'll see about your insulin after I've seen how your leg's getting on'.
'The doctor says you should take one of these tablets three times a day . . . I don't think you understand – I'll say that again . . . We want you to take one of these tablets three times a day . . . Oh dear . . . (louder) . . . DOCTOR SAYS YOU TAKE TABLET THREE TIMES A DAY'.
'I'll leave this list of foods for you. There are ticks and crosses on it to show you what you can eat and what you should not eat. Do you understand? Your son can read English, can't he?'
Using the guidelines in points 1–8 in Box 10.1:

■ identify what is unhelpful about the way the district nurse speaks to the patient
■ suggest better alternatives.

Non-verbal Communication

Non-verbal communication includes all the ways by which people communicate with each other except the words they use, and is sometimes called body language. The main categories of non-verbal communication are as follows.

Bodily Contact

Bodily contact is people touching each other, how much they touch, and which parts of the body are in contact. Shaking hands, holding hands, or putting an arm around someone's shoulders, for example, all convey a meaning from one person to another.

Some health promoters, such as nurses, obviously touch patients frequently in the course of their work, whereas others, such as environmental health officers, rarely do so. Touching people is surrounded by 'rules' dictated by cultural expectations and taboos, and by expectations of 'professional distance', which may be barriers to the positive use of touch. For example, a handshake can say 'I'm glad to see you – welcome' and touching a distressed person can say 'I'm here for you'.

Proximity

Proximity is how close people are to each other. Different messages are conveyed to a bed-ridden patient by someone who talks to him from six feet away at the foot of the bed and by someone who comes closer and sits on the bed or a chair. However, people vary in the amount of 'personal space' they need, and feel uncomfortable when others come too close.

Orientation

How individuals position themselves in relation to other people and objects is known as orientation. A useful example is to consider the messages conveyed by the lay-out of a room where a small group of people are meeting. Chairs in rows facing one separate chair (perhaps with a table in front of it) imply that one person will dominate and control the meeting, whereas chairs placed in a circle without a table to act as a barrier imply that everyone is encouraged to join in, and that no one individual is expected to dominate.

Level

This refers to differences in height between people. Generally, communication is more comfortable if people are on the same level; so it feels better to bend down or sit down to talk to a child or a person in a wheelchair, for example. Talking to someone on a different level can leave one or both parties feeling disadvantaged. Sometimes this is done deliberately; for instance, not offering a chair to someone entering an office conveys a message that the visitor is not welcome to stay.

Posture

Posture is how people stand, sit or lie. For example, are they upright or slouched, arms crossed or not? Posture can convey a message of tension and anxiety, for example, by being hunched up with arms crossed, or one of welcome by being upright with arms outstretched.

Physical Appearance

All kinds of messages may be conveyed by physical appearance, such as a person's social standing, personality, tidy habits or concern with fashion. Physical appearance can be very important to health promoters because of the messages it conveys. A uniform may convey an impression of professional competence, but may also convey an unwelcome image of authority. Casual dress in a formal committee may convey the impression (perhaps a false one) that the committee's work is not being taken seriously.

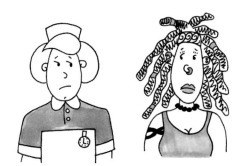

All kinds of messages can be conveyed by physical appearance

Facial Expression

Facial expression can obviously indicate feelings, such as sadness, happiness, anger, surprise or puzzlement.

Hand Movements and Head Movements

Movements of the hands and head can be very revealing. Nods and shakes of the head obviously convey agreement and disagreement without the need for words. (But beware of the fact that movements of the head do not convey the same meaning in all cultures.) Clenched fists, fidgeting hands (and sometimes tapping feet) reveal stress and tension, whereas still, open hands usually denote a relaxed frame of mind. Mental discomfort, such as confusion or worry, is often shown by putting hands to the head and playing with hair, stroking a beard or rubbing the forehead.

Direction of Gaze and Eye Contact

Whether people are 'looking each other straight in the eye' is significant. As a general rule, a speaker looks away from the listener for most of the time when talking (because she is concentrating on what she is saying), and looks directly at the listener when she wants a response. The general rule is that the listener will look the speaker straight in the eye while he is paying attention to what she says, but will look elsewhere if his attention has wandered. This is particularly important if you work with people on a one-to-one basis: a person who is talking to you will infer that you are not listening if you are looking anywhere other than at the speaker. It is critical when counselling someone in distress; the counsellor needs to be giving the client full attention, and if the client looks up and sees the counsellor gazing elsewhere the implication is that the counsellor is not listening.

Non-verbal Aspects of Speech

Consider how many ways a word like 'no' can be said. The way in which it is said can convey meanings such as anger, doubt or surprise. Tone and timing are two non-verbal aspects of speech which convey messages to the listener.

Raised awareness of non-verbal communication can help you to improve communication between you and the people you work with. For example, a person who says 'Yes, I understand' in a doubtful tone of voice, with a puzzled frown or with clenched fists, clearly requires further help. Words alone are only part of a message, and can be misleading. Non-verbal communication is an area worth further study.

Exercise 10.6   Non-verbal Communication in Your Work[9]

Work through the following questions and exercises with a partner.

1. **When do you touch people at work, if at all?**
    What 'rules' govern when it is acceptable/unacceptable to touch them?
    Would people you work with be helped if you touched them more?

2. Carry on a conversation with your partner, first standing too close for comfort, then standing too far away.
    What does it feel like? What is the most comfortable distance?
    What implications does this have for your work?

3. When you talk to an individual in the course of your work, where do you sit or stand in relation to that person? For example, is furniture a barrier between you?
    If you talk to people in groups, how do you seat them?
    Do you think communication could be improved by making changes? If so, what changes?

4. Have a conversation with your partner with one of you sitting and the other standing. Both describe your feelings.
    Do you ever work with people who are on a physically different level from you? What are the implications?

5. Practise tense and relaxed postures, then welcoming and rejecting postures.
    Which do you normally adopt with people?

6. Identify a few people you work with whom you know fairly well. Think back to your first impressions of these people.
    Do you think that your first impressions were right?
    What were the important features of their appearance which led to your first impressions?
    What is the importance of physical appearance in your health promotion work?
    If you wear a uniform, or a white coat, how do you think it affects your relationships?

7. Look around at other people in the room.
    What can you infer from their facial expressions, hand and head movements?
    What is the importance of noticing facial expression, hand and head movement in your job?

8. Hold a conversation with your partner while staring into each other's eyes all the time, and then without looking at each other at all.
    Describe your feelings.
    Watch two people talking.
    Do they look directly at each other or do they frequently look away?
    Do they look more at each other when speaking or listening?
    How important is eye contact in your job?

9. Say 'I don't know' in as many ways as possible, trying to convey a different feeling each time, such as despair, confusion and irritation.
    How important is it for you to pick up on non-verbal aspects of speech in your health promotion work?

Written Communication

See also Chapter 8, section on writing reports.

Writing is a craft, as well as an art, which all health promoters need to develop. The 12-point guidelines in Box 10.2 may help.[10]

Box 10.2	Guidelines on Writing

1. The point of writing is clear communication, not showing how clever you are. On the whole, the more simply and briefly you write, the more effective your writing is likely to be.

2. Think about what kind of document you are writing. For example, is it a paper for a formal committee, a memo to your manager, or a letter to a client? This will help you to know what style to write in: formal in a set lay-out for a committee, brief and to the point for a manager, business-like but friendly to a client.

3. Think about who is reading what you write, and what sort of communication they will welcome: how long should it be, how detailed, how formal or chatty, first person or third person?

4. Use clear, simple language, and avoid long or obscure words if you can find shorter or more familiar ones.

5. Avoid technical terms if you can. If you must use them, explain them in the text or a footnote the first time you use them.

6. Keep sentences short.

7. Break the text up with paragraphs. A paragraph should usually deal with one point and its immediate development. A new point needs a new paragraph. In formal papers and reports use headings and subheadings to break up the text and guide the reader through.

8. Use active rather than passive verbs where possible, as this sounds stronger and simpler. For example, write 'the nurses covered the patients with bedclothes' rather than 'the patients were covered with bedclothes by the nurses'.

9. Make sparing use of adjectives and adverbs. The sparer your writing the more striking it will be. For example, 'the patient was really very upset, cried and sobbed a lot and said she would never, ever come back to the clinic again' (23 words) could be better expressed as 'the patient was in tears and said she would never return to the clinic' (14 words).

10. Use language accurately. If in doubt check with a guide to English usage.[11] A common inaccuracy is to confuse *it's*, which is a shortened form of 'it is' ('it's raining'), and *its*, which is the possessive of 'it' ('the cat had its flea collar on'). Another common inaccuracy is to confuse apostrophes around the letter s. *Cats* is plural ('two cats'), *cat's* is possessive ('the cat's flea collar'), *cats'* is the plural possessive used instead of saying 'cats's' ('both the cats' flea collars were lost').

11. If you have difficulty with spelling and punctuation, use a spell and grammar checker on a word processor or ask someone to check your writing for you.

12. If you have the time, finish a piece of writing and then put it aside for a few days. This gives your subconscious mind a chance to think about it, and you can take a fresh look and edit it. Check for clarity, simplicity and structure.

PRACTICE POINTS

- The quality of your relationships with your clients is at the heart of your helping role. It is important to review and consider how your attitudes and values are reflected in your relationships.

- Good communication is fundamental to these relationships. It is not just a matter of common sense but involves specific skills such as active listening.

- Words, whether verbal or written, are only a small part of communication, and it is important to consider all aspects of a communication.

- You are responsible for communicating effectively with your clients, and it helps if you make it clear to them that you accept this responsibility (through asking them to help you by giving you feedback).

- Skills of written communication are important in health promotion, and need to be reviewed and developed.

Recommended Reading

On Communication and Counselling Skills

➤ Burnard P 1997 Effective communication skills for health professionals. London: Nelson Thornes
➤ Burnard P 1999 Counselling skills for health professionals. London: Standard Publishing
➤ Burnard P 1999 Practical counselling and helping. London: Routledge
➤ Faulkner A 1998 Effective interaction with patients. Edinburgh: Churchill Livingstone
➤ Hargie O D W (ed.) 1997 The handbook of communication skills, 2nd edn. London: Routledge. (Includes one-to-one and group communication, non-verbal communication, questioning and listening.)
➤ Hargie ODW, Morrow NC, Woodman C 2000 Pharmacists' evaluation of key communication skills in practice. Patient Education and Counselling 39 (1), 61–70
➤ Katz J, Peberdy A, Douglas J (eds) 2001 Promoting health: knowledge and practice, 2nd edn. Part 2: Communicating and educating for health. Basingstoke: The Open University in association with Palgrave
➤ Williams D 1997 Communication skills in practice – a practical guide for health professionals. London: Jessica Kingsley. (Practical advice and guidance on developing communication skills for the health professional. Includes verbal and non-verbal behaviours, clinical interviews, working with interpreters.)

On Listening

➤ Burley-Allen M 1995 Listening: the forgotten skill: a self-teaching guide, 2nd edn. New York: Wiley

On Assertiveness

➤ Burley-Allen M 1995 Managing assertively: how to improve your people skills: a self-teaching guide, 2nd edn. New York: Wiley
➤ Ferguson J 1999 Perfect assertiveness. London: Arrow Books

See also the assertiveness website: www.assertiveness.com

On Self-esteem

➤ Lindenfield G 2000 Self esteem, 2nd edn. London: Thorsons
➤ Sorensen M J 1998 Breaking the chain of low self-esteem. Sherwood, OR: Wolf

On Communication and Child Development

➤ Gottman J, DeClaire J 1997 The heart of parenting: how to raise an emotionally intelligent child. London: Bloomsbury. (Explains how children can learn emotional lessons that will enable them to communicate their feelings and have flourishing relationships.)

On Racism and Working with People from Different Ethnic Backgrounds

➤ Douglas J 1997 Developing health promotion strategies with black and minority ethic communities which address social inequalities. In Sidell M, Jones L, Katz J, Peberdy A (eds) Debates and dilemmas in promoting health, Chapter 27. Basingstoke: Macmillan/Open University Press. (Explores the role of health promotion in opposing the impact of race and racial discrimination and discusses lessons learnt from health promotion work in Smethwick and Sandwell.)

➤ Henley A, Schott J 1999 Culture, religion and patient care in a multi-ethnic society: a handbook for professionals. London: Age Concern Books. (Available from Age Concern, Astral House, 1268 London Road, London SW16 4ER. Deals with needs of people of all ages but has a special focus on the needs of older people. Covers an overview of culture, racial discrimination, illness and health care, generic issues about providing care in a multi-ethnic society, communication, dealing with specific health issues, and briefings on specific cultures and religions.)

➤ Kaj J 1999 Valuing diversity: a resource for effective health care of ethnically diverse communities. London: Royal College of General Practitioners

➤ Peberdy A 1997 Communicating across cultural boundaries. In: Sidell M, Jones L, Katz J, Peberdy A (eds) Debates and dilemmas in promoting health,

Chapter 10. Basingstoke: Macmillan/Open University Press

On Written Communication

➤ Burnard P 1996 Writing for health professionals: a manual for writers, 2nd edn. London: Chapman & Hall

➤ Cutts M 1995 The quick reference plain English guide. Oxford: Oxford University Press

➤ Jay R 1999 How to write proposals and reports that get results. London: Financial Times Prentice Hall.

➤ Maslin-Prothero S (ed.) 1997 Baillière's study skills for nurses. London: Baillière Tindall/Royal College of Nursing, Chapter 12.

➤ The Plain English Campaign produces information and runs courses on writing plain English. Contact: The Plain English Campaign, PO Box 3, New Mills, High Peak SK22 4QP. Tel: 01663 744409. Website: www. plainenglish.co.uk. E-mail: info@plainenglish.co.uk

Notes and References

1   For reading that aims to develop awareness of the ways we communicate in order to lead to changes for the better, see:

Hargie O D W 1997 The handbook of communication skills, 2nd edn. London: Routledge

2   Many of the ideas in this section are adapted from: Habeshaw T 1983 Empowering the learner. Bristol Polytechnic (unpublished).

3   For a discussion of the concept of self-empowerment, see:

Kendall S 1998 Health and empowerment. London: Arnold

Tones K, Tilford S 2001 Health education: effectiveness, efficiency and equity, 3rd edn. Chapter 1, The empowerment model of health promotion. Cheltenham: Nelson Thornes, p. 49

4   Faulkner M 1996 Negotiating a contract. In Hodgsan K, Hoile R W (eds) Managing health service contracts, Chapter 6. London: Saunders

5   See:
Beavers R 1990 Successful families. New York: Norton

Skynner R, Cleese J 1993 Life and how to survive it, Chapter 1. London: Methuen

6   Gottman J, DeClaire J 1997 The heart of parenting: how to raise an emotionally intelligent child. London: Bloomsbury

7   Figure adapted from Rollnick S, Mason P, Butler C 1999 Health behaviour change – a guide for practitioners. London: Churchill Livingstone. (Reproduced with kind permission.)

8   Material in this section is largely based on:

Henley A 1979 Asian patients in hospital and at home, Chapter 12. King Edward's Hospital Fund for London. (Reproduced by permission of King Edward's Hospital Fund for London.)

9   Adapted from teaching materials produced by Sue Habeshaw, Bristol Polytechnic. (Reproduced by kind permission of Sue Habeshaw.)

10   These are adapted from a number of sources, including: Legat M 1986 Writing for pleasure and profit. London: Robert Hale

Maslin-Prothero S (ed.) 1997 Baillière's study skills for nurses. London: Baillière Tindall/Royal College of Nursing

11   Such as:

Greenbaum S, Whitcut J 1991 Longman guide to English usage. London: Longman

11 Using Communication Tools

SUMMARY

In the first part of the chapter we suggest some principles governing the choice of health promotion communication tools and a summary of the uses, advantages and limitations of the main types of teaching and learning resources. In the next section we outline points for making the most of display materials, for producing written materials (including guidance on non-sexist writing), and for presenting statistical information. The following section is about mass media: identifying the key characteristics of mass media, the variety of ways in which mass media are channels for health issues, what mass media can be expected to achieve, and how they can be used effectively. We give practical guidelines for health promoters working with radio, television and local press. We include a case study on the use of mass media advertising, and exercises on writing plain English, preparing and presenting material on television and radio, writing a press release, and writing a letter to the editor. We finish the chapter with a section on using information technology for health promotion.

In this chapter we look at a range of communication tools used by health promoters in their work: written materials such as leaflets and handouts; and audiovisual materials such as posters, displays, videos and CD-ROMs. These materials are often collectively referred to as *health education* or *health promotion resources*. We also discuss the use of mass media in health promotion: television, radio, newspapers and the Internet.

These communication tools are used extensively, but are they always used effectively? In this chapter we aim to give you information and guidelines to help you to choose and use them with maximum effectiveness, and to create your own where appropriate. Throughout, it is vital to bear in mind that these tools will be useful only if they are used with skill; *how* they are used is as crucial as the quality of the resources themselves.

First we look at how to select health promotion resources such as leaflets, posters or videos that can be used for displays, group teaching, or for use with individual clients.

Health Promotion Resources: Criteria for Choice

There is a huge range of material available, with a constant turnover as items become out of date or out of print and new ones come on the market. You could find yourself with the task of selecting a leaflet, poster, display or video from a range of possibilities. Or you may find that there is very little available, and you have to decide whether the one item you have found is suitable.

The following guidelines are designed to help you select the most appropriate and useful resources. The guidelines apply to selecting any kind of material, such as leaflets, posters or videos, and you can also use them when you are producing your own.

Guidelines for Selecting and Producing Health Promotion Resources

Is it Appropriate for Achieving Your Aims?

See Chapter 14, section Stages of Change Model.

Think about the item in the context in which you intend to use it: for example, if you are working with a group of young smokers who are not motivated to stop, a leaflet or video on how to stop smoking is unlikely to be helpful. Materials to trigger discussion with the aim of challenging attitudes might be better.

Is it the Most Appropriate Kind of Resource?

Will something else be cheaper and just as effective (e.g. photographs instead of a video)? Could you use the real thing instead of portraying it with a teaching aid (e.g. parents in person talking about their experiences of a new baby instead of appearing in a video, a real baby instead of a doll, actual foods instead of pictures or models)?

Is it Consistent with Your Values and Approach?

See section Exploring Relationships with Clients in Chapter 10.

If your approach is to work in a non-judgmental partnership with your clients, the materials you use should reflect your values. You need to avoid material that is patronising, authoritarian or scare-mongering, for example.

The resource should not be 'victim blaming'. That is, it should not attribute blame to individuals experiencing ill health when that ill health is rooted in their social circumstances, for example low income or poor housing.

Is it Relevant for the People You are Working With?

Does it reflect the values and culture of your clients? Does it reflect their concerns? Does it take into account their age, ethnic group, sex, and social and economic circumstances?[1] Does it reflect local practice and conditions, and health services available?

Obvious examples of irrelevance are videos portraying American lifestyles, or homes of affluent middle-class families, which are unhelpful if you are working with people in the UK who are not well off. Materials designed for one ethnic group may not be appropriate for another, not just because of language but because some aspects (such as sexual behaviour or attitudes to bereavement) are seen differently in different cultures.

Is it Racist or Sexist?

See Further Reading on racism and working with people from different ethnic backgrounds at the end of Chapter 10.

All resources should be non-racist. Racist material is that which stereotypes people into racial types, attributing certain roles or character attributes based on ethnic group alone. Implicit in this are the assumptions that one ethnic group (usually white or European) is superior to another, and one ethnic group (usually white), represents the desired 'norm'.[2]

All resources should be non-sexist. Sexist material is that which stereotypes men and women into certain roles or character attributes based on gender. In particular, it is any portrayal of women as sex objects for the gratification of men, any trivialisation or demeaning of women as second-class citizens, dependent on their relationships with men for social status, and any assumption that male equals desirable norm whereas female equals undesirable deviant. Resources should also not make assumptions about sexual orientation.

Guidance on non-sexist writing is provided later in this chapter.

Resources should reflect the fact that we live in a multi-racial society where the roles of men and women have changed and continue to do so. Strong, positive messages and images should be provided of people of all ethnic groups and both sexes.

Will it be Understood?

There is more about writing plain English later in this chapter.

Is it written in plain English, which people will readily understand? Are there any incorrect assumptions about the level of literacy or existing knowledge? Does it need to be produced in other languages, to make it accessible to people from minority ethnic groups? Do leaflets need to be produced in other formats so that they are accessible to people with disabilities, such as in large type or Braille, or (for videos) with a sign language insert on the screen?

Is the Information Sound?

Is information in the materials accurate, up to date, unbiased and complete? Or does it contain half-truths, one-sided information on controversial issues, and out-of-date or incomplete messages?

Does it Contain Advertising?

Commercial companies such as drug companies, baby food manufacturers or makers of safety equipment produce much material. Leaflets and posters, for example, usually carry the name of the company or its products, or include advertisements. Using these resources can imply that you (or your employer) are endorsing the product. It may also damage your image as a credible source of unbiased health information, and lead people to doubt the value of the information ('they're just trying to sell me something').

For these reasons, resources containing company names, products and advertising should be avoided whenever possible. However, the item may be just what you want, and there may be no alternative. In this case, we suggest that:

- The product or service advertised must be ethically acceptable as 'healthy' and 'environmentally friendly'. This excludes tobacco, alcohol and confectionery advertising, for example.
- The advertising content must be low key. The company name on the front or back cover is acceptable, but constant references to named-brand products are not.

The Range of Health Education Resources: Uses, Advantages and Limitations

A wide range of resources is available for health education sessions with groups or individuals. Two points are worth emphasising by way of introduction:

■ Educational resources are aids, and not substitutes for the educator. Leaflets can be distributed by the thousand with no thought of targeting the audience or using leaflets in conjunction with face-to-face discussion.[3] Videos can be easily misused by being presented without introduction or follow-up discussion, shown just because 'it's a good video'.

See the section on teaching and learning in Chapter 12.

■ It takes time and practice to become familiar with all the teaching aids available, and it takes courage to try new things – but it is worth it.

Table 11.1 summarises key points about the uses, advantages and limitations of the main types of teaching aids.

Table 11.1	Resources to Use in Health Education Sessions	
Type of resource	**Uses and advantages**	**Limitations**
Leaflets and handouts	Clients can use at their own pace and discuss with other people. Educator and client can work through together. Can be easy and cheap to produce basic written information. Can reinforce points in a talk, and add further detailed information.	Commercially produced leaflets can be expensive and may contain advertising. Mass-produced leaflets are not tailored to everyone's needs. Not durable, easily lost. Mass distribution can be wasteful.
Posters and display charts	Can raise awareness of issues. Can convey information and direct people to other sources (addresses, tel. numbers, 'pick up a leaflet'). Simple posters and information displays can be cheap to produce.	High quality is expensive to make or buy. Get tatty quickly unless laminated. Need to ensure any writing is big enough to be read at the distance most people will see it. Displays need changing frequently to attract attention.
Blackboards and whiteboards	Good for building up information, explaining particular points. Cheap, re-usable.	Educator needs to turn back to audience to write on board. Image too small for large groups.
Flip-charts	Good for brainstorming and involving groups in producing ideas which can be stuck up round the room for discussion. Useful for recording notes to be written up later. Can be prepared in advance. Useful where no blackboard or white board available.	Educator needs to turn back to audience to write on board. Flip-chart paper easily torn and dog-eared.
Videos	Can be used to convey real situations otherwise inaccessible (e.g. childbirth), convey information, pose problems, demonstrate skills, trigger discussion on attitudes and behaviour. Can be used for self-teaching. Can be stopped, started or replayed to allow discussion.	Normal TV-size screen too small for large audiences. Educator relies on equipment working properly. Equipment expensive and not easily transported. May need partially darkened room.
Slides	Useful in large halls or lecture theatres with a big screen. Complex information (such as graphs) can be seen clearly.	Needs slide projection equipment and screen, and blackout.
Audiocassette tapes	Good for certain skills development, e.g. relaxation, exercise routines. Equipment cheap, easy to use and transport.	Lack of visual material requires extra concentration to hold attention.

Overhead projector transparencies	Cheap and easy to produce. Can build up information by overlaying one or more transparencies. Use with large or small audiences. Equipment relatively cheap, and portable models easy to transport.	Educator dependent on equipment working properly. Need special sloping screen to avoid image wider at the top than the bottom, with uneven focus. The lens part of the projector, and the person using the projector, can obstruct the audience's view of the screen.
Projection of computer-generated images	Standard office software can enable text and sophisticated, complex images to be prepared in advance and produced on large or small screen.	Requires a portable PC and special projector. May need some blackout.
CD-ROMs	These are popular with young people and are interactive. They are a fun way of raising awareness and conveying information. They are comparatively cheap to produce.	They can only be used with individuals and not everyone will have the necessary equipment.
Health websites	Websites have the potential of reaching a worldwide audience and are useful for raising awareness of health issues, conveying information and delivering self-help materials.	There is an enormous amount of health information that can be accessed on the Internet and no control over the quality. A Quality Information Checklist for children and young people can be found at www.quick.org.uk, a site owned by the Health Development Agency.

Producing Resources

See also Chapter 10, section on written communication, and Chapter 12, section on improving patient communication.

Most resources, particularly posters, leaflets and audiovisual materials, come ready made, but you might want to work with a community group to help them to produce their own materials, or produce some yourself.

We have not attempted to give a comprehensive guide on how to produce materials, but approaching the task in a systematic way using the planning and evaluation flowchart in Chapter 5 may be helpful. If you are producing a resource such as a leaflet, you will need to consider who will write the draft, who will edit it, whether and how to pilot the draft, what it will cost, and whether you need the services of a desktop publisher, designer, illustrator, translator, or printer.

We have identified some important points for making the most effective posters, displays and written materials as follows.

Making the Most of Display Materials: Posters, Charts, Display Boards and Stands

Be brief and to the point Keep the objective firmly in mind. Do not include material that is irrelevant – it will only distract from the main message.

Emphasise the key point(s) Use size of lettering, style or colour to achieve this. Place them just above the centre of a display, which is the point of maximum visual impact.

Use language the audience understands Explain any unfamiliar technical terms. If possible, express the message in both pictures and words. Test it out on a few people to ensure that you have no unexpected ambiguities in your message (e.g. does the phrase 'beating heart disease' refer to information about how to avoid getting heart disease, or is it information on a health problem known as 'beating-heart disease'?)

Be bold   Words and pictures should be as large as possible.

Make the most of colour   It can create continuity; for example, a repetition of background colour can link a series of posters. Colour can be used to identify parts of a diagram or highlight important information. Choose colours with care, because responses to colour are emotional (e.g. blue is cool, green is soothing), and because colours may be associated with certain messages, images and places (e.g. red for danger, purple for funerals, white for clinical cleanliness).

Improve the display site   If all you have is a blank wall or a wall covered with distractingly patterned wallpaper, fix a rectangle of coloured card to the wall as a background display board. If a display board has a rough or marked surface, give it a coat of paint or a covering of coloured paper, hessian or felt.

Use the display site to best advantage   Busy corridors can only be useful sites for posters with immediate appeal and few words. More information can be conveyed in a waiting area, and it may be possible to supplement displays with leaflets to take away. Ensure that writing on displays is at eye level and large enough to read without people having to move from the queue or their chair.

Be aware of lighting   Daylight is unreliable; spotlights directed on to a display are ideal.

Making the Most of Written Materials: Instruction Sheets and Cards, Leaflets and Booklets

Always test materials on a sample of consumers   Do not assume that you know what they like, want or need – *ask them.*

Use colour, layout and print size to improve clarity   Large print may be helpful for older people.

Use plain English   Use everyday words; avoid jargon and explain any technical or medical words. Use short sentences: aim for an average sentence length of 15–20 words. Use active verbs rather than passive ones, for example, say 'change the bandage . . .' rather than 'the bandage should be changed . . .'

Do a readability test   on your written materials. Many word-processing packages are able to give readability statistics as well as the average sentence length and the percentage of passive sentences used. They give a rough measure of readability for adult readers based on the principle that, by and large, the combination of long sentences and long words is harder to comprehend. But note that many other factors that affect readability are not taken into account, such as how the text is laid out, the use of illustrations and the size of print.

Non-sexist Writing

We have already discussed the importance of material being non-racist and non-sexist, but using language in a non-sexist way presents particular challenges. One is the use

---

Exercise 11.1   **Writing Plain English**

Write 'plain English' versions of the following. The first three are very similar to the instructions found on the packages of medication bought over the counter in chemist shops. The last three are very similar to passages in health education leaflets.

1. *Wheezoff* paediatric syrup is specially formulated for children. It is indicated for the relief of cough and its congestive symptoms and for the treatment of hay fever and other allergic conditions affecting the upper respiratory tract. Contraindications, warnings, etc. Hypersensitivity to any of the active constituents. If symptoms persist consult your doctor.
2. *Notwinge* cream – directions for use.
    Apply a sufficient quantity of balm to the part affected. Massage lightly until penetration is complete.
3. *Soothe* vapour rub – how to apply.
    Rub on chest, throat and back. Then spread it thick on chest. Repeat at bedtime. Leave bedclothes loose around the neck so that the decongestant antiseptic vapours may be inhaled freely. For severe nasal catarrh, head colds, coughs and bronchitis, melt some *Soothe* in boiling water and inhale the intensified decongestant antiseptic vapours.
4. If the room has a solid fuel, oil or gas-burning appliance ensure adequate ventilation.
5. The baby lies curled up in what is called the fetal position. It lies in a bag of water and the membranes which make up this fluid-filled balloon are enclosed in the womb.
6. Vitamin B1, also called thiamin, is required for the functioning of the nervous system, digestion and metabolism. Insufficient vitamin B1 can cause anorexia and fatigue.

---

of 'man' as a generic term for 'human being'. For example, people talk about 'manning' an exhibition stand when it is just as likely to be 'manned' by a woman. And 'man-power resources' are assumed to include both men and women, with the hidden assumption that women are second-class resources. Many job titles end with 'man' and date from the time when only men performed these duties, for example postman. So it is important that, today, we choose words which reflect the reality of our situation. For example, instead of 'housewife' we can say 'houseworker'. Table 11.2 provides some more suggestions.

Table 11.2   **Non-sexist Writing**

Change from:	To:
Foreman	Supervisor
Salesman	Sales associate, salesperson
Repairman	Repairer
Manpower	Workforce, staff, personnel
Manning	Staffing
Ambulancemen	Ambulance staff
Newsman	Newscaster, reporter

When *man* comes in the middle of a word, finding a one-word alternative can be difficult. Fortunately synonyms can usually be found; for example, instead of 'the carpenters did a workmanlike job', say 'the carpenters did a skilful job'.

Another problem is the generic use of the pronoun 'he'. For example, 'each doctor presented a case from his own practice', assumes that all the doctors are men. Although it may seem clumsy to say 'he or she', it can sometimes usefully emphasise that both sexes are involved. An alternative is to turn the singular into a plural and use the words 'they' or 'their': 'The doctors presented cases from their own practices'. Similarly, instead of: 'A health promoter must be a fluent communicator. He must also be a good listener.' say: 'Health promoters must be fluent communicators. They must also be good listeners.'

It may be possible to rephrase a passage to eliminate the pronouns altogether. So, instead of 'Information given to a social work agency is confidential in the same way as communications between a doctor and his patients' say 'in the same way as communications between doctors and patients.'

Another way is to use 'you' instead of 'he', 'she' or a noun that implies male or female. For example, in a leaflet on parenting, you could change 'A mother often finds difficulty in persuading her two-year-old to eat' to 'You may find difficulty in persuading your two-year-old to eat' or 'Parents may find difficulty ...' This avoids the implication that only mothers (not fathers) have a parenting role.

Or avoid 'he' by finding another noun. Thus, in 'You may find it difficult to persuade your two-year-old to eat. He may prefer throwing his food around instead' you could say ' ... A child at this age may prefer throwing food around instead.'

Sometimes, though, it seems impossible to avoid saying 'he' because the alternatives are clumsy or unclear. When we have found that to be the case in this book, we have chosen to use 'she' to denote a health promoter rather than 'he'. Many writers do this, thus challenging the tradition of using 'he' when meaning 'he or she'.

It is also important to avoid sexism when speaking as well as writing. So, for instance, a consultant who refers to the women who attend for breast cancer screening (mammography) as 'the ladies' and the female radiographers as 'the girls' may intend no insult, but it could affront both groups. It is far better to refer to the radiographers as 'the staff' ('girls' are women who have not yet grown up) and to the women who attend as 'women', 'patients' or 'clients'. A test is to think how it would seem to use male equivalents (would you refer to men attending a clinic for testicular cancer as 'the gentlemen' and the staff attending them as 'the boys'?).

For further discussion of language barriers, see the section on overcoming language barriers in Chapter 10.

Presenting Statistical Information

Numbers are useful for answering questions that begin how much? how many? how long? what's the risk? But numbers can be indigestible and meaningless unless they are carefully presented in a visual way. The increasing availability of desktop publishing and computer graphics means that it is becoming easier to produce information in ways that are visually arresting and easy to understand. NHS organisations and local authorities are likely to have the equipment and expertise to do this quite easily.

Figures 11.1–11.4 show how to bring statistics to life. The article from *The Guardian* (Figure 11.1) is an example of concise and well-illustrated statistical information from a survey.[4] Figures 11.2–11.4 show statistics from a health survey of over six thousand schoolchildren in England in 1995.[5]

Fig 11.1   **Effective Use of Graphics to Illustrate Statistical Information[4]**

Junk food 'winning war'

What's for tea?

Children's food markets sales by sector, 1995

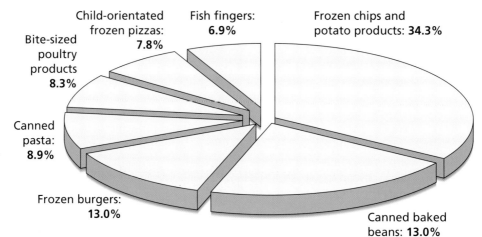

Child-orientated frozen pizzas: **7.8%**

Fish fingers: **6.9%**

Frozen chips and potato products: **34.3%**

Bite-sized poultry products **8.3%**

Canned pasta: **8.9%**

Frozen burgers: **13.0%**

Canned baked beans: **13.0%**

Chips with everything

Changes in children's food markets, current prices, 1991 – 95

Frozen chips and potato products	**39%**
Bite-sized poultry products	**28%**
Canned pasta	No change
Frozen beef burgers	**-2%**
Fish fingers	**-13%**
Canned baked beans	**-21%**
Child-orientated frozen pizzas	**-36%**

Source: Mintel

| Fig 11.2 | This Figure Uses Bar Charts to Show the Proportions of all Children, then Boys and Girls Separately, who Assess Themselves as 'Very Healthy', 'Quite Healthy', or 'Not Very Healthy'[5] |

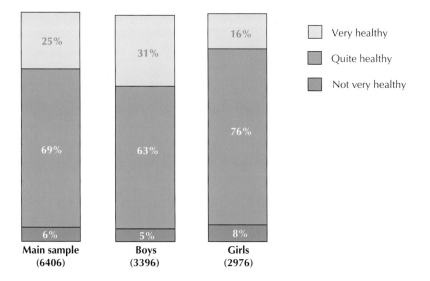

| Fig 11.3 | This Figure Uses a Graph to Show what Proportion of Boys and Girls Desire to Change their Physical Appearance and How this Desire Increases with Age (base: all main sample – 6406)[5] |

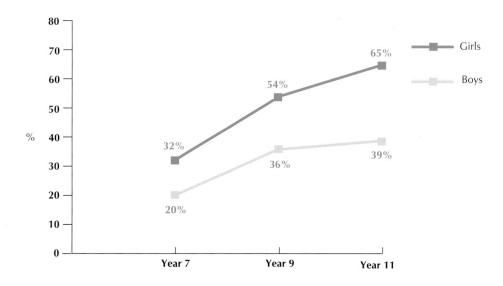

Using Mass Media in Health Promotion

The mass media are channels of communication to large numbers of people: television, radio, the Internet, magazines and newspapers, books, displays, and exhibitions.

| Fig 11.4 | **This Figure uses a Bar Chart to Show which Topics Children Wanted More Lessons on, with Drugs and Sex Education Being the Most Common Requests, and Smoking and Food/Diet the Least Requested[5]** |

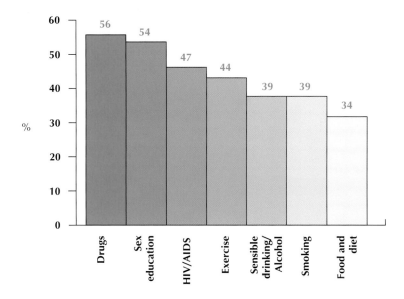

Leaflets and posters are also mass media when they are used on a 'stand alone' basis, as opposed to use as a learning aid in face-to-face communication with an individual or a group. However, usually when people talk loosely about 'the media' they mean television, radio and newspapers.

Health promoters are most likely to become involved with mass media when undertaking health promotion programmes or campaigns with the public, or when a health issue becomes a news item. Probably most involvement will be with local newspapers and local radio or television. However, it is useful to put this into a wider context, and to appreciate the range of ways in which health issues and messages are portrayed via mass media.

Mass Media as Channels for Health Issues

Health messages and information are sent through the mass media in a number of different ways:

■ Planned, deliberate health promotion, e.g. displays and exhibitions on health themes, Department of Health advertisements on television and in newspapers, Open University community education programmes on health. In discussion about using mass media in health promotion, people are generally thinking of this kind of promotion, mainly advertising on television and radio, or via posters or advertisements in newspapers and magazines.

■ Health promotion by advertisers and manufacturers of 'healthy' products and services – for example advertisements for wholemeal bread or toothpaste, educational leaflets on 'feeding your baby', or guides to 'healthy eating establishments' that also promote relevant products or services.

- Books, documentaries and articles about health issues, e.g. television programmes and magazines about food, AIDS, pollution or physical fitness. Often issues will feature in the media because of new research reports or government publications; they may be distorted with attention-grabbing headlines. (See the example in Figure 11.5, which illustrates that when a research report on teenage pregnancy was published a newspaper wrote about it under the headline 'Birth control urged for 11-year-olds', which was a great distortion of the information in the report.[6])
- Discussion of health issues as a by-product of news items ('Rock star dies from drugs overdose') or entertainment programmes, notably 'soaps' where a character has a health problem, such as being abused as a child or suffering from cancer.[7]
- Health (or anti-health) messages conveyed covertly or incidentally, e.g. well-known personalities or fictional characters refusing cigarettes or, conversely, chain-smoking. The portrayal of alcohol on television, for example, conveys a norm of heavy drinking and associates consumption of alcohol with benefits rather than costs.[8]
- Planned promotion of anti-health messages (probably denied or rationalised as not anti-health!) such as advertisements for tobacco, sweets and chocolates.
- Sponsorship of health-promoting events and services by organisations or commercial companies, such as sponsorship of sporting events by cigarette manufacturers or health promotion events by commercial companies. By associating with a health-promoting event or service, the sponsor's product or service is brought to the public eye with an implied stamp of approval and a sense that it is somehow associated with health.

Using Mass Media for Effective Health Promotion[9]

The fact that the message is sent via a medium (such as television) makes it difficult to obtain immediate feedback and modify the message to respond to the needs and characteristics of the audience. There can be some two-way communication through audience phone-ins and by talking to people at exhibitions, but mostly it is one-way. One-way communication has major implications. For example, it is not possible for the sender to repeat, clarify or amplify the message, so in general it is best to use the mass media for conveying simple, rather than complex, messages.

Many research studies have shown that the direct persuasive power of mass media is very limited.[10] Expectations that the mass media alone will produce dramatic long-term changes in health behaviour are bound to lead to disappointment. A particular problem is that mass media campaigns can be an easy response to many health problems, with the characteristic of being high profile. Many health campaigns in the media are driven by the need to do something, and to be seen to be doing it, even though there is evidence that a media campaign on the issue is likely to be useless.

So it is important for you to know what success you can realistically expect when you use mass media in your health promotion work. We can summarise the research evidence that tells us how mass media can be used effectively, and what it cannot be expected to achieve, as follows.

Mass media *can* be an effective health promotion tool if it fulfils the following criteria:

1. The information is perceived as relevant ('for people like me').
2. The information is backed up with other methods such as one-to-one advice.
3. The information is new and presented in an emotional context.

| Fig 11.5 | Often Issues will Feature in the Media Because of New Research Reports or Government Publications, Sometimes Distorted with Attention-grabbing Headlines[6] |

FEBRUARY 1997   VOLUME 3 NUMBER 1   ISSN: 0965-0288

Effective Health Care

Bulletin on the effectiveness of health service interventions for decision makers

NHS Centre for Reviews and Dissemination, University of York

CHURCHILL LIVINGSTONE

Preventing and reducing the adverse effects of unintented teenage pregnancies

■ Teenage pregnancy is associated with increased risk of poor social, economic and health outcomes for both mother and child.

■ A factor strongly associated with deferring pregnancy is a good general education.

■ The health and development of teenage mothers and their children has been shown to benefit from programmes promoting access to antenatal care, targeted support by health visitors, social workers or 'lay mothers' and provision of social support, educational opportunities and pre-school education.

■ School-based sex education can be effective in reducing

teenage pregnancy especially when linked to access to contraceptive services. The most reliable evidence shows that it does not increase sexual activity or pregnancy rates.

■ Contraceptives when used properly are highly cost-effective and can result in significant savings.

■ Increasing the availability of contraceptive clinic services for young people is associated with reduced pregnancy rates.

■ Contraceptive services should be based on an assessment of local needs and ensure accessibility and confidentiality.

When this research report was published, *The Times* ran an article with the following headlines:

Target the young, say NHS advisers

**Birth control urged
for 11-year-olds**

4. The aim is to:

- raise awareness of health and health issues (for example, to raise awareness that the budget for running the NHS is not bottomless and difficult choices have to be made about what to spend it on; or to raise awareness about the link between over-exposure to the sun and the risk of skin cancer)
- deliver a simple message (for example, that babies should sleep on their backs not their tummies; that there is a national helpline for people who want to stop smoking)
- change behaviour if it is a simple one-off activity that is easy (for example, phone for a leaflet) and which people are already motivated to do.

5. The use of mass media is part of an overall strategy that includes face-to-face discussion, personal help and attention to social and environmental factors that help or hinder change. For example, mass media publicity is just one strand in a long-term programme to combat smoking.[11]

What mass media *cannot* be expected to do is:

1. Convey complex information (for example, about transmission routes of HIV).
2. Teach skills (for example, how to deal assertively with pressure to have sex without a condom or take drugs).
3. Shift people's attitudes or beliefs. If a message challenges people's basic beliefs, they are more likely to dismiss the message than change their belief (for example, 'my dad drank six pints a night till he died at 80, so saying I shouldn't have more than two pints a day is rubbish').
4. Change behaviour unless it is a simple action, easy to do, and people are already motivated to do it. For example, it will not change the eating, drinking or exercise habits of people who do not want to change them or find it difficult to change.

Exercise 11.2   Using Mass Media to Stop Young People Taking Drugs

A Department of Health mass media campaign in 1985/86 costing £2 million directed at heroin misuse was widely criticised.[12] Although it was very successful at penetrating the market (young people aged 13–20), and thus demonstrated the effectiveness of the mass media in raising awareness, it had little or no influence on drug-related behaviour.

Ten years later, in 1995, the tragic death of Leah Betts from taking one Ecstasy tablet on her 18th birthday led to a charitably funded poster campaign. Many experts believed this to be a well-meant but ineffective approach.

The Independent, on 8th December 1995, put it this way in an article entitled 'Drugs: ads are not the answer':[13]

All will sympathise with the Betts family's attempts to use their daughter's awful death to warn others. But Mark Gilman, director of research at the drugs organisation Lifeline, doubts whether the campaign (like many others) will work. 'These posters may make some people feel like they're doing something, but all they do is compound the fears of parents and serve to reinforce those young people who have decided to say no already. It won't put anyone else off'.

Talking to young regular users of Ecstasy about the Betts case, Gilman found that they saw it as undeniably sad 'but a tragedy like any other – like a friend being killed in a car crash'.

Fear has been the main weapon in the long and losing ad and media war against drugs over the last two decades... In the meantime, drug use among the young has become almost the norm... 16-year-olds... know that the use of soft drugs such as cannabis or – for the vast majority of users – Ecstasy does not result in death... 'When you're young, you think you're immortal. You know that having sex can kill you, that driving over the speed limit can kill you, that almost everything else your parents disapprove of can kill you. But you do it anyway – because it's fun.

This has now been tacitly acknowledged by the Department of Health, which has passed on the responsibility for its antidrugs crusade to the Health Education Authority. Its new campaign is designed primarily to promote the National Drugs Helpline, a daytime phone line staffed by trained counsellors offering non-judgmental advice.

What does this example tell you about how mass media can be used effectively and ineffectively?

What does *The Independent* article illustrate about the role of newspapers in health promotion?

Creating Opportunities

Even though most health promoters are motivated to use the mass media, they may have misgivings and identify the need for further training.[14] For example, you may feel apprehensive of interviews with reporters from the local news media (local newspapers, radio and television). You might feel 'They'll misquote me'; 'I'll dry up if I'm interviewed'; 'they'll sensationalise the issue'; or 'I'll get into trouble with my manager'.

There may be more than a grain of truth in these fears, so what can be done to overcome them and make useful alliances with journalists? Firstly, many NHS organisations and local authorities now employ public relations specialists with a background in journalism, and employees can enlist their help.

Another way forward is to establish personal contact with local journalists. Do not wait for them to ring you – you ring them. Establish an informal, personal relationship; get to know how they work and what their special areas of interest are, which will help to establish mutual trust and understanding. You can then approach them if you wish to give exposure to a particular topic, or if you wish to discuss how the media are portraying a current issue. The benefits are mutual; journalists will be more likely to approach you to get help with an item of health news.

Also, remember that it is in both your interests to have good skills in communicating via the mass media, so why not ask for help with training needs? Many local radio and television journalists are happy to help with training. Short courses on using the media may also be available at local colleges and universities.

Keep a record of what you find out about local media, and update it regularly. Include information on names and special interests of journalists and the 'copy dates' for each of the media in your area. The 'copy date' is the deadline for submitting written information ('copy'). For example, note the last day for submitting copy to a regular fortnightly magazine or local weekly paper. The daily newspapers should be able to respond immediately to a press release; radio often needs a few days to prepare coverage; television may need longer advance notice to allow time for booking a film crew.

This information will help you to be prepared when opportunities for useful media coverage arise.

The following sections give practical guidelines on working with radio, television and local newspapers. Having this information may also help to overcome fear of working with the news media.

Working with Radio and Television

Using a spot on radio or television effectively requires research, preparation and skill. The following checklists are prepared to help you get your health promotion story to the right person and have the best chance of getting coverage. You need to listen to your local radio and watch television to see which programmes might be interested in your kind of news.

Basic Information

- What hours do they broadcast?
- What region do they cover?
- Who are the listeners? Does the profile alter according to the time of day?

The Programmes

- What is covered on the news items?
- How many minutes of current affairs and local interest items?
- Are interviews used, or straight reporting?
- What are the different kinds of programmes, and what is the proportion of time they occupy (news, current affairs, weekly events, phone-ins, music, etc.)?
- Which programmes use guests or 'experts'?
- Is there any local programme that regularly covers health issues?
- Is there a round-up of events in the week ahead? What is the deadline for information?
- How much detail do they give? What sorts of events are covered?

Interviews

- Which programmes use interviews?
- How many minutes?
- What is the tone (bland, chatty, aggressive)?
- How long is the average answer before the next question? Time it!
- Are they on location or in the studio?
- Are they recorded or live?
- Who are the presenters or interviewers on the programmes who might be interested in health? What is their style?

Finding Out About a Specific Programme

- What programme is it? What sort of approach does the programme have? How long is it? When is it transmitted? What kind of audience does it have?
- Why is your topic of interest *now*? Is there some local or national controversy or news item that sparked off interest? If so, do you know all about it?

- How are you going to be presented: an information spot, an interview or a discussion panel?
- If you are going to be interviewed, who will do it? Will it be in the studio, on location (perhaps in your workplace or outdoors) or 'down the line' (where you are in one studio and the interviewer in another)?
- If you are going to take part in a discussion, who else will be taking part?
- Will it be broadcast live or recorded first?
- How much time are you likely to have on the programme?
- When and where is the broadcast or recording to take place?

Preparing the Message

- Do your homework. You may know a lot or a little about the subject, but in either case you need to identify exactly what it is you want to get across, and to have this very clearly in your mind *before* you are 'on the air'.
- Be positive. Emphasise the good news, *not* a series of don'ts. Tell people what they *can* do and emphasise the benefits.
- You should have two or three key points to put across, and *no more*. You can expand on these and describe them in different ways but do not overload your audience with too much detail or too many points. They will not remember the additional information anyway, and may even forget the key points.
- Use anecdotes and analogies to illustrate what you mean; simple messages do not have to be bald and boring. Tell stories (short ones!) and use real-life experiences. Put complex points over with everyday analogies, e.g. 'Use too much fertiliser and you'll kill the plants – use the right amount and they'll grow strong and healthy. The same applies to food and people.'
- Avoid technical terms (unless these are essential, in which case use them and explain them) and jargon, but do not be patronising. It helps to pitch the level right if you imagine that you are talking to an intelligent 14–15-year-old whom you have never met.

Presenting Your Message

- Accept that you are nervous and regard it as a good thing because it means that you will be keyed up to do your best. Remember that the interviewer is there to help you tell your story and to put you at ease.
- Perform with liveliness and conviction. Be alert and (if you are on television) look alert at all times. Always assume that the camera is on you even when you are not talking. Make sure your eyes look convincing and involved.
- Speak with your normal voice; if you have a regional accent this will make you more interesting to listen to. Speak clearly and distinctly, and (especially on radio) vary the pitch and speed.
- Make sure you say what *you* want to say. You do not have to follow the line of the interviewer's questions if, for good reason, you do not wish to. Provided you stick to the broad framework of agreed subjects, you have every right to steer the interview or discussion in such a way that you get over what you want to say. Regard the questions as springboards from which to make your points. For example, if you do not like a question you can say:
'I can't really answer that question without explaining first that . . .'

'The real problem behind all this is ...'

'We don't know the answer to that at the moment, but what we do know is ...'

- When the interview is over, sit still, keep alert and keep quiet until you are *told* it is over.
- On television, wear what makes you feel comfortable and good. Avoid wearing blue or bright red, predominant stripes, small patterns or flashing jewellery. As you will appear as a 'talking head' for most of the time, pay special attention to what you wear in the neckline area.

Exercise 11.3   **Looking Good and Sounding Good on Television and Radio**

1.   Prepare Your Message

Select a health promotion topic that you are familiar with, e.g. slimming, eating health-giving food, sensible drinking, feeding your baby, keeping fit, avoiding home accidents, living with stress.

Identify *three* key points you would want to put across in a five-minute radio or television interview. Be clear in your mind:

- what the three key points are
- how you will explain them in an interesting way – what illustrations, analogies or anecdotes you could use
- how you will develop your points further if you have time.

2.   Practise Your Presentation

Get a partner to act as your interviewer, and record your interview on an audio or a videotape. Ask a third person to be an observer. Play the tape back and assess your performance.

- Did you sound/look lively, alert and convincing?
- Was your voice clearly understandable? What did it sound like for speed and pitch?
- Did you get your key points across? Did you do so in an interesting way?
- Were you able to deal with 'difficult' questions?

Working with the Local Press

Local newspapers are an excellent medium for health promotion in a local community. Local journalists will be interested in newsworthy health issues and it is worth studying the newspapers to see who writes about health topics. This is a checklist of what to look for when researching a paper.

Basic Information

- When is it published?
- What are the deadlines for copy?
- What locality does it cover?
- How many readers, and who are they?

The Copy

- What is the style (bright, sober, campaigning, etc.)?
- What is the average length of articles (often different for news, business, features)?
- What percentage of articles have photos?
- How many photos per page?
- How are photos used generally?
- How are quotes used?

The Subjects

- What sorts of stories are used (local, jolly, controversial, educational), and how are they treated?
- What is the ratio of coverage for news, features, business, diary, etc.?
- How long and how full is the 'events ahead' section?
- Are there special sections or supplements on health, education, women, etc.? How long and on what day?
- Are there regular columnists? What are their special interests?

The Language

- What is the average length of sentences?
- What is the average length of paragraphs?
- What kind of language is used (multi-syllabic, slangy, turgid, lively, short and simple)?

Your Special Interests

- Anything in the papers that may be of special use to you or to your organisation?

This may seem a lot to cope with, especially if you have a number of local and regional newspapers. Gradually build up expertise, with a fact sheet on each one. This will be indispensable for targeting your press releases.

How to Write a Press Release[15]

To write a press release (sometimes also called a 'news release') you need:

A good text   Use a title to grab attention. The guts of the story must be in the first short paragraph. However complex the subject there will be one outstanding thing that makes it newsworthy. Start with a bang by spelling this out. Make your points in order of importance. (A story is cut from the bottom up.) Use short sentences and easy language, with no abbreviations or jargon. Using quotes can bring a piece to life. Do not be afraid of making up things that you or your group might have said (but check first with the people concerned). For example, 'Mrs Gloria Slim, the chief hospital dietitian, said "I am delighted at the number of hospitals which now offer patients choices of vegetarian and traditional ethnic dishes on the menu".'

A short text   Keep it brief – one page if possible. If longer, type 'More follows. . . .' at the bottom right hand corner. Do not carry over paragraphs or sentences to the next page. Type 'ends' after the last line of the release. Sentences must be short, paragraphs brief.

A local angle for a local paper News is people and local news is local people. So focus on people rather than making generalised statements or quoting dry statistics. For example, say: 'Last week three Bloggsville children were admitted to the Royal Infirmary after accidentally swallowing weedkiller. This brings the number of children accidentally poisoned this year to over 100. Sister Florence Nightingale, in charge of the Accident and Emergency Department, said: "It is heartbreaking to see the needless distress this causes" . . .'

Good timing Your news will not be newsworthy on the day of election of a new prime minister! Yesterday's news is dead, today's may still be of interest, but tomorrow's has the best chance of being printed. Alert newspapers a few days in advance so that they can send reporters to cover an interesting event. For example, contact on a Friday or Monday is usually best for a weekly paper published on the following Friday. If you want to launch a story at a particular time, use the 'embargo' system. This means writing, for example, 'Not for use until Wednesday July 2nd 2003' or 'Embargoed 6 p.m. July 2nd 2003' across the top of the press release.

Good presentation Use A4 paper, headed with a logo if possible. Colour catches the eye, so a coloured heading or coloured paper will make your release stand out.

Good technique Journalists work at speed, so make their task easier by:

- using only one side of the page, placing the text centrally on the page
- using a lay-out with double spacing
- leaving at least one inch (2–3 cm) margin on either side
- putting a release date or embargo date at the top
- giving names and telephone numbers of people in your organisation for further information (including an after-hours telephone number)
- sending it to a named journalist if possible
- not underlining any words (because this gives printers instructions to use italics; use **bold** for emphasis instead).

A big photo If you are sending a photo, a 7" × 5" or 10" × 8", generally black and white, is preferred, with a full label on the back giving names and details. Don't forget to include the names of everyone on the photo ('the picture shows, left to right, June Bloggs, Sam Smith . . .') and explain what they are doing ('presenting Healthy Eating awards at 3 p.m. on Tuesday March 10th at Bloggsville Town Hall'). Never write directly on the back of a photo, as this will destroy its quality. Photos should be eye-catching and clear.

Good communication Send a copy of the press release to everyone who will be affected, including your organisation's press officer, and to everyone mentioned or otherwise involved in the story.

A final check Before you send it, ask yourself if this would tell you:

- What?
- Who?
- When?
- Where?
- Why?
- How?

Fig 11.6   Local News is Local People

NEWS

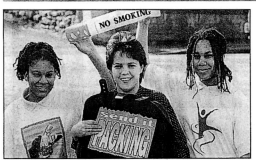

Stub it out, pupils urged

SCHOOL nurses are marking No Smoking Week by urging children in Bath not to take up cigarettes.

Pupils have been entering anti-smoking poster competitions and a contest to see how many cigarettes they could pack away in suitcases.

Bath Health Promotion Unit runs anti-smoking training courses for health visitors, practice nurses and school nurses.

No Smoking Day events are continuing throughout the week. Health promotion spokesman Donna Smith said: "We teach the skills needed for people to give up smoking. The training is vital for one-to-one counselling or group work.

"And it also teaches how to recognise if a smoker is truly motivated to quit."

Pupils Debbie Russell, and Shanna Fields, both aged 14, were involved in an anti-smoking workshop held at Hayesfield School, Bath yesterday.

● **PACK IN: Nurse Sam Shrubsole pictured putting the message across to Debbie Russell, left, and Shanna Fields.**

Reproduced with kind permission of the Editor, Bristol Evening Post.

Example 11.1   Press Release

KOFFCOUNTY DISTRICT HEALTH AUTHORITY
PRESS RELEASE 1st October 2002
SMOKERS HOTLINE LAUNCHED

Koffcounty's Smokers Hotline got off to a flying start this week, when Dr Jo Goodheart, a specialist in heart disease at Kofftown General Hospital, launched the service.

The hotline has been set up as part of Koffcounty Heart Week (2nd–9th October), to help people who want to stop smoking. Anyone ringing 1234 567 890 will be sent a free pack of useful ideas to help them give up, including tips from ex-smokers and information about local stop-smoking groups.

'I smoked myself when I was younger and I remember what a struggle I had to stop. Many of my patients with heart trouble also find it incredibly difficult', said Dr Goodheart. 'That's why I'm delighted to launch this scheme. The pack has lots of useful information to help people over the difficulties.'

Smokers have a two to three times greater risk of having a heart attack than non-smokers. At least 80% of heart attacks in men under 45 are thought to be due to cigarette smoking. Stopping smoking could lead to 150 fewer deaths each year of men and women under 65 in Koffcounty.

For further information, please contact:
Sally Prohealth, Senior Health Promotion Officer, Central Health Clinic, People's Lane, Kofftown KT1 2YZ

Telephone 1234 246 802 (day) or 1234 135 790 (evenings)

Writing Letters to the Editor

Another way of using the local paper as a medium for health promotion is by writing letters to the editor. This can keep an issue in the public eye for some time, and provides good opportunities for public debate of controversial issues. Letters to the editor should be short (some newspapers restrict length), to the point, and be on one topic only.

Exercise 11.4	**Writing for the Local Paper**

1. Write a press release about a public health issue you are currently concerned about or working on (for example, school meals, traffic congestion around local schools, drug taking by young people in local clubs, lack of play facilities for young children, or poor public transport).
2. Write a letter to the editor supporting a current health education campaign or drawing attention to a specific need for health promotion.

Using Information and Communication Technology for Health Promotion

See Chapter 7, section Evidence-based Health Promotion.

The Internet has revolutionised the way in which people – public health professionals, health promoters from all backgrounds, and the public – can gain access to health information. It is estimated that there are 70,000 websites disseminating health information.[16] In the UK, there has been substantial investment in information technology; in the NHS, it is linked to the national strategy *Information for Health*.[17]

We can describe the use of information and communication technology in health promotion under three headings, each discussed in more detail below:

- supporting evidence-based health promotion practice
- disseminating resources and information to other health promoters
- providing information and support to the public.

Supporting Evidence-based Health Promotion Practice

The Internet provides the means of accessing research evidence on the effectiveness of health promotion. The Health Development Agency has a website called HealthPromis,[18] which is a national bibliographic database of health promotion materials. It provides easy access to the best available information on what works to improve health and reduce inequalities, and includes effectiveness reviews that can be downloaded.

Through the secure NHS 'information superhighway' NHSnet, health care professionals can access the National Electronic Library for Health, which aims to provide accredited reference material to develop evidence-based practice. Other electronic databases that can be accessed through the Internet include the Cochrane Library, CINAHL and Medline.[19]

Disseminating Resources and Information to Other Health Promoters

A number of local health promotion services have developed their own websites, and use them to disseminate reports of local projects and locally produced health promotion resources. Leaflets and teaching packs are often available in PDF format so that visitors to the website can download the materials for their own use.

The Health Development Agency has a number of websites for teachers and parents to use with children and young people.[20]

Providing Information and Support to the Public

A key objective of the national strategy *Information for Health* is to 'provide fast, convenient access for the public to accredited multimedia advice on lifestyle and health, and information to support public involvement in, and understanding of, local and national health service policy development'.

As a result, NHS Direct and NHS Direct on-line[21] have been set up, and on-screen consultations with an NHS nurse through digital television are being piloted.

Websites are used for health promotion, with information from organisations such as the national health promotion agencies and local health organisations. For example, the Health Development Agency and the Health Education Board for Scotland have websites, as do a number of local health promotion services.[22] Most sites are 'read-only', that is, used to publish information for the user – a one-way process. But some also allow the user to interact. For example, users may supply information such as survey questionnaire responses or play 'games' on a health theme. There are also sites that offer self help guides such as the Department of Health site to help people stop smoking (www.givingupsmoking.co.uk).

Computer programs giving tailored advice on lifestyle issues are also becoming more widely used and there are ever-widening possibilities for the future, as more people have computers at home, and computers (some with 'touch screen' facilities) become available in schools, libraries, GP practices and other public places. There is a growing body of research supporting the effectiveness of computer-generated interventions.[23]

CD-ROMs are also available, using interactive games and questionnaires to get messages across. Many of these are designed specifically for use with young people. CD-ROMs are comparatively cheap to produce and young people are often keen to design and develop this type of resource themselves.

Assessing the Quality of Information on the Internet

Not all the information found on the Internet is accurate and there is no governing body checking the quality of Internet websites.[24] It is therefore important that you evaluate for yourself the quality of any website you use before trusting the information it provides. The following guidelines may be useful.[25]

1. **Is it clear who has written the information?**
    Who is the author? Is it an organisation or an individual person? Is there a way to contact them?
2. **Are the aims of the site clear?**
    What are the aims of the site? What is it for? Who is it for?
3. **Does the site achieve its aims?**
    Does the site do what it says it will?
4. **Is the site relevant to me?**
    List five things you want to find out from the site.

5. **Can the information be checked?**
   Is the author qualified to write the site? Has anyone else said the same things anywhere else? Is there any way of checking this out? If the information is new, is there any proof?

6. **When was the site produced and last updated?**
   Is it up to date? Can you check to see if the information is up to date, and not just the site?

7. **Is the information biased in any way?**
   Has the site got a particular reason for wanting you to think in a particular way? Is it a balanced view or does it only give one opinion?

8. **Does the site tell you about choices open to you?**
   Does the site give you advice? Does it tell you about other ideas?

PRACTICE POINTS

- Communication tools useful for health promoters are written materials such as leaflets and handouts, audiovisual materials such as posters, displays and videos, and the mass media of television, radio and newspapers. You need to select and use them with skill in order to be effective.

- When you select materials such as leaflets and videos, ensure that you consider the criteria they should meet.

- Consider the range of advantages, uses and limitations of each kind of resource and audiovisual aid you are thinking of using.

- Create effective displays by considering factors such as site, colour, language, and style.

- Make written materials in plain English, with attention to other issues such as non-sexist writing.

- Ensure that materials are accessible to everyone you want to reach by producing them in, for example, ethnic minority languages, large type or alternative formats such as audiotape instead of written materials.

- Present statistical information with appropriate use of graphics to bring it to life.

- Mass media of television, radio and newspapers are used to convey both deliberate and unplanned health messages, images and information. You can use mass media successfully to raise awareness of health issues, deliver simple messages and encourage one-off actions that are easy to do. You are unlikely to be successful if you try to use mass media to teach complex information or skills, or lead to shifts in attitudes, beliefs or lifestyle.

- In order to work effectively with local journalists on newspapers, radio and television, you need to research potential opportunities, and know how to prepare presentations and press releases.

- Consider the possibilities for using information and communication technology in your work.

Recommended Reading

On Writing Plain English

➤ Burnard P 1996 Writing for health professionals; a manual for writers, 2nd edn. London: Chapman and Hall. (Covers the basics of writing, buying and writing with a computer, keeping databases, writing essays, dissertations, articles, books and reviews.)

➤ Cutts M 1995 The quick reference plain English guide. Oxford: Oxford University Press. (A short, practical guide on writing more clearly.)

➤ The Plain English Campaign produces information and runs courses on writing plain English. Contact: The Plain English Campaign, PO Box 3, New Mills, High Peak SK22 4QP. Tel: 01663 744409. Fax: 01663 747038. Website: www.plainenglish.co.uk E-mail: info@plainenglish.co.uk

On Using Mass Media in Health Promotion

➤ Boyd A 1999 How to handle media interviews. Chalford: Management Books. (A clear practical guide to working with the media; wider content than the title suggests. Includes how to get publicity, making contacts, producing news releases, interviews on TV, radio, newspapers and magazines, putting yourself across.)

➤ Katz J, Peberdy A, Douglas J (eds) 2000 Promoting health: knowledge and practice, 2nd edn. Chapter 11, Educating and communicating through the mass media. Basingstoke: The Open University in association with Palgrave. (Covers use of mass media, social marketing, and interactive multi-media health education.)

➤ Naidoo J, Wills J 2000 Health promotion: foundations for practice, 2nd edn. Chapter 12, Using the mass media in health promotion. London: Baillière Tindall. (Covers the role of mass media, using mass media, effectiveness.)

➤ Reid D 1996 How effective is health education via mass communications? Health Education Journal 55, 332–344. (Reviews effectiveness and cost-effectiveness of mass communications.)

➤ Tones K, Tilford S 2001 Health education: effectiveness, efficiency and equity, 3rd edn. Chapter 8, The mass media in health promotion. Cheltenham: Nelson Thornes. (A detailed review of the effectiveness of mass media in health promotion.)

On Information and Communication Technology

➤ Bernhardt M M 2000 Health education and the digital divide: building bridges and filling chasms. Health Education Research 15 (5), 527–531. (Discusses concern about access to health education for those not connected to the Internet – 'the digital divide'.)

➤ Catford J 1997 The mass media is dead: long live multimedia. In Sidell M, Jones L, Katz J, Peberdy A (eds) 1997 Debates and dilemmas in promoting health, Chapter 34. Basingstoke: Macmillan/Open University Press. (Looks at new possibilities in the ever-expanding world of new technology in the mass media, and the challenges and opportunities this presents for health promotion.)

➤ Cline R J W, Haynes K M 2001 Consumer health information seeking on the Internet: the state of the art. Health Education Research 16 (6), 671–692. (Discusses how the Internet offers widespread access to health information with the advantages of interactivity, information tailoring and anonymity.)

➤ Eysenbach G, Ryoung Sa E, Diepgen T I 2001 Towards the millennium of cybermedicine. In: Heller T, Muston R, Sidell M, Lloyd C (eds) Working for health, Chapter 35. London: The Open University in association with Sage Publications

➤ Fotherinham F M, Owies D, Owen N 2000 Interactive health communication in preventive medicine: Internet-based strategies in teaching and research. American Journal of Preventive Medicine 19 (2), 113–120. (On using Internet-based strategies in preventive medicine.)

Notes and References

1 For resources to use with older people, see: Squire A 2002 Health and well-being for older people: foundations for practice. London: Baillière Tindall in association with the Royal College of Nursing, Chapter 12

2 The issue of promoting health with black and minority ethnic communities is much wider than simply ensuring that materials are non-racist. See:

Douglas J 1995 Developing anti-racist health promotion strategies. In: Bunton R, Nettleton S, Burrows R (eds) The sociology of health promotion, Chapter 6. London: Routledge. (This chapter outlines, reviews and provides a critique of health promotion approaches to promoting health with black and minority ethnic communities in the UK.)

3 For examples of research on the use of leaflets, see:

Hart A R et al 1997 The effect on compliance of a health education leaflet in colorectal cancer screening in general practice in central England. Journal of Epidemiology and Community Health 51, 187–191

Little P, Griffin S, Kelly J, Dickson N, Sadler C 1998 Effect of educational leaflets and questions on knowledge of contraception in women taking the combined contraceptive pill: randomised controlled trial. British Medical Journal 316, 1948–1952

Macfarlane J et al 2002 Reducing antibiotic use for acute bronchitis in primary care: blinded, randomised controlled trial of patient information leaflet. British Medical Journal 324, 91

Murphy S, Smith C 1993 Crutches, confetti or useful tools? Professionals' views and use of health education leaflets. Health Education Research 8(2), 205–215. (This study on the views and use of health education leaflets by health professionals showed that they thought leaflets were important and used them extensively, but at the same time they did not believe that they were particularly effective; there were contradictions between how leaflets were used and their perceived effectiveness. For a full report, see: Murphy S, Smith C 1992 Crutches, confetti or useful tools? Good Health Wales Technical Report Number 3, Health Promotion Authority for Wales.)

Sowden A J, Arblaster L 2001 Mass media interventions for preventing smoking in young people. Cochrane Review. (Cochrane Reviews can be obtained from the Cochrane Library. See note 19 for how to access the Cochrane Library.)

4 Article in The Guardian 6.8.96. (Reproduced with kind permission of The Guardian.)

5 Reproduced with kind permission of the Health Education Authority from Turtle J, Jones A, Hickman M 1997 Young people and health: the health behaviour of school-aged children – summary of key findings. London: Health Education Authority

6 Title of article from The Times, reproduced with kind permission of The Times. Front cover of Effective Health Care Bulletin reproduced by kind permission of Churchill Livingstone.

7 The following exploratory study indicated that medical dramas could prove a useful tool for disseminating health promotion messages:

Davin S 2000 Medical dramas as a health promotion resource – an exploratory study. International Journal of Health Promotion and Education 38 (3), 109–111

8 Hansen A 1986 The portrayal of alcohol on television. Health Education Journal 45, 127–131 Institute for Alcohol Studies 1985 The presentation of alcohol in the mass media. Report of a seminar, January 1985. Institute for Alcohol Studies, 12 Caxton Street, London

9 Some of this section is based on Naidoo J, Wills J 2000 Health promotion: foundations for practice, 2nd edn. Chapter 12, Using the mass media in health promotion. London: Baillière Tindall

Examples of using mass media in public health campaigns:

Friend K, Levy D T 2002 Reductions in smoking prevalence and cigarette consumption associated with mass media campaigns. Health Education Research 17 (1), 85–98

Miles A, Rapoport L, Wardle J, Afuape T, Duman M 2001 Using the mass media to target obesity: an analysis of the characteristics and reported behaviour change of participants in the BBC's 'Fighting Fat, Fighting Fit' campaign. Health Education Research 16 (3), 357–372

Smith B J, Ferguson C, McKenzie J, Bauman A, Vita P 2002 Impacts from repeated mass media campaigns to promote sun protection in Australia. Health Promotion International 17(1), 51–60

Wimbush E, MacGregor A, Fraser E 1998 Impacts of a national mass media campaign on walking in Scotland. Health Promotion International 13, 45–53

10 Tones K, Tilford S 2001 Health education: effectiveness, efficiency and equity, 3rd edn. Chapter 8, The mass media in health promotion. Cheltenham: Nelson Thornes

11 Reid D J, Killoran A J, McNeill A D, Chambers J S 1992 Choosing the most effective health promotion options for reducing a nation's smoking prevalence. Tobacco Control 1, 185–197. (This article reviews all the options for health-promotion interventions to reduce smoking. It highlights the importance of creating unpaid publicity in the media, and that the effective use of mass communications is crucial to the success of the whole campaign.)

12 Tones B K 1986 Preventing drug misuse: the case for breadth, balance and coherence. Health Education Journal 45, 223–230

13 Reproduced by kind permission of The Independent.

14 Flora J A, Wallack L 1990 Health promotion and mass media use: translating research into practice. Health Education Research 5, 73–80.

15 This section is based partly on:

Association of Community Workers 1986 Talking Point 74, June 1986. (Association of Community Workers, Colombo Street Sports & Community Centre, 25 Colombo Street, London SE1 8DP.)

16 Cline R J W, Haynes K M 2001 Consumer health information seeking on the Internet: the state of the art. Health Education Research 16 (6), 671–692

17   NHS Executive 1998 Information for health (www.doh.gov.uk/ipu/strategy)

18   Health Development Agency's website HealthPromis: http://healthpromis.hda-online.org.uk

19   Medline can be accessed on www.ncbi.nlm.nih.gov/PubMed

     More information about accessing the CINAHL database can be found on www.cinahl.com

     The Cochrane Library can be accessed through the National Electronic Library for Health website www.nelh.nhs.uk

20   The Health Development Agency owns or maintains a number of websites, including: www.welltown.gov.uk (Key stage 1), www.galaxy-h.gov.uk (Key stage 2), www.lifebytes.gov.uk (Key stage 3), and www.mindbodysoul.gov.uk (Key stage 4), which are for teachers and parents to use with children and young people. They are educational tools that aim to help young people make informed choices about their health.

21   NHS Direct is a telephone helpline (tel: 0845 4647) intended to become a home-based gateway to information and services covering the whole area of NHS activity. NHS Direct on-line is an Internet-based service.

22   Health Development Agency website: www.hda-online.org.uk

     Health Education Board for Scotland website (HEBSWeb): www.hebs.scot.nhs.uk

     Other useful websites for access to health information:

     Health on the net: www.hon.ch

     Medical World search: www.mwsearch.poly.edu

23   For example, see:
     Aveyard P et al 1999 Cluster randomised controlled trial of expert system based on the transtheoretical ("stages of change") model for smoking prevention and cessation in schools. British Medical Journal 319, 948–953

     Graham W et al 2000 Randomised controlled trial comparing effectiveness of touch screen system with leaflet for providing women with information on prenatal tests. British Medical Journal 320, 155–160

     Revere D, Dunbar P J 2001 Review of computer-generated outpatient health behaviour interventions: clinical encounters "in absentia". Journal of the American Medical Informatics Association 8, 62–69

     For a study of the development and implementation of health promotion software packages using behaviour theory, see:
     Rhodes F, Fishbein M, Reis J 1997 Using behavior theory in computer-based health promotion and appraisal. Health Education and Behavior 24 (1), 20–34

24   One study simulated a typical search for information on coronary heart disease by a member of the public. The study cautiously concluded that, at present, the quality of health information accessible via the Internet should not be a major cause for concern, but this may not always remain the case and users need to be vigilant.

     Eachus P (1999) Health information on the Internet: is quality a problem? International Journal of Health Promotion and Education 37 (1), 30–33

25   Based on the QUality Information ChecKlist (QUICK website) produced by the Health Development Agency and the Centre for Health Information Quality www.quick.org.uk and reproduced with kind permission of the Health Development Agency.

12 Helping People to Learn

SUMMARY

In the first section of this chapter we discuss the principles of adult learning. We then use an exercise to analyse the qualities and abilities of a good teacher, and outline some principles of helping people to learn. Subsequent sections contain guidelines on giving talks, strategies for patient education and teaching practical skills. We include a role-play exercise on skills of patient education.

This chapter is about the skills and methods of helping people to learn, when the aims are primarily educational, concerned with helping people to acquire knowledge or skills. Examples are: giving a talk on a health topic to a large community group; teaching an adult education class in food hygiene and safety; running cardiac rehabilitation classes for patients recovering after heart attacks; giving information to a patient on a one-to-one basis about diagnosis, treatment and self-care; or teaching a small group of colleagues about the techniques and procedures used in a screening programme.

Principles of Adult Learning

Other relevant chapters are 10, 11, 13 and 14.

We will focus on selected aspects of education, teaching and learning that we identify as especially relevant for health educators and health promoters who are working with adults. This chapter is certainly not comprehensive, and further reading is recommended at the end.

Health promoters and health educators generally have credibility because of their training and expert knowledge. This is likely to be valued and respected by clients, but expertise alone does not make a good health educator. Effective educators get results in the form of measurable learning achievements by the individuals and groups with whom they work, such as greater retention of information, and better application of the learning in learners' own lives.

To be effective, health educators need to understand key principles of adult learning, which are based on extensive research. Authorities like Malcolm Knowles[1] and many others have been emphasising for years that adult learners do best when they are involved and are treated with respect and dignity. They do not want merely to sit and listen, to be talked down to, to be bored, or to be bombarded with theory without opportunities for practical application. Effective educators therefore appreciate the importance of participative learning methods and use them. As Carl Rogers said:[2]

I know I cannot teach anyone anything. I can only provide an environment in which he can learn.

One of the most significant findings from research about adult learning is that when adults learn something naturally (as distinct from being taught in a formal way) they are highly self-directing. Furthermore, what they learn on their own initiative is learnt more deeply and permanently than what they are taught through traditional educational methods. Good educators also take account of brain research about the right and left brain, which reveals that people are not only logical and rational (left-brain thinking) but also have the capacity to be spontaneous and creative (right-brain thinking). The basic principles of adult learning are summarised in Box 12.1.

The next section is concerned with identifying the qualities and skills of a good educator.

Box 12.1	Principles of Adult Learning

- It is important for adults to direct themselves – they learn most effectively when they identify their own learning needs and set their own goals.
- The teacher's role is thus to enable or facilitate learning rather than to direct it. Teachers who adopt this approach often refer to themselves as 'facilitators'.
- Adult learners are generally most ready to learn things that they can apply immediately to existing problems or to their own situation. They do not, on the whole, learn for distant possibilities.
- Adult learners bring with them a wealth of life experience, which should be seen as a resource and to which new learning should be related.
- Adult learners can help each other, because of their experiences, and should be encouraged to do so.
- Adults learn best by being active (not passive), by doing and experiencing, for which they need a safe environment where they feel accepted.
- Adult learners should be encouraged to carry out continuous evaluation of their own learning. Teachers should use this evaluation to fit the learning process to the learners' needs.

What Makes a Good Teacher?

Every health promoter has spent many hours on the receiving end of other people's teaching, and this in itself is a useful learning experience. Exercise 12.1 will help health promoters to identify factors that have helped and hindered their own learning, and to assess their own qualities and abilities.

We do not suggest that health promoters set out to change their personalities. The aim of identifying strengths and weaknesses is to provide a basis for developing skills.

Exercise 12.1	**What Helps and Hinders Learning?**

Think of two occasions when you have been a learner, such as when you were a student in class, or in the audience listening to a talk, or when you were being taught on a one-to-one basis. These occasions need not have been connected with work (for example, listening to an art lecture or taking a driving lesson). One should be when you felt, overall, that the teaching session was *good* and the other when it was *bad*. The aim of the exercise is to identify the factors that made them good or bad for you.

In each of your two situations in turn identify factors that helped you to learn, and factors that hindered your learning. Think of these factors in three categories:

1.   Those to do with the *environment* (e.g. too hot? noisy? hard chairs? a spacious, comfortable room?)
2.   Those to do with the *qualities of the teacher* (e.g. sense of humour? appeared bored? contagious enthusiasm? seemed unfriendly?)
3.   Those to do with the *presentation* (e.g. talked too long? used relevant illustrations? involved audience? muddled? used words you didn't understand? used audiovisual aids effectively?)

Enter these factors on the chart:

	Environment	Teacher	Presentation
Factors that helped			
Factors that hindered			

If you are working in a group, compare your chart with those of other people.

- What have you learnt about the importance of the environment?
- What qualities of a good teacher do you think you already possess?
- What helpful points about presentation do you think you already use in your own teaching?
- What points about your own qualities or presentation would you like to improve?

Some Principles of Helping People to Learn

Here we identify some basic principles, which should be borne in mind in all health education teaching, whether working with individuals or groups.

Plan Your Session

It is vital to put thought and time into preparation. It is an easy mistake to assume that you do not need to prepare a teaching session because you know your subject. Even if you are very skilled and knowledgeable, you still need to think through what you aim to achieve and prepare how you are going to introduce and develop your session, how you will involve your audience and so on. Preparation is especially important when teaching is new to you, but even the most experienced and self-confident teacher needs to spend some time in preparation.

It is also a fallacy to think that the educator can give less attention to planning if the learners are going to be active. Active participation is a more complex process and will require greater attention to planning.

Work from the Known to the Unknown

Your starting point is what people know already; this is obviously common sense, but is frequently overlooked. The result is that time is wasted in teaching people something they know already or by talking over their heads. You need to find out as much as possible about what your clients already know. If you cannot do this in advance, spend some time at the beginning of the session asking a few questions. If you have a mixed audience with varying degrees of knowledge, it may be best to acknowledge that some people know more than others, and you will have to make a decision about the level at which to pitch your information: 'Some of you will probably know this, but I'll talk about it briefly because it will be new to others . . .'.

Your aim is build new information, or new skills, on to what is already known.

Aim for Maximum Involvement

People learn best if they are actively involved in the learning process, not just passively listening.

First, try to involve your clients in deciding the aim and content of the teaching. If you are running a course, such as a series of antenatal classes or one on food hygiene, you might begin by explaining your aims, asking for comments and suggestions, and then going on to discuss the content. This will help to increase motivation by including clients' own interests and, hopefully, stimulating them to think about new areas. It also helps clients to recognise that they are responsible for their own learning. The goals and content of one-to-one teaching can always be established by mutual agreement at the beginning of a session.

As a general rule, it is worth considering how much room for negotiation there is in your teaching, and spending time to find out what people really want. Ask yourself 'is what I teach what *I want to teach* or what *my clients want to learn?*'

Secondly, keep your clients involved as much as possible during teaching sessions. This is a challenge if you are giving a talk or a lecture to a large audience, but there are possibilities, such as asking people to respond to a question, e.g. 'I'd like you to put your hand up if you made a New Year resolution to take more exercise this year'. Or ask them to respond to a series of statements; for example, as an introduction to a talk on nutrition, ask the audience to stand up, then ask them to sit down if they: usually eat white bread . . . add sugar to tea and coffee . . . regularly eat fried food . . . add salt at the table . . . Most of them will be sitting down by now but will feel alert and involved. Another way of keeping an audience involved is to give them time to talk. This can be done by having question-and-answer sessions, or by allowing short breaks when they can talk about something in groups of two or three for a few minutes. In a talk on passive smoking, for example, you could give your audience a couple of minutes to tell their neighbours how they are affected by other people's smoke.

You can also keep people involved with eye contact. Look members of your audience in the eye, and make sure that you look round at everybody, not just the people immediately in front of you.

Vary Your Learning Methods

It is natural to consider teaching from the teacher's point of view but it may be more helpful to look at it from the learner's point of view. For example, talking for half an hour demands concentrated effort and total involvement on your part; but all your audience is doing is listening, which involves only one of their senses and is highly unlikely to hold their full attention.

Variety can be brought into health teaching in many ways, including strategies that can be used with individuals, groups, large audiences, children or adults – see Table 12.1.

Table 12.1	Learning Methods Involving Clients	
	Client involvement	**Materials and methods**
	Listen	Lectures, audiotapes
	Read	Books, booklets, leaflets, handouts, posters, black/white board, flipchart, overhead projector transparency
	Look	Photographs, drawings, paintings, posters, charts, material from magazines (such as advertisements)
	Look and listen	Films, videotapes, tape-slide sets, slides with commentary, demonstrations
	Listen and talk	Question-and-answer sessions, discussions, informal conversations, debates, brainstorming
	Read, listen and talk	Case studies, discussions based on study questions or handouts
	Read, listen, talk and actively participate	Drama, role-play, games, simulations, quizzes, practising skills
	Read and actively participate	Programmed learning, computer-assisted learning
	Make and use	Models, charts, drawings
	Use	Equipment
	Action research	Gathering information, opinions, interviews and surveys
	Projects	Making health education materials – videos, leaflets, etc.
For discussion of some of these methods, see Chapters 13 and 14; for discussion on the use of audiovisual aids, see Chapter 11.	Visits	To health service premises, fire station, sewage works, playgroups, voluntary organisations
	Write	Articles, letters to the press, stories, poems

Devise Your own Learning Activities

Activities are the means by which you help learners to think through what is being said and act on it, in their own way. Listening is passive; activities are active! It is not sufficient to ask a group of learners 'What do you think?' at the end of a talk or after viewing a video; planned activities are necessary to help people to explore ideas, feelings, attitudes and behaviour. It is important to have a mix. Activities specifically tailored for a particular group of learners will be most effective, so it is important to develop the skill of devising your own activities rather than relying on learning aids made for general audiences. There is an almost infinite range of possibilities. Some of the more common types of activity are set out in Table 12.2. There are more ideas in the exercises we use in this book.

Table 12.2	Common Types of Learning Activities
Type of activity	**Example**
Guidelines for discussions with particular people about particular topics	Guidelines on 'what to do if you think your child is offered drugs' for discussion at a parent–teacher meeting.
Analysing and discussing diary records	Ask people to keep a diary or write down what they ate or drank in the last 24 hours. Ask them to talk about what they are pleased about and not pleased about.
Sentence completion	Ask people to complete a sentence such as 'I feel really stressed when . . . '
Using checklists	Have a list of 'ways to be green' such as keeping a compost heap, recycling newspapers and bottles, using biodegradable detergents, and discuss how many you use.
Identifying your own thoughts/ feelings/behaviour in particular situations	Ask people to think about and discuss what they feel when visitors to their home ask if they can smoke, and how they respond.
Generate lists	Ask a group to make a list of all the ways they could deal with a toddler who won't settle down to sleep.
Answer sheets	A quiz with yes/no or multiple answers on 'How much do you know about sensible drinking?'
Drawing charts or bubble diagrams	Draw a stick-person picture of yourself in a supermarket in the middle of a page. Draw bubble thoughts about all the things that influence what food you buy.
Writing instructions	Ask a group learning about food hygiene to write down instructions for someone else on how to store food safely in a fridge.
Practical skills development	Practise bathing a baby using a doll or a real baby.

Ensure Relevance

When teaching you should ensure that, as far as possible, what you say is relevant to the needs, interests and circumstances of the clients. For example, recommendations about health-promoting activities that cost money may be helpful to a relatively well-off audience, but not of much use to an audience which has no money for 'extras'. A discussion on vaccination may be irrelevant to a pregnant woman whose over-whelming concern is the birth itself; she may not relate to an issue that will not affect her until afterwards.

You will help your clients to see the relevance of your subject if you use concrete examples, practical problems and case studies to explain and illustrate your points. Abstract generalisations and quotations of high figures are difficult to relate to. For example say 'one person in ten' instead of 'X million people in this country', tell the story of a home accident rather than describe a list of risk factors, and describe 'increasing the risk' by saying 'It's like driving a car with faulty brakes – there's no guarantee that you will have an accident, but your chances of having one are greater'.

Identify Realistic Goals and Objectives

See Chapter 5, section Stage 2 Set Aims and Objectives.

We discussed in Chapter 5 the importance of clearly identifying health promotion aims and objectives, but it is worth emphasising again that it is essential to be clear about what you are trying to do (raise awareness of a health issue? give people more health knowledge?) and what you want your clients to know, feel and/or do at the end of your teaching session. As we mentioned above, your clients may be involved in these decisions.

A common mistake is to attempt too much – three or four key points are all that you can ever expect people to remember from a teaching session. Teaching more than that does not mean that they learn more; it usually means that they forget more. For example, if you are asked to give a talk on a huge theme, such as food for health, avoiding accidents, first aid or pollution, you will need to select what you feel to be the few points most relevant for your audience, and avoid the temptation to give an everything-you-ever-wanted-to-know-about talk. A well-moved molehill is better than an abortive attempt to shift Everest.

Use Learning Contracts

In traditional education the learner is told what objectives to work towards. This conflicts with the adult's psychological need to be self-directing and may induce resistance, apathy, or withdrawal. Learning contracts are an agreement between the learner and teacher about what is to be learnt. Teacher and learner (or group of learners) decide it together. By participating in the process of diagnosing needs, formulating goals, choosing learning methods, and evaluating progress, learners develop a sense of ownership of the plan, and feel committed to it.

We describe the stages of developing a learning contract below.

Step 1. Diagnose Learning Needs with the Learners

First, decide the competencies required to carry out the actions, or behaviour, or role that the learners want to learn (for example, the competencies required to be the parent of a new baby at an antenatal education class). A competency can be thought of as the ability to do something, and it is a combination of knowledge, understanding, skills, attitudes, and values.

For instance, 'the ability to ride a bicycle from home to the shops' involves knowledge of how a bicycle works and of the route from home to the shops; understanding of the dangers inherent in riding a bicycle; skills in mounting, pedalling, steering and stopping. It is useful to analyse competencies in this way, even if it is crude and subjective, because it gives the learners a clearer sense of direction.

Next, assess the gap between where learners are now and where they should be in regard to each competency. Learners may wish to draw on the observations of friends, family or experts to make this assessment. Each learner will then have an idea of the competencies needed, that is, a profile of their learning needs.

Step 2. Specify the Learning Objectives of Each Learner

Translate the learning needs identified in step one into objectives that describe what each learner wants to *learn*. All learners should state their learning objectives in terms most meaningful to them. For example, in order to ride a bicycle from home to the shops, learners may decide that they need knowledge of how to work the bicycle gears and improved skills of steering and stopping safely.

Step 3. Specify Learning Methods

Review the learning objectives of the learner or (if you are working with a group of learners) all the members of the learning group, perhaps through listing them on a flip-chart and identifying shared objectives and areas of difference. Now think about how you could go about accomplishing these objectives. Specify the methods you would use. In the bicycle example, you could specify that practical demonstration followed by supervised practice in a traffic-free area would be the way to learn. Ask learners to suggest the methods they prefer.

Step 4. Evaluate Learning

See also Chapter 5, section Stage 5 Plan Evaluation Methods.

Now describe what evidence you will need to show that these objectives have been achieved. For example, knowledge can be tested through quizzes; understanding can be tested through solving problems; skills can be tested through demonstrations of performance; attitudes can be tested through role-play and structured activities; values can be tested through structured activities and value-clarification exercises.

See Chapter 14, section on strategies for increasing self-awareness, clarifying values and changing attitudes.

An example of a learning contract for a group is provided in Box 12.2. Individuals in a group can have their own personal version of the learning contract.

Box 12.2	Learning Contract for Mary's Young Parents' Group

Group members said they wanted to know more about how to cook cheap, interesting, healthy meals for their families, as a change from the usual fish fingers, beans, chips, etc. Mary and group members worked out the following learning contract.

Learning objectives	Learning methods	Evaluation of achievement of objectives
Know what to eat to be healthy	Keep food diaries for two days. Mary to produce guidelines and members discuss how far their food matches up to guidelines	Be able to say what sort of food each member should aim to eat more or less of
Know where to buy good cheap food	Group members share experience of where they buy food, its price and quality	Two weeks later, members identify changes in where they buy food, and whether it is better quality and value for money
Be able to cook healthy meals that their families enjoy eating	Mary and group members bring recipes, choose some to try out and cook together	Have cooked new healthy meals at home

Organise Your Material

Whether you are talking to a group or teaching an individual, it helps if you organise your material into a logical framework, and tell your client(s) what this is, both at the beginning and during your teaching session.[3] For example, with an individual patient, say:

'I am going to tell you:

- what we have found to be wrong with you
- the treatment I am going to suggest for you
- how much time you will need off work.

First, what we have found out is that ...
Secondly, I think that the best treatment for you is ...
Finally, about taking time off work, I think that you will probably need ...'

The same principle applies if you are talking to a group. The old adage is: 'Tell 'em what you're going to tell 'em; tell 'em; then tell 'em what you've told 'em'. This is sound advice, because it helps both you and the audience to know where you are and where you are going. 'Flagging' where you are at intervals is helpful: 'That's all I've got to say on the benefits of yoga; now, to move on to how you can get started ...', or 'Now I'd like to move on to my third and final point, which you may remember I said was about ...'

Evaluation, Feedback and Assessment

See Chapter 5, section Stage 5: Plan Evaluation Methods, and Chapter 10, section on asking questions and getting feedback.

As we emphasised previously, it is important to get feedback on your teaching, so that you can assess how much your client is learning and improve your own performance in the future.

Three aspects to consider are:

- how you will assess your own performance as an educator/facilitator (self-assessment), and record how well you feel the session went, and what could be improved
- how you will get feedback from your learners on how well they think the session went
- how you will assess the extent to which your learners are achieving the planned learning outcomes.

We now consider each of these.

Assessing Your Own Performance

You need to ask yourself what went well, what didn't, why, and how things could be improved next time. You may find it helpful to use a simple form to record your thoughts. This is especially useful if your session is part of a course with a team of people involved. An example is given in Box 12.3 – a form used by a group facilitator to record issues after a group session on healthy eating and cooking.

Getting Feedback from Learners

You could include oral feedback as part of your session. For example, at the end ask people to do a round of sentence completion:

Box 12.3	Nutrition and Cooking Project Monitoring Form[4]

Session no:
Date:
Course leader:
Number of attenders:
Number in crèche:
Activity:
Positive outcomes:
Negative outcomes:
Feedback/comments from participants:
Crèche issues:
Issues needing further action:
Action plan:
Completed by:

'The thing I liked best about today's session was . . .'
'The most important thing I am taking away from this session is . . .'
'The thing I liked least about today's session was . . .'
   However, people may find this intimidating, and might not feel comfortable with expressing what they feel directly to the educator. You may wish to use a written evaluation form, and we give two examples in Boxes 12.4 and 12.5.

Box 12.4	Evaluation Form A

Title of session:

Date:

Please help me to get the session right for you by completing the following sentences about how you feel. Thank you.

It helps me when . . . .

It is difficult for me when . . . .

I would like more of . . . .

I would like less of . . . .

Assessing the Learning Outcomes

Assessing learning outcomes is an important aspect of evaluation in teaching and learning situations. It is the process of measuring the extent and quality of your clients' learning: judging how successful they have been in progressing towards goals which they set themselves. It may be carried out very informally through getting appar-

Box 12.5	**Evaluation Form B**

Title of course:

Date:

We would like your views to help us assess this course and make plans for similar courses in the future. All your comments will be valued and used, and treated confidentially.

	Yes	No	Partly
1. Overall, have you found this course beneficial? (please tick)	☐	☐	☐
2. What did you expect to gain from the course?			

	Yes	No	Partly
3. Did the course match up to your expectations?	☐	☐	☐

Please comment:

4. Which parts of the course have you found most beneficial?

5. Which parts of the course have you found least beneficial?

6. How do you think the course could be improved?

7. Do you have any other comments you would like to make?

Please write your name here (or leave blank if you prefer to remain anonymous). Thank you very much for filling this in.

---

ently casual feedback from clients about how they have applied the learning to real-life situations, or it may involve setting tests in formal situations. Here are two examples of ways in which health promoters assess how well they are doing:

- Sandra teaches yoga. She does not feel it appropriate to assess her students formally, so she uses the British Wheel of Yoga standards to check on their performance and give them feedback.
- Marleen teaches cookery and healthy eating to adults with learning difficulties. She keeps records of their progress in relation to their previous level of competence in choosing healthy menus and cooking healthy meals.

Monitoring students' progress by keeping records of achievements can be valuable for helping them to see what they have achieved. If your teaching is geared towards people learning to change behaviour, it can help to keep diary-type records of what they ate or drank, or how much physical activity they did. If they are learning practical creative skills, photographic records can help. For example, on a course designed to help people cook and eat healthier food for their families you could give them a single-use camera to make a pictorial record of the dishes they cooked and their family enjoying the meals.

Guidelines for Giving Talks

Giving a talk, or perhaps a formal lecture, is a frequent feature of a health promoter's work. There are considerable disadvantages in this method: a talk is largely a one-way communication process with little opportunity to assess how much people are learning or understanding, and with only a small proportion of it likely to be remembered at the end (and still less a few days later).

Despite these limitations, talks and lectures can be valuable for several reasons. A talk can be used to introduce a subject by giving a bird's-eye view of it, and this may lead people to take further action. For example, an introductory talk on first aid may lead people to enrol for a first aid course. A talk may awaken a critical attitude in the audience, for example, by drawing their attention to issues such as pollution or the lack of understandable information on food labels. Many people do not read books and articles, or habitually watch documentary programmes on television; for them, a talk may be an important source of health information. Giving talks is also a relatively economical way to use a health promoter's time, since large numbers of people can be addressed at one time.

In addition to the general principles discussed in the last section we now discuss some specific points which may help you to plan, and deliver, a successful talk.

Check the Facilities

If possible, visit the place where you are going to give your talk and check the seating, lighting and audiovisual equipment, including electric power points and extension leads. On the day of the talk, arrive in good time so that you can arrange chairs, open windows, and check that the equipment is working. Get your video player or overhead projector ready for use. If you need blackout, check that you can turn the lights on and off quickly so that you do not lose rapport with the audience while they are left in the dark.

Make a Plan

It can be useful to make an outline plan of your whole session, indicating the sections, times and any audiovisual aids you are using. This is particularly useful if you are sharing a teaching session with a colleague, so that you are both clear what you are doing – see the example in Box 12.6. You can either use this as a skeleton overall plan to guide you when you make detailed notes to speak from (see section below) or it might be enough to enable you to speak from the plan itself.

Making and Using Notes

It is generally best to give a talk from notes written on paper or cards. The more experienced you are the fewer notes you are likely to need, unless your talk is full of technical detail or likely to be taken down and quoted verbatim (for example, by the press). However, very few people can give a successful talk with no notes at all, and beginners may find it helpful to write out a talk in full before they transfer the main points to notes.

If you are writing out your talk in full to begin with, it is useful to know that a 50 minute lecture consists of about 5000 words, allowing for pauses and an estimated speed of delivery of about 110 words per minute. You can then try transferring the key points as notes to cards or paper.

Box 12.6	**Plan for Giving a Talk**

TALK ON 'SENSE IN THE SUN – PREVENTING SKIN CANCER'
Bloggshire Secondary School Parent–Teachers Meeting
21.5.2002 ¾ hour at the end of the business meeting, 8.00–8.45 p.m.
Mrs N (school nurse) & Mr DH (deputy head)
AIM: to give parents basic information on risks and prevention of skin cancer

Time	Section	Content	Audiovisual aids (OHT = overhead projector transparency)	Who
8.00	Intros	Intro Mrs N & Mr DH Why we are now concerned about skin cancer – rising incidence	OHT graph showing rise in skin cancer in UK	Mr DH
8.05	What is skin cancer?	Different types of skin cancer How you spot it Who is most at risk (fair skin, sunburn, etc.)	OHT key points	Mrs N
8.15	Prevention	Key message: respect the sun – avoid exposure at hottest times, use good sunscreen, cover up with sun hats and light clothing Be a mole-watcher	Examples of sun hats, light clothing (big, long-sleeved, cotton shirts etc.) Examples of sunscreen creams	Mrs N
8.25	What the school can do	Encourage the use of cover-up and sunscreen creams in outdoor PE Include topic in health education and science teaching	Main points on OHT	Mr DH
8.30	Summary	Aim for school and parents to work together Main points to remember: Care in the sun, Cover up, use sunscreen Creams	OHT: 3 C's to remember: Care in the sun Cover up Creams Leaflets to take away.	Mrs N
8.35	Any questions?			Mrs N

Never give a talk by writing it out in full and then reading it. Unless you are an exceptional orator who can 'act' the lines, it will sound flat and stilted. Furthermore, you will find it difficult to look at your audience, because you will need to keep your eyes on the notes, and once you look up you are likely to lose your place.

Prepare Your Introduction

Secure the attention of your audience with your opening words. Some ways of doing this are:

- state a startling fact
- ask a question that has no easy answer
- use a visual image to trigger interest
- get the audience to do something active (some suggestions are discussed in the earlier section on aiming for maximum involvement)

■ tell a joke, if you have the confidence to do it successfully.

Establish eye contact with your audience and, if necessary, ask them whether they can see and hear you.

State your aim and theme at the beginning of your talk ('Tell 'em what you're going to tell 'em'). It should be a brief statement, not a complex summary of the whole talk. For example, say 'I'm going to talk about what to do if someone is unconscious, not breathing, bleeding or in a state of shock', but do not go into detail at this point about what the correct actions should be; save that for the main part of the talk.

By the time you have finished the introduction, you should have:

■ established your aim and theme with the audience
■ obtained their interest and commitment
■ ensured that they can hear and see you clearly. ·

Prepare the Key Points

See Chapter 11, on using and producing audiovisual materials, including leaflets, handouts and videos.

Identify the three or four main points you wish to make, and prepare your talk around each point in turn. Illustrate and support your points with evidence from your experience or from research, with examples, audiovisual materials, and so on.

Plan a Conclusion

You need to plan how you will end your talk in order to avoid rambling on or trailing off. Some ways of ending are:

■ a very brief recapitulation (not a boring repetition) of what you've said – e.g. 'We've now covered the basics of life-saving first aid'
■ a statement of what you hope the audience will do with the information you have given them – e.g. 'I hope that you can confidently do the right thing next time you have to help someone who's had an accident'
■ a suggestion for further action – 'If you'd like to learn more please come to see me afterwards'
■ a question – 'Don't you think that basic first aid is so simple and so important that it should be taught to every child in school?'
■ thanking the audience for their attention and/or participation.

Ask for Questions

If possible, include a question-and-answer session in your talk. It gives you feedback, and gives the audience a chance to participate.

When you ask for questions, allow people time to think; do not assume that there are to be no questions just because one is not instantly forthcoming. When a question is asked, it is often helpful to repeat or summarise it. This gives you a little time to consider the question, and ensures that everyone else in the audience has heard it. Never ignore or refuse to answer a question – if you don't know the answer say so, and ask whether anyone else in the audience does. In any case, this helps to involve the audience; you could also ask for comments on answers 'Does anyone else have suggestions which could help the person who asked that question?'

Work on Your Presentation

Important points about presentation include pace and timing, which usually means consciously having to slow down your rate of speaking; the nervous beginner finds the silence of pauses to be threatening and wants to get the whole thing over! Other factors are looking at the audience and using notes appropriately.

Thorough preparation will help you to feel confident, but however nervous or inexperienced you may feel, do not apologise for being there. For example, if you have been asked to give a talk about your work, *do not say* 'I'm going to talk about the work of health visitors, but I'm afraid I've only been qualified for a year so there's a lot I don't know yet'. Instead, present yourself positively 'I'm going to talk about the work of health visitors. I've been qualified for a year now, and I'd like to share my experience of the work with you'.

The way to improve presentation is practice. Practise giving your talk out loud, or to friends or colleagues. Ask a trusted colleague to sit in when you give a talk, and to give you feedback afterwards. It is even more helpful to see yourself on video, so that you can assess your own strengths and weaknesses.

Plan for Contingencies

A major fear when giving a talk is that you might 'dry up' or lose your place. If this is a possibility, it is better to face it and think beforehand about what you will do if it should happen. It is best to acknowledge that you have a problem rather than leave an embarrassing silence. For example, say 'Sorry, my mind seems to have gone blank' or 'I've lost my place'. Then remember that an audience is likely to be friendly rather than hostile and will probably want to help you. So let them help by asking for time: 'Would you mind if I took a minute to get myself together?' or 'Excuse me for a moment while I look through my notes'.

See also section on dealing with difficulties in Chapter 13.

Another fear is that audiovisual equipment will break down. You cannot insure against this, so it is best to have a contingency plan ready. For example, 'As we can't see the sequence on the video as I'd hoped, I'll write the stages up on the blackboard and talk through them instead'.

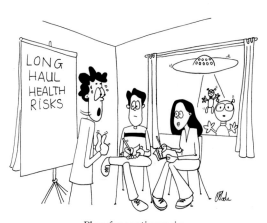

Plan for contingencies

Improving Patient Education

Research over many years has shown that patients want information but have difficulty in understanding and remembering what they have been told by their doctor, nurse, or other health worker. Substantial numbers of patients feel dissatisfied with the communications aspect of their encounters with health professionals, and are reluctant to ask for more information. Furthermore, a large proportion of patients do not comply with the advice and treatment prescribed for them.

There are many reasons for these apparent failures, but certainly some of the cause lies in the way in which information, advice and instructions are given to patients. Often the circumstances are less than ideal, because patients are distressed or feeling unwell, and there may be little time in a busy surgery, outpatient clinic, or hospital ward. Therefore, there is all the more reason to ensure that the best possible use is made of the time and opportunities for patient education.

All the basic communication skills discussed in Chapter 10, and the principles of helping people to learn outlined earlier in this chapter, are important. There has also been considerable research in the field of patient education and information.[5] Some particular principles that have been found helpful in patient education are set out in Box 12.7.[6]

Exercise 12.2 is designed to help you practise the skills of patient education we have discussed here, as well as the basic communication skills outlined in Chapter 10. Another useful way of learning to improve communication skills is to video an interview with a patient and analyse it.

Box 12.7	Some Principles of Patient Education

- Say important things first: patients are more likely to remember what was said at the beginning of a session, so give the most important advice and instruction first whenever possible.
- Stress and repeat the key points: patients are more likely to remember what they consider to be important, so make sure they realise what the really important points are. For example, say:

    'The most important thing for you to remember today is . . .'
    'The one thing it's really essential to do is . . .'
    Repetition of key points also helps people to remember them.
- Give specific, precise advice: sometimes it is appropriate to give general guidance, but specific, precise advice is more likely to be remembered than vague guidance. For example, say:

    'I advise you to lose five pounds in the next month' rather than 'I advise you to lose weight'
    'Try to take an hour's rest with your feet up every afternoon' rather than 'Get more rest' or 'Take things easier'.
- Structure information into categories: this means telling the patient headings and then categorising your material under these headings as you present it.

See Organise Your Material above.

See Chapter 11 on using communication tools.

- Avoid jargon and long words and sentences: if you need to use medical terms or jargon, make sure the patient understands what they mean. Never use a long word when a short one will do. Use short sentences.
- Use visual aids, leaflets, handouts and written instructions.
- Avoid saying too much at once: three or four key points is all that you can expect someone to remember from one session.

See Ensure Relevance above. See the section on asking questions and getting feedback in Chapter 10.

- Ensure advice is relevant and realistic in the patient's circumstances.
- Get feedback from patients to ensure that they understand.

Exercise 12.2   Skills of Patient Education

Work in groups of three, taking each role in turn.

The **first person** takes the role of the health promoter. She selects the topic to be taught, drawing on her own experience, and tells the 'patient' his medical history before role-play starts.

The **second person** plays the patient. This patient should have one of the following sets of characteristics:

- intelligent, but with very limited understanding of spoken English, no ability to read or write English, and no one available to translate
- extremely worried, tense and anxious about his medical condition and prognosis
- has some learning difficulty, finds great difficulty in understanding and remembering instructions although he tries hard to be cooperative.

The **third person** takes the role of the observer, using the observer's checklist below.

Role-play the scene in which the health promoter is teaching the patient for ten minutes. The observer keeps time. Then give constructive feedback as follows:

- firstly, the 'health promoter' assesses herself, saying what she felt she did well, and identifying points she feels the need to work on in the future.
- secondly, the 'patient' describes how it felt to be the patient, identifying what the health promoter did or said which made him feel at ease/put down/ anxious/reassured/ more confused, and so on.
- finally, the observer gives feedback using the checklist as a guide.

Communication Checklist

1. Non-verbal aspects of communication, e.g. tone of voice, posture, gestures, facial expression, use of touch.
2. Sequence and structure of key points, e.g. important things first, logical sequence, information in categories.
3. Choice of language, e.g. appropriately simple and short, use of jargon/idioms, medical terms.
4. Two-way communication, e.g. encourage patient to talk and express feelings, get feedback about how much is understood, open/closed/biased/multiple questions.
5. Amount of information, e.g. too much or too little.

6. Clarity of objective(s).
7. Use of repetition.
8. Use of emphasis to stress important points.
9. Any assumptions made but not checked, e.g. about previous knowledge, facilities for carrying out instructions, willingness to comply.
10. Anything else?

Teaching Practical Skills

Health promoters are often called upon to teach practical skills, such as relaxation or keep-fit exercises, how to bath a baby or change a nappy, and how to give an injection or test urine.

All the communication skills we have discussed are relevant, but a few additional points are useful. Teaching a skill is not just about achieving 'knowing' and 'doing' objectives; that is, it is not *solely* concerned with giving the client information and teaching new practical skills. It is also necessary to pay attention to what clients *feel*. If people are afraid to do something because they are worried about looking foolish or doing it incorrectly, they are unlikely to succeed: encouragement and step-by-step progress are needed. Confidence-building is as important a part of the health educator's role as developing practical skills.

In order to develop clients' ability to perform a skilled task, a three-stage approach is most effective:

Stage 1. Demonstrate.

Stage 2. Rehearse.

Stage 3. Practise.

Clients will be watching and listening in stage 1, but they become actively involved in *doing* in stages 2 and 3.

It may be useful to begin by using a dummy, for example, when teaching safe lifting techniques, or to use an orange instead of a person when teaching injection techniques. As skills develop, the techniques can be tried in real-life situations (lifting people, for example) and perhaps under more difficult circumstances.

Individual learners need to progress at their own pace and build up confidence at each stage. For this reason teaching practical skills needs time and patience, but it is worth the investment to get the right skills programme from the beginning. People who have lost confidence in their ability to do something are even more difficult to help than a new learner.

- To be successful in health education with adult clients you need to understand principles of adult learning and factors that help and hinder learning. Key principles include paying attention to planning, involving learners in the learning process as much as possible, ensuring material is relevant and structured into a logical sequence, and having realistic objectives. You may find it helpful to use informal learning contracts.

- If you are giving talks, you need planning, preparation and practice.

- You can help patients to understand and remember more if you take account of some key principles of patient education.

- It is best to use a three-stage approach of demonstration, rehearsal and practice when you are teaching practical skills.

Recommended Reading

On Health Education

➤ Katz J, Peberdy A, Douglas J (eds) 2000 Promoting health: knowledge and practice, 2nd edn. Chapter 10: Educating for Health. Basingstoke: The Open University in association with Palgrave. (Historical and contemporary approaches to health education.)

On Adult Learning

➤ Castling A 1996 Competence-based teaching and training. Basingstoke: City and Guilds/Macmillan

➤ Rogers J 2001 Adults learning, 4th edn. Buckingham: Open University Press

➤ Sotto E 1994 When teaching becomes learning. London: Cassell

On the Nurse's Role as a Teacher

➤ Hinchcliffe S (ed.) 1992 The practitioner as teacher. London: Baillière Tindall. (Looks at the nurse's role as a teacher and examines the skills and methods that help the nurse become a more effective teacher.)

➤ Jarvis P, Gibson S 1997 The teacher practitioner and mentor in nursing, midwifery, health visiting, 2nd edn. Cheltenham: Nelson Thornes.

On Giving Talks

➤ Stanton N 1996 Mastering communication, 3rd edn. Chapter 2. Basingstoke: Macmillan.

➤ Stevens M 1996 How to be better at giving presentations. London: Kogan Page/Industrial Society

➤ Williams D 1997 Communication skills in practice – a practical guide for health professionals. Part Four: Presentation skills. London: Jessica Kingsley Publications

On Running Workshops

➤ Brooks-Harris J, Stock-Ward S 1999 Workshops; designing and facilitating experiential learning. Thousand Oaks: Sage Publications

On Patient Education

➤ Coates V 1999 Education for patients and clients. London: Routledge

➤ Pestonjee S F 2000 Nurses' handbook of patient education. Springhouse: Springhouse Corporation

Notes and References

1   A 'classic' text is:

Knowles M 1978 The adult learner: a neglected species, 2nd edn. Houston, Texas: Gulf

2   Rogers C 1969 Freedom to learn. Merrill: Ohio. (This is another classic text.)

3   One early study found that the use of this technique improved patients' recall by 17%:

Ley P et al. 1973 A method for increasing patients' recall of information presented by doctors. Psychological Medicine 3, 217–220.

4   Form used by Hartcliffe Health and Environment Action Group and health visitors from Hartcliffe and Withywood, Bristol, in their 'Feed Your Face' project on nutrition and cooking. Reproduced with their kind permission.

5   The Cochrane Library has a number of reviews on patient education on particular health issues:

Limited (information only) patient education programs for adults with asthma

Self-management education and regular practitioner review for adults with asthma

Patient education for mechanical neck disorders

Patient education for preventing diabetic foot ulceration

Abstracts of the Cochrane Reviews can be obtained from the Cochrane Library which can be accessed through the National Electronic Library for Health (www.nelh.nhs.uk). Cochrane Reviews are updated regularly.

Other research reviews:

Arthur V A M 1995 Written patient information: a review of the literature. Journal of Advanced Nursing 21(6), 1081–1086.

Kok G, van den Borne B, Mullen P D (1997) Effectiveness of health education and health promotion: meta-analyses of effect studies and determinants of effectiveness. Patient Education and Counselling 30(1), 19–27. (Research showing effectiveness of health education and pointers to effective practice.)

Vahabi M, Ferris L 1995 Improving written patient education materials: a review of the evidence. Health Education Journal 54, 99–106. (Discusses evidence on how to improve written patient education material.)

The Centre for Health Information Quality has been commissioned by the NHS Executive to develop guidelines for written health information. Training on the use of the guidelines is offered by the Centre. More information can be found on their website (www.hfht.org/chiq), or by writing to the Centre for Health Information Quality, Highcroft, Romsey Road, Winchester.

6   This section was originally based on:

Ewles L, Shipster P 1981 One-to-one health education. East Sussex Area Health Authority, and

Ley P 1988 Communicating with patients – improving communication, satisfaction and compliance. London: Croom Helm

13 Working with Groups

SUMMARY

This chapter is about working with clients in groups. We begin by considering the range of groups in health promotion, potential benefits of group work, and when it is appropriate to use it. Next we look at group leadership – styles and responsibilities – then turn to group behaviour. The last part of the chapter focuses on the competencies needed for working successfully with people in groups: the practicalities and skills of setting up a group, getting groups going, discussion skills, and dealing with difficulties. We include exercises on identifying the benefits of joining a group, looking at your leadership style, and planning a group meeting.

See Chapter 9.

Health promoters work with many different kinds of groups in a variety of settings. We looked at working with groups of colleagues in Chapter 9; in this chapter, we focus on the health promoter's work with groups of clients, but it is worth saying that many of the skills we discussed in Chapter 9 (such as coordination, teamwork, and working effectively in meetings and committees) may also apply when working with clients.

Group work can be seen as part of the movement away from clients as passive recipients of services, towards clients as people actively involved with their own health issues and active within their communities. Many of the groups with which health promoters are involved will already exist, where members have come together for a common purpose and health issues form part, or the whole, of the agenda. The role of the health promoter may vary widely, from leading a one-off session to facilitating the development of a new group, or leading a group with a defined lifespan. Whatever the role, competencies in group work are needed, and this chapter sets out some of the basic ones. (We are excluding leading therapeutic groups from our discussions; therapy requires in-depth professional training in a range of possible approaches, outside the scope of this book.)

Specialist training in group work is recommended to develop skills and confidence further.[1] Group work may be given only a brief introduction in basic professional training courses and in-service professional development; consequently many practitioners feel ill equipped for the task. For further reading, see the suggestions at the end of the chapter.

First, we discuss the kinds of groups that exist for different purposes.

Kinds of Groups

Groups are not random collections of individuals; group members have a sense of shared identity, common objectives, defined membership criteria, and their own particular ways of working. Groups are formed for a variety of purposes. The term *group work* can be applied to a range of activities such as group therapy, social action, or self-help. We suggest that groups in the context of health promotion are usually formed for one or more of the following purposes.

For raising awareness: to increase members' interest in, and awareness of, health issues through group discussion. This may be a group already in existence, such as a women's group, which may agree to discuss a health issue.

For mutual support: to support members in difficult decision making, to help each other to cope with shared problems/disabilities, or to change a health-damaging behaviour. Examples are self-help groups such as groups of people living with HIV, patients' associations, tenants' associations, and Alcoholics Anonymous.

For social action: to use the collective power of the group to campaign for social change, for example tackling a local problem of drug misuse, housing standards, or community facilities.

For education: to impart skills, offer information and sometimes to prepare members for specific life events, for example becoming a parent.

For group counselling: to help members to find solutions through exploring a shared problem with a counsellor, for example a group of menopausal women.

Being clear about the purpose of a group is important. Confusion can result if the tasks of a group are changed, especially if this means that individual members have to adopt different roles. For example, an individual will have difficulty if she attends a group to obtain support, and finds the task has changed to campaigning. A new group is required for the new task.

The type of task will determine the most effective size for the group; for example, educational groups may be larger than support groups.

Different kinds of groups may also require the health promoter to take on different roles, and use different skills. Leading or facilitating groups requires special skills and methods; later in this chapter we discuss group leadership and the skills you need.

Potential Benefits of Group Work

It is important that a group leader or facilitator considers the benefits for the individual client of using a group as a medium for help.[2] The *process* of being part of a group is often as important as the intended outcome of the group; for example, a young parent may gain friends and social skills by being part of a parenting group as well as learning parenting skills.

In addition to thinking of potential benefits for the group as a whole, the group facilitator needs to think about which benefits are relevant to individual group members. Different group members may benefit in different ways. Exercise 13.1 is designed to help you think about what joining a group could mean to a client.

When to Use Group Work

See also Chapter 5, Stage 3 – Decide the Best Way of Achieving the Aims.

Health promoters can be unsure about when it is appropriate to use a group work approach to health promotion. We suggest that group work is appropriate when your plans fulfil the following criteria:

Exercise 13.1   How Can Joining a Group Help?[3]

Think of a group that you have:

- set up in the past, or
- intend to establish in the future, or
- belonged to yourself.

Consider the list of potential benefits below. Which ones could apply to members of your group?

Trying out new behaviours that are better for the group members or other people they have contact with.

Gaining new knowledge, becoming better informed.

Learning new ways of doing things and acquiring new skills.

Finding better ways of coping with everyday life.

Feeling less isolated, reducing the sense of being alone with an illness or problem or in particular circumstances and that nobody else really understands.

Developing more confidence, with group members having a more positive view of themselves.

Group members recognising that they do not have to go on as they have always done: they can see new possibilities.

Revising previously held assumptions group members had about themselves and/or others; they think differently about themselves and others.

Developing an understanding, or a fuller and more accurate understanding, of how past experiences have, until now, influenced group members.

Feeling able to work with other people to take action about something group members feel strongly about.

Can you think of any other benefits?

- You have looked critically at what other health promotion opportunities exist, and you have concluded that group work is needed to meet the particular needs of specific groups of people.
- You have evidence that group work is effective for this particular client group, for example that group work is an effective approach to the education of young mothers.[4]
- You are going to be working with a defined group of people over a period of time, which will allow the group to build up trust and be able to help each other, for example a group of prospective parents, a 'self-help group' of patients who are recovering after heart attacks, or people who have been diagnosed as HIV positive.
- You have access to a comfortable, private and relaxed environment in which to run the group, for example a community centre.

■ You have access to support and supervision in order to provide you with support when you need it and help you to develop your group work.

In some circumstances group work may be particularly helpful. Examples are:

■ you are planning to work with people who are already in a close-knit small group, and possibly already used to group work, for example a group of young people who are in a residential drug rehabilitation setting
■ you are starting a long-term relationship with a number of people who have a common interest, and wish to develop an equal and respectful partnership with them, for example a group of people with mental health problems who have recently moved into a group home
■ you want to work with a particular ethnic minority community but you do not come from that group yourself and are faced with issues of differences in culture and language. In this case, it could be helpful to run a group to look at health issues in partnership with a link worker or health advocate, who can offer culturally sensitive help and skills in translation and interpretation.

There are times when it may not be advisable to embark on group work, or to continue to run an existing group. These may include situations when:

■ you have not consulted with prospective clients to establish their needs
■ group members are from such a diverse range of backgrounds that they have little in common and feel uncomfortable with one another
■ the cultural background of the group will make it difficult for them to adapt to group work; for example older people who are uncomfortable with informal group work methods, or groups from some ethnic minority communities
■ the group will meet only once or twice, which means that people will not have long enough to get to know and trust one another
■ the membership of a group is not stable and people are constantly leaving or joining
■ your aim is solely to transmit information, so that a talk with questions and answers would be better
■ the aim of the group is to encourage a change towards a healthier lifestyle but the people concerned do not have the opportunity to make changes because of lack of money, skills, support or facilities
■ you do not have suitable accommodation for meetings; for example you have access only to a large, tiered lecture theatre
■ you do not yet have the skills or confidence to embark on group work, or access to training and support.

Group Leadership

Two aspects of group leadership are useful to consider. One is your leadership style and the other is your responsibilities as a group leader.

Leadership Style

It is important that all the members of the group are agreed on who is the leader, and support the leader in this role. The leadership style needs to be compatible with the group members, especially if the group has to work together to complete complex

Case study 13.1   **Good Practice in Group Work[5]**

45 Cope Street in Nottingham is a health project which works with mothers between 16 and 25 years. It is complementary to the existing health services, which provide antenatal and postnatal education. The aim of the project is to work in partnership with parents to improve the health of the child and the family. It is based on the principle that people learn best from others who have been in the same situation as they are. The group work is designed to be self-empowering and stresses the importance of self-confidence as an outcome. Evaluation of the intervention was to do with increased self-confidence and improved health.

tasks. For example, a group of highly motivated and trained professionals will work best with a leader who encourages participation and shared decision making. It is essential for leaders to be aware of which style members prefer, and to develop the ability to adjust their style if the situation demands it.

A key dimension of leadership style is where the leader stands on a continuum from authoritarian to participative.

authoritarian └─────────────────────┘ *participative*

An **authoritarian** style is directive, with the group leader acting as a 'director', who is a source of expertise. If you adopt this approach, you rely on your status, credibility and expertise to ensure acceptance of your views and leadership role.

The *strength* of this style is that children and vulnerable people (such as those who are sick or distressed) may feel secure, reassured and protected from harm.

The *weaknesses* of this style are that clients may become fearful, anxious and reluctant to take independent action; it does not develop their ability to take responsibility for their own decisions and actions. Furthermore, clients may respond by rebelling and rejecting your guidance.

A **participative** style involves shifting power from the group leader so that it is shared between the leader and the group members. This means using all the skills and knowledge of the group members as well as the leader, who is more likely to choose the title of 'facilitator'. As a facilitator, you will need to show warmth and empathy, encourage group members to express their feelings, and provide counsel and encouragement. You will need to be tolerant of different viewpoints, showing fairness and impartiality. You will need skills and ability to confront difficult issues and resolve conflict using a problem solving approach.

See Section in Chapter 9 on understanding conflict and Exercise 9.3 on your conflict resolution style.

The *strength* of this style is that clients learn to trust their own judgments and at the same time to appreciate other people's rights and opinions.

The *weaknesses* of this style may be that strong feelings are uncovered and distress experienced by the client; this may also be distressing for you as the leader and hard for you to cope with. Also, clients who are used to being told what to do may feel confused and dissatisfied because they are not receiving the advice and direction they want. They will need to have the approach explained to them and be given suitable learning experiences to show them that it works.

There is no 'right' or 'wrong' style, and indeed most leaders probably operate somewhere between the two extremes, providing some authoritative leadership while also encouraging a degree of participation.

It is commonly assumed that groups will be more effective with a participative rather than authoritarian leadership style, but research and experience do not always support this conclusion.[6] Rather, we suggest that the reality of leadership is more complex, and that successful group leadership depends on a variety of factors such as:

- The leader's preferred style of operating and personality. For example, if you have been used to being perceived as the 'expert', with the authority of professional knowledge that you want to pass on, you will probably feel (and look) uncomfortable if you try to switch to a 'facilitator' style without sufficient training, and this will produce tension in the group.
- The group members' preferred style of leadership in the specific circumstances of the group. For example, if group members are low in confidence, they may need you to be more authoritarian to start with, so that they feel secure. You can then gradually encourage participation and adopt a more facilitative style as members learn to trust you and each other, and feel confident enough to join in.
- The group's objectives and tasks. For example, a group that has the objective of learning new skills (such as an exercise class) will need a more authoritarian leader who will tell them how to do the exercises properly, whereas a group of parents in a support group that aims to help them recover from the death of a child will need a facilitator to help members to express and work through their grief.
- The wider environment, such as the culture of the group members, and of the organisations they belong to. For example, the culture of some ethnic minorities may be such that members (especially women) are brought up to be passive, and will not only lack confidence about active participation in groups but may also perceive it as 'wrong'.

See Chapter 3, section 9: Analysing your Aims and Values; Five Approaches.

You need to consider these factors and how they might be modified in order to achieve the 'best fit'. The easiest thing to modify in the short term should be your own style, but in the long term it may also be possible to make other changes, for example to develop the group members' confidence so that they are willing to take on more responsibility and participation.

The participative style fits best with the self-empowering client-centred approach to health promotion. However, many health promoters will have been trained by people operating in an authoritarian style and will have modelled themselves on this experience. If this is true in your case, you will need to learn how to work in a participative style, and this could be fundamental to becoming more effective in empowering your clients.

Finally, a participative style must be distinguished from a permissive style. A permissive style lets clients come to their own conclusions and aims to avoid conflict and keep everyone happy. Helping the clients to enjoy the educational experience is more important to the leader than achieving the goals of the group. Difficulties and conflict are not confronted and the clients may feel neither secure nor cared for. Group leaders may need to build up their own assertiveness skills in order to avoid an overly permissive approach.

Leadership Responsibilities

The responsibilities of group leaders will depend on the role they take; for example, whether they are responsible for the practical organisation such as booking a venue. But whatever the role, a leader's responsibilities will probably include:

Exercise 13.2   Looking at Your Leadership Style

The following questions aim to help you to examine your own leadership style. Put a tick in the appropriate box.

	Never	Sometimes	Usually	Always
1. **Do your clients say what they feel?**	☐	☐	☐	☐
2. **Do clients finish what they are saying before you respond?**	☐	☐	☐	☐
3. **Do you think you are able to see things from your clients' point of view?**	☐	☐	☐	☐
4. **Do clients disagree with you?**	☐	☐	☐	☐
5. **Do you explore with your clients the consequences of alternative actions?**	☐	☐	☐	☐
6. **Do you help clients to discuss painful memories or sensitive issues?**	☐	☐	☐	☐
7. **Do you share all the information at your disposal?**	☐	☐	☐	☐
8. **Do you help clients to discover their own strengths?**	☐	☐	☐	☐
9. **Do you respect your clients' right to reject your advice?**	☐	☐	☐	☐

What leadership style – authoritarian, participative or permissive – do you think you usually use?

What influences led you to develop this style?

Can you identify any advantages in using alternative leadership styles in your work?

Can you identify any aspects of your leadership style that you would like to change?

- helping members to identify and clarify their interests and needs, and what they would like to gain from the group in the short and long term
- helping to develop a relaxed atmosphere in which members feel able to be open and trusting with each other, and able to participate freely
- offering her expertise to the group on the understanding that members are free to accept or reject the offer
- accepting and valuing all contributions from group members.

But it is not only the group leader who has responsibilities: group members have them too. They will probably include:

- participating in clarifying the aims of the group
- choosing whether and how much to participate
- identifying their own goals and concerns

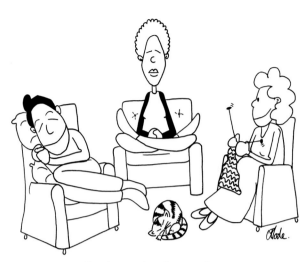

Develop a relaxed atmosphere

■ deciding which challenges and risks they are prepared to take. For example, how much are they prepared to expose their own weaknesses and vulnerability to other people in the group?

Group Behaviour

Health promoters will be able to work with a group more effectively if they are aware of the ways in which people are likely to behave when they come together in groups (sometimes called 'group dynamics'). We focus on three aspects of group behaviour that you may find particularly useful: the pattern of behaviour that usually develops in a group's life, the different roles group members may perform, and the concept of 'hidden agendas'.

Group Development

Groups tend to show a particular pattern of behaviour as they mature and develop. This developmental cycle has been categorised as having four stages:[7]

1. **Forming** The group is forming. People meet each other, and get to know one another, with individuals establishing their own identity and role within the group. The group's purpose and way of working are established.

2. **Storming** Most groups go through a conflict stage when the leadership and ways in which the group is working are challenged. For example, people may question how things are being done and what the leader's role is, and may get into heated discussions with each other. This can be a difficult period for both leader and members, but it is a vital stage in the group's maturing process, rather like the period of rebelling and questioning during adolescence. Successful handling of this period leads to the development of open communication, trust and shared responsibility for achieving the purposes of the group.

See section in Chapter 9 on understanding conflict.

3. **Norming** At this stage the group settles down, with the norms and accepted practices of the group established.

4. **Performing** The group is fully effective at this stage and is able to concentrate on its tasks.

When the developmental process fails in some way, backstage politicking and attempts to sabotage the group may occur. It is thus worth investing time and effort to help new groups to develop successfully.

Many groups have a limited life, meeting for a set number of sessions or until a particular task has been completed. At the end of a group's life, it is natural for members to feel a sense of loss. It may be helpful to have a final 'rounding up' session, which could give group members an opportunity to express their appreciation of each other, their sadness at parting, and perhaps arrange a follow-up or 'reunion'.

Group Members' Roles

Studies of the characteristics of members of groups have concluded that a mix of nine roles is needed for fully effective groups.[8] These roles are outlined in Box 13.1.

Each person may play a variety of these roles in a group, and most people have their preferred roles. If one or more of these roles is lacking, a member or leader can help to make a group more successful by consciously adopting a new role herself, or helping someone else to do so.

Box 13.1	Nine Roles Needed for Effective Groups

The Coordinator – clarifies goals, promotes decision making, delegates well to enable the group to work effectively.
The Shaper – is action oriented and encourages the group to get on with its tasks.
The Plant – is the creative source of ideas and proposals.
The Monitor/Evaluator – is good at analysing and criticising.
The Resource Investigator – has a good network of contacts and liaises with other people and agencies.
The Company Worker – is good at organising and administration.
The Team Worker – supports the members of the group and is a good listener.
The Specialist – provides specialist knowledge and skills.
The Finisher – contributes foresight and perserverance to ensure that the group completes its tasks.

Hidden Agendas

People will have their own individual reasons for joining a group, which may be in addition to, or instead of, the reason expected. For example, a woman may attend a women's health group because she is lonely and sees the group as way of meeting people; she has not joined because she is particularly interested in health issues. Or a group member may seek a prominent position in a group, such as being the Chair or Secretary, to fulfil her need to be valued and useful; she may or may not also be committed to the work itself and the aims of the group. In these examples, fulfilling these personal objectives are 'hidden agendas'.

Most people bring their own 'hidden agendas' to groups, in addition to the agreed group objectives; these commonly include meeting the need for social contact, or making a particular alliance. Members will work together best when there is communication about individual objectives and agreement about shared objectives. Otherwise members may promote their own interests at the expense of the group's. You will be more effective as a group leader if you are aware of the hidden agendas in the group and can find ways of dealing with them.

Setting up a Group

See also Chapter 5 on the basic planning and evaluation process.

Planning and preparation are essential for successful group work. The sections below take you step by step through the thinking and planning you need to do when setting up a group.[9]

Why are You Proposing to Run the Group?

- Are you reacting to a demand from clients, other professionals, a community, or your own observations?
- Are you trying to develop your health promotion role and see this group as a way of progressing?
- Are you aiming to provide advice and support, to supply information, or to help people to change health-related behaviour?
- Are you aiming to satisfy your own needs or your clients' needs? (Your reasons can include both, but it is helpful to distinguish between them.)

Who Will the Members Be?

- Will the members be referred to the group (from their GP, for example), will they be coerced into joining, or will membership be entirely voluntary?
- Have you given everyone an equal opportunity to join (e.g. by ensuring facilities for wheelchairs, disabled toilets, signing for those hard of hearing, hearing loops, translation into appropriate minority languages)? Have you made provision for people to let you know of any special needs?
- How will you identify the potential members of your group – from individuals requesting a group, from local or national registers, from people with shared characteristics (such as age, sex, lifestyle, culture, job, health concern), or by other means?
- How will you recruit your members? Do you need to advertise?
- How many members do you aim to have? What is the ideal number, bearing in mind the purpose of the group and any constraints imposed by your location?

What are the Group's Aims and Objectives?

- Are these within the realistic abilities of yourself and the members?
- Can all the potential membership understand them?
- Are you clear about your own objectives in setting up the group, and whether these are different from the members' objectives?

■ Are all members clear about their individual objectives, i.e. the specific outcomes they hope to achieve through attending the group?

Where Will the Group Meet?

■ Is the location appropriate? For example, a health centre or hospital could appear clinical and cold and remind people of illness. 'Neutral' territory, such as a room in a pub or community centre, or someone's house, may be more relaxing and inviting.
■ What is the seating like? If you are aiming for participative group work, seating people in a circle is best (see Figure 13.1, p 262), with physical barriers to communication such as tables or desks removed. Can you put chairs in a circle, where all group members can see each other?
■ What are the facilities like? Is there enough space for the activities you plan? Is the floor covering suitable for the purpose? Is the temperature suitable and adjustable if necessary? Are the facilities adequate for the purpose (for example, access for pushchairs, toilets, catering facilities, washing/shower rooms, crèche)? Are there facilities for people with special needs (for example, wide access for wheelchairs, disabled toilets, hearing loops, signs in minority languages)?
■ Is access good? Is the venue accessible by local transport? Do you have transport for members who cannot manage on public transport? Are parking arrangements satisfactory?
■ What are the security arrangements? Where are the fire extinguishers and what is the fire drill? In case of an emergency, who do you contact? Do you need insurance cover?

What Resources do You Need?

■ Do you need any special equipment, for example video equipment, power points? Are you familiar with the equipment and confident you can operate it? Does the equipment have to be booked in advance? If so, are you familiar with the booking system?
■ Do you need any additional resources such as videos, leaflets, posters, books, outside speakers? If so, have you made all the necessary arrangements in advance?
■ Do you need money to pay for anything? If so, have you identified a source of funding (for example, a charge to the group members, a trust fund or a sponsor)?

When Will the Group Meet?

■ Is the time you have chosen the best one for the clients, or have you chosen it to suit yourself? Does the length of meetings suit members and take into account their other commitments? Have you consulted potential members about timing and tried to satisfy the majority?

How Will the Group be Run?

■ Will it be a self-help group and directed by the members, or leader led?
■ To what extent will the structure be flexible and the content negotiable?
■ Will the group be open (anyone can join at any time) or will there be restrictions on admitting new members once the group has started?

| Fig 13.1 | (a) Seating in a Circle – Best for Group Work; (b) Traditional Seating in Rows – Not Suitable for Group Work |

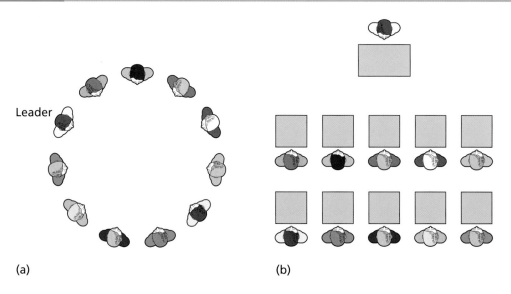

(a)   (b)

How Will the Group be Evaluated?

See also the section on evaluation, feedback and assessment in Chapter 12.

- At the end of each meeting? At the end of the group? Or both?
- Verbally, or in writing, or both? How will you ask questions in order to obtain accurate feedback from members (for example, by providing opportunities for anonymous feedback)?
- How will you know that the agreed group objectives have been achieved? How will you know whether your own objectives have been achieved? How will you know whether individuals have achieved their objectives?
- Were there any unplanned outcomes of the group? Were these desirable or undesirable? What caused them?
- What have you learned? What would you do differently next time?

Getting Groups Going

Almost everyone feels nervous about going to a group meeting for the first time, especially if they are unlikely to know anyone else there. The initial task for the group leader is to 'break the ice' and help people to feel at ease.

Before the First Meeting

If you know in advance who is coming to a group meeting, it may be helpful and welcoming to confirm by letter or telephone that you are expecting them, and the time and place. If anyone has let you know they have special needs, contact them in advance to discuss their needs and let them know what facilities will be available.

On Arrival

It helps if clients can be greeted personally, introduced to other people or given something to do: 'Help yourself to a cup of tea', 'There are some books and leaflets on the table if you'd like to look at them till everyone has arrived'. Ensure that anyone with special needs has appropriate facilities and assistance (e.g. with mobility or hearing loops).

Getting to Know Each Other

Knowing each person's name and something about them is the first step towards constructive group work because it helps them to feel valued as a member of the group, and is the beginning of openness and trust between members.

There are many ways of going about this, some of which are as follows.[10]

Introduction in Pairs

Ask each person to sit next to someone they have not met before. One person in each pair then 'interviews' their partner. After a few minutes (the leader keeps the time) the partners swap roles. Then, in turn, each member of the group introduces their partner by name and says something about them. You may like to remind people that no one has to answer any questions if they do not wish to.

The leader could also suggest appropriate questions. For example, in groups for prospective parents the leader could suggest that partners find out if this is the first baby, where the mother goes for antenatal check-ups, or where she is booked to have her baby.

Name Games

Group members sit in a circle and you, the leader, take an object, such as a pen, and hand it to the person on your left, saying 'My name is A and this is a pen'. You ask the person who now holds the pen to say 'My name is B and A says that this is a pen'. B then passes the pen to the person on his left, who says 'My name is C and B says that A says that this is a pen'. This continues until the pen gets back to the beginning. If group members forget someone's name the rest of the group can prompt them. This helps to establish a cooperative and supportive atmosphere as well as helping people to learn each other's names. Any tension and embarrassment is relieved by laughing and ice is effectively broken.

At subsequent group meetings, it is often helpful to do a quick round of names at the beginning, for example 'Who would like to have a shot at naming every member of the group?' or 'I'm going to try to see if I can remember everyone's name'.

You might like to set the tone by suggesting how people are addressed – by first names or more formally by Mr, Mrs, etc. The important thing is to encourage people to use whatever feels comfortable: 'My name is Ann Jones, and I'm happy for you to call me Ann'.

Sharing Initial Feelings and Expectations

People may be helped to relax if they know that others also feel nervous or shy. So ask 'What did you feel about coming here today? Did anyone feel nervous? Did anyone almost *not* come?' This can open the way for people to express their anxieties. You can also encourage them to say why they have come to the meeting and what they expect to gain from it. It might help to ask members to complete a checklist, ticking statements that are true for them. Such statements could include:[11]

- I'm afraid I won't have anything to say.
- I'm afraid I'll talk too much.
- I'm worried I'll make a fool of myself.
- I'll be too embarrassed to join in.
- I'm afraid I might get upset.
- I'm afraid I may be bored.
- I want to meet other people in the same boat.
- I enjoy talking to others.
- I enjoy a good argument.
- I want to get out of the house.
- I want to go somewhere different.
- I enjoy listening to other people.

People can then compare their list with that of one or two other people, and then it may be helpful to share what has been discovered with the whole group.

Setting Ground Rules

People joining a group will have different expectations and assumptions about how the group will run. Problems can arise if these are not brought out in the open and clarified at the beginning. For example, people may assume that what they say in a group will be treated confidentially, and then be upset if they find that another member did not realise this and had discussed the issue elsewhere; or some members might expect the group leader to take all the responsibility for organising the group, and may feel let down if they later discover that the leader expects them to do some of the work.

To prevent these difficulties, it is often helpful to establish a clear 'contract' or set of 'ground rules'. So early on in the group's life members need the opportunity to explore their expectations, and reach agreement about issues such as:

- How members are expected to behave in the group. For example, is smoking allowed?
- Are any rules and sanctions to be set, for example about non-attendance at group meetings or whether members can join in if they arrive late?
- What is confidential to the group?
- Can new members join at any time, or is the group 'closed' to new membership?
- How will the leader and the members exercise control in the group?
- Who has responsibility for the practical aspects of running the group, such as bringing refreshments along or booking the room?

For example, in a self-help group, mutual rights and responsibilities will be agreed on the basis of equality of leader and clients but in reality the power balance will not be completely equal and a contract will help with power sharing. In a counselling group the power of the counsellor is much greater than that of the clients and the leader has a duty to respect the members and to promote their autonomy.

Exercise 13.3	Planning a Group Meeting

1. Identify a health promotion opportunity that you have encountered or are likely to encounter, where informal group work would be appropriate

For example, this could be a group of food handlers, a pre-retirement group, an antenatal group, a group of patients in hospital recovering from a heart attack, a stop-smoking group or a group for healthy eating and weight control.

Assume that your group consists of about 12 people who do not know each other, and that this is the first of several meetings.
What do you think would be the best place and time to meet, and the best physical features of the meeting room?
What are your aims for the first meeting?
What are your objectives for your group members for the first meeting?

Complete the following:
At the end of the first meeting, each group member will:
    1. . . . . . .
    2. . . . . . .
    3. . . . . .
    etc. . . . . . .

2. Make a plan for what you will do

- As people start to arrive.
- To get people to know each other.
- In the main part of the group meeting.
- To round off the meeting at the end.
- To evaluate whether you have achieved the objectives you set.

Discussion Skills

It is a fallacy to believe that a discussion will just happen by putting a group of people together and saying 'Let's discuss . . .'. Discussion needs planning and preparation, and there are many ways of triggering it off and providing structures that will help everyone to participate. Some of these are as follows.

Trigger Materials

Discussion can be triggered by providing a focus, preferably a controversial one. This can simply be a question ('What do you think about the decision to close the hospital?'), but it might also be a leaflet, a poster, a videotape, or an item in a newspaper or magazine ('What do you think the makers of this cigarette are trying to convey in this advertisement?'). Choose something that people are likely to have strong views about.

Some health promotion videos are specially made as trigger materials, presenting situations for people to talk about. Helpful notes for group leaders often accompany such videos.

Brainstorms/Think Sessions

Brainstorming is a useful way to open up a subject and collect everyone's ideas. Ask an open question to which there is no single right answer (e.g. 'Why do people drink?', 'What do you feel you need to know before your baby is born?'). Accept every suggestion, without comment or criticism, and write them down in a list on a flipchart or blackboard. Ask the group not to start discussing the ideas until everybody has finished. You can make your own suggestions and write them down along with everyone else's.

In this way all members' contributions are equally valued and everyone has a chance to participate. Encourage shy members by asking 'Anything else?' and allowing silent pauses while people think.

Then you can set the group to work by asking them to put the ideas into categories, and to identify the key features of each category. For example, people might categorise reasons for drinking into a 'constructive' category ('It helps me to socialise', 'It helps me to relax, to feel good') and an 'escape' category ('I can forget my problems', 'It stops me from feeling upset').

Rounds

A 'round' is a way of giving everyone an equal chance to participate. You invite each group member, in turn round the circle, to make a brief statement. You might like to start the round yourself or to join in when your turn comes in the circle. For example, ask everyone to make a brief statement about one of the following:

'My first feelings when I knew I was pregnant were . . .'

'What I think about jogging is . . .'

'The main reason why I can't lose weight is . . .'

'The thing that has helped me most is . . .'

There are four essential rules for successful rounds, which must be explained, and gently enforced if necessary. These are:

- No interruptions until each person has finished his statement.
- No comments on anybody's contribution until the full round is completed (no discussions, praise, interpretation, criticism or 'I think that too' remarks).
- Anyone can choose not to participate. Give permission, clearly and emphatically, that anyone who does not want to make a statement can just say 'pass'. This is very important for reinforcing the principle of voluntary participation.
- It does not matter if two or more people in the round say the same thing. People should stick to saying what they had intended even if someone else has said it already; they do not have to think of something different.

Rounds are also useful ways of beginning and ending sessions. For example:

'One thing I've put into practice since last week is . . .'

'The main thing I've got from today's session is . . .'

'One thing I'm going to find out by next time we meet is . . .'

It is also a useful way of getting feedback. For example:

'One thing I really liked about today's session was . . .'

'One thing I didn't like about today's session was . . .'

'One thing I wish we'd done is . . .'

Buzz Groups

Buzz groups are small groups of two to six people who discuss questions or topics for short periods, usually about ten minutes. It is especially useful for large groups to be divided up in this way, as it gives everyone more chance to talk. Form the groups first of all, then say what you would like each one to do ('Make a list of the times when you want a cigarette' or 'Talk about the things you find helpful when you feel stressed'), and how long they have in which to do it. If you want people to share ideas with the rest of the group as a whole afterwards, it may be helpful to provide large sheets of paper and felt-tip pens, so that 'posters' can be put up for everyone to see and discuss.

Safe Revelations

Sometimes people may hesitate, or refuse to say what they really feel for fear of looking silly, being embarrassed, or getting upset. One way of overcoming this is to give everyone a piece of paper and ask them to write down, for example, what their biggest worries are, or what they really want to know. All the papers are then folded and put in a receptacle, such as a waste-paper basket or a shopping bag. Each person in turn picks out one piece of paper and reads aloud what is written on it. Tell people not to say if they happen to pick out their own piece of paper, and that, of course, nobody needs to identify themselves as the author of any of the statements.

The aim is to find out the concerns of the group members in the security of anonymity. Make sure that everyone listens and does not comment until all the papers have been read out. Then you can discuss what was discovered.

Dealing with Difficulties

Group workers often find the prospect of group work daunting, and anticipate being unable to cope with problems. A way forward is to acknowledge and face these fears, and work out strategies for coping should the problem actually arise. Some common fears and possible strategies for coping are as follows.

Silence

Are you afraid that you may be left with your group in an awful silence? If so, remember that silence can be useful; it can be time that group members need to think. Silence often does not feel as threatening to group members as it may do to you; however, you may find it helpful to:

- run a group with a partner, so that you can help each other out if either of you gets stuck

- ensure thorough preparation, so that you have planned activities and questions. Write down a plan, and a list of questions to ask (e.g. at the end of a video) and don't be afraid to refer to it in front of the group
- have a 'spare' activity ready to use if the reason for the discussion 'drying up' is that what you have planned does not seem to be working.

Disasters

Unexpected 'disasters' include such things as getting lost and arriving late, or finding that too few or too many people have turned up. There is no blueprint strategy to cope with the unexpected, but it will help if you acknowledge what has happened and share it with your group ('I'm delighted that so many of you have come along, but I wasn't expecting such a crowd, so we may be a bit squashed this week'). Also share your plans for dealing with the 'disaster' ('I'm going to try to get a bigger room next time'... 'I'm going to start 10 minutes late'). Sharing the problem and enlisting cooperation can have the positive benefit of encouraging mutual support; *not* sharing it can leave your group feeling angry.

Distractions

Distractions can take many forms: noises outside the room (e.g. road works), noises inside the room (e.g. crying babies, coughing), people coming in late or leaving early, or interruptions. Distractions can also be caused by group members themselves, for example by someone becoming very angry or upset.

As a rule, there are three choices for you as group leader:

- **Ignore them.** This is seldom a good idea, as it leaves people wondering whether you are going to do anything, and this in itself is a distraction.
- **Acknowledge and accept them.** This is generally best with things you cannot change ('I know the traffic is really noisy, but there's nothing we can do about it, so I think we'll just have to put up with it').
- **Do something about them.** It is preferable to involve the group in the decision ('As so many of you found it difficult to get here by 2 o'clock, shall we start at 2.15 next week?' 'Do you think it would be helpful if you took it in turns to look after the babies in the next room?').

  If someone is showing emotion, such as crying, acknowledge it ('I can see that you're upset'), offer reassurance that it is OK to show emotion ('There's no need to be embarrassed... we don't mind if you cry...'), and offer the opportunity to talk about it ('Would you like to tell us what is upsetting you?') or to take some time away from the group, accompanied by you or someone else ('Shall we go outside for a few minutes?'). Do not put any pressure on people in distress. Help them to do what they want to do, whether it is cry, talk, keep silent, stay, leave or be by themselves. But *do not* ignore a show of emotion; ignoring it will only cause tension and embarrassment.

Difficult Behaviour

How group members behave can pose difficulties for the leader. There are two broad categories of difficult behaviour: non-participation and talking too much. The latter category takes many forms: the know-all who always chips in with all the 'answers', people who launch into long stories, people who interrupt, people who do not let other people get a word in edgeways, people who talk off the point, people who always disagree, and people who always crack jokes. Note that people often change their behaviour as they get to know others and feel more comfortable in a group, but here are some points about dealing with people who talk too much, and about encouraging quiet members.

- Think about why dominant people are behaving like this. Are they nervous, threatened or worried? Are they desperately in need of attention? If you can deal with the underlying cause, the situation is likely to improve.
- Try getting people to work in pairs or small groups, which can help quiet members to join in and give others a break from the constant talker.
- Use structures in your discussion such as 'rounds', or make a point of asking for other people's opinions ('Would someone else like to say what he thinks?' 'Would you like to give us your opinion, Ann?').
- Finally, it may be necessary to confront a person who talks too much (but not in front of the rest of the group!). For example, you could say: 'I've noticed that you contribute a great deal to the group discussions. That makes me concerned about whether other people are getting enough chance to talk. I'd like to suggest that you keep your comments to just a couple of sentences. Would you feel OK about doing that?'

PRACTICE POINTS

- Group work covers a range of activities, and in health promotion groups are useful mainly for raising awareness of health issues, mutual support, social action, education and group counselling.

- Group work has a wide range of potential benefits for individual group members.

- Group work is not always the most appropriate health promotion method to use; you need to be sure that it is right for your particular clients and circumstances.

- You need to develop skills of group leadership, appreciate the range of leadership styles, understand the roles and responsibilities of group leaders and members and the way in which groups develop over time.

- Thorough planning and preparation are essential for successful group work, which includes having a clear rationale and aims, and paying attention to recruitment, venue, facilities, resources, timing, and evaluation.

- If you run groups, you will find it helpful to develop a range of skills and strategies for getting groups going, encouraging discussion, and dealing with difficulties.

Recommended Reading

A Comprehensive Introduction to Group Theory and Practice

➤ Johnson D W, Johnson F P 1999 Joining together: group theory and group skills, 7th edn. Boston MA: Allyn and Bacon

On the Working of Groups

➤ Douglas T 2000 Basic groupwork. London: Routledge
➤ Ringer TM 2002 Group action: the dynamics of groups in therapeutic, educational and corporate settings. London: Jessica Kingsley

Groups From the Viewpoint of the Group Members

➤ Douglas T 1995 Survival in groups: the basics of group membership. Buckingham: Open University Press

On Working with Groups of Adults

➤ Wlodkowski R 1998 Enhancing adult motivation to learn. A comprehensive guide to teaching all adults, 2nd edn. New York: Jossey Bass

On Informal Education with Children, Young People and Adults

➤ Jeffs T, Smith M K 1999 Informal education and health promotion. In: Perkins E R, Simnett I, Wright L (eds) Evidence-based health promotion. Chichester: Wiley, pp 206–215.

Notes and References

1   Short courses on working with groups are often run by health promotion departments in the NHS.

2   Stock Whitaker D 2001 Using groups to help people, 2nd edn. Hove: Brunner-Routledge

3   Adapted from Stock Whitaker D 2001 Using groups to help people, 2nd edn. Hove: Brunner-Routledge

4   Mackeith P, Philipson R, Rowe A 1991 45 Cope Street: young mothers learning through group work: an evaluation report. Nottingham Community Health, Old Basford Health Centre, Nottingham

5   Rowe J, Mahoney P 1993 Parent education: guidance for purchasers and providers. London: Health Education Authority

6   Handy C B 1993 Understanding organisations, Chapter 6. Harmondsworth: Penguin Business Library

7   Tuckman B W 1965 Developmental sequence in small groups. Psychological Bulletin 63, 384–399. (This is a classic study of group work.)

8   Belbin R M 1981 Management teams: why they succeed or fail. Oxford: Butterworth–Heinemann. (This is a classic work on team roles.)

Belbin R M 1993 Team roles at work. London: Butterworth–Heinemann

Sharpe S 2001 Using team roles to improve performance. Modern Management 15(4), 38–40

9   We acknowledge, with thanks, that much of the material in this section is derived from a checklist produced by Louise Walker and Margaret Douglas, Health Promotion Officers, Bristol & Weston Health Authority, August 1990.

10   There are many more structured activities ('games') for group leaders in:

Brandes D, Phillips H 1978 Gamesters handbook. London: Hutchinson

Brandes D 1983 Gamesters two. London: Hutchinson

Brandes D 1998 Gamesters three. Cheltenham: Stanley Thornes

11   Adapted, with kind permission, from:

Open University 1983 Community education group notes. Buckingham: Open University Press, p 10

14 Helping People Towards Healthier Living

SUMMARY

This chapter is about helping people towards healthier lifestyles and changing their health-related behaviour. In the first section we look at models of the process of changing health-related behaviour. In the next section we discuss working with a client's motivation and how to work towards client self-empowerment before outlining strategies for increasing self-awareness, clarifying values and changing attitudes. Strategies for decision making and for changing behaviour follow. The chapter ends with principles for using strategies effectively and summarises key points. It includes exercises, examples and a case study.

In this chapter we look at the competencies you need when you are helping people to change their health-related behaviour and lifestyles. Much health behaviour appears to have developed without conscious decision making; it has 'just happened' in response to individual and group circumstances and external events. Active control of behaviour is different because it involves committing time and effort (yours and your client's) to understanding the factors that influence health choices and behaviour, and to taking considered decisions and actions.

See Chapter 10, section Exploring Relationships with Clients.

However, it has to be accepted that people may prefer to carry on with behaviour that seems 'unhealthy' to you. To a client, it may not seem 'unhealthy' as the benefits outweigh the risks. Respect for people's right to their own point of view and their right to choose are fundamental to establishing relationships between health promoters and their clients.

On the other hand, you also have to consider that a person's right to individual freedom of choice has to be balanced against the effect of that choice on other people; for example, choosing to drink and drive could affect many others as well as the driver.

Furthermore, choosing a 'healthy' behaviour does not automatically lead to practising it. Changes such as taking more exercise, practising relaxation, going for screening tests, wearing ear protectors in noisy surroundings, eating different foods and stopping smoking can be hard work, and these changes in themselves may be stressful. Social or economic circumstances can also prevent people from carrying out new health behaviours, even if they would like to.

However, despite these limitations, it can be very rewarding to help people to look at their motivations, beliefs, values and attitudes, and to make and carry out decisions that will lead to improved health and well-being. We first turn to the theory of behaviour change and how you can use it in your practice.

Models of Behaviour Change

Models are simplified ways of describing reality. Models provide frameworks and routes to help you make sense of a situation, know where to start and what to do. Health-related behaviour change is a very complex process involving a web of psychological, social and environmental factors. So using behaviour change models will help you to clarify your thinking and make your practice more effective. Several models have been used by health promoters,[1] and suggestions are made for further reading at the end of the chapter. Here we describe two useful models: the Health Action Model and the Stages of Change Model.

The Health Action Model

The Health Action Model (HAM) was devised by Tones[2] and emphasises the important influence of self-esteem on behaviour. It assumes that someone with high self-esteem and a positive self-concept is likely to be more motivated towards ways of healthier living. Furthermore, it suggests that people with low self-esteem may feel that they have limited control over their behaviour and that they are victims of bad luck or fate. Many health promoters, particularly those working in the field of drugs, have used this model, through concentrating on boosting people's self-esteem and their skills in resisting peer group pressure. According to this model, learning 'life skills' such as how to be assertive may be essential before someone is ready to change their lifestyle.

The HAM identifies a variety of psychological, social and environmental influences which research and practice have shown to be important determinants of a number of health-related choices. The model offers an explanation about how these influences work. It suggests that health decisions and actions are influenced by our beliefs, our values, our motivation, our expectations of how other people will react to our actions, and our self-concept and self-esteem (see Figure 14.1).

The HAM is concerned with empowerment – with increasing the control people have over their lives. It suggests that health promotion should not just focus on the provision of information and the pros and cons of particular behaviours. More important than this is helping people to feel good about themselves, to value themselves, and to acquire the skills to assert themselves. Equally important is the provision of environmental circumstances that facilitate healthy choices, rather than acting as barriers. And at a broader level, national and local policy needs to address basic environmental determinants of health, such as poverty and deprivation.

Stages of Change Model

A helpful way of thinking about how people make health-related decisions and change their behaviour is to consider all the stages in the process, and how people move from one stage to another. A useful model has been developed by Prochaska and DiClemente.[4] It is rooted in extensive research and integrates the understanding drawn from a range of psychological theories. It provides a valuable conceptual framework for how people naturally change their behaviour. However, it remains to be established whether this can successfully be translated into an intervention programme in the UK. Randomised controlled trials in the West Midlands suggest a small benefit from using this approach, which is not explained by chance.[5] Research elsewhere shows that strategies based on this model can be used for changing a range of health-related

Fig 14.1   The Health Action Model[3]

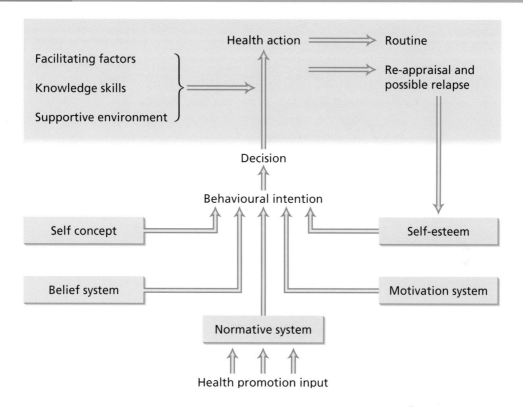

behaviours, such as alcohol and drug abuse, smoking, taking more exercise, weight control and accepting the offer of various types of screening.

The model identifies a number of stages that a person can go through during the process of behaviour change. It takes a holistic approach, integrating factors such as the role of personal responsibility and choices, and the impact of social and environmental forces that set very real limits on the individual potential for change. It provides a framework for a wide range of potential interventions by health promoters, as well as describing the process individuals go through when acting as their own agents of change; for example, when someone stops smoking without any professional support. The main stages identified in the model are set out in Figure 14.2.

The key to the model is to regard the cycle in the centre as a series of stages that people go through in the process of changing health behaviour, such as stopping smoking, taking more exercise regularly or adopting healthier eating. A crucial point is that the cycle can be thought of as a 'revolving door', because people usually go round more than once before emerging to a permanently changed state. It is also important to recognise that some people may never get as far as entering the revolving door.

Pre-contemplation stage The stage that precedes entry into the change cycle is referred to as 'pre-contemplation'. At this stage a person has no awareness of a need for change, or does not accept it, and has no motivation to change habits or lifestyle.

Fig 14.2   **Stages of changing health behaviour[6]**

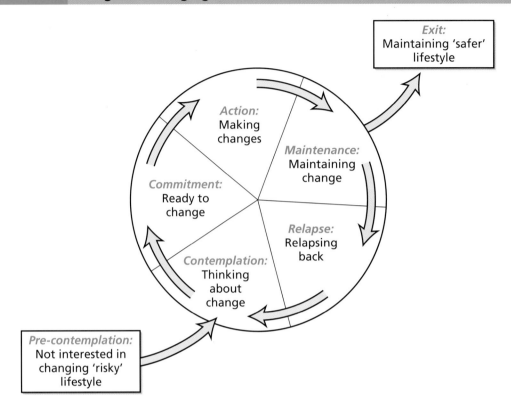

Contemplation stage This stage is the way in to the 'revolving door' cycle of stages of change. People enter this stage when they have enough motivation to contemplate seriously changing their habits – the entry stage is therefore called 'contemplation'.

Commitment stage If people continue to progress round the cycle they enter the 'commitment' stage, in which they make a serious decision to change the particular habit concerned, such as stopping smoking or taking more exercise.

Action stage They next enter the 'action' stage as they actively begin to change the habit.

Maintenance stage At this stage people struggle to maintain the change and may experiment with a variety of coping strategies.

Relapse stage Although individuals experience the satisfaction of a changed lifestyle for varying amounts of time, most of them cannot exit from the revolving door the first time around. Typically, they relapse; for example, they start smoking again. Of great importance, however, is that they do not stop there, but move back into the contemplation stage, engaging in the cycle all over again. Prochaska and DiClemente have found that on average successful former smokers take three revolutions of change before they find the way to become fully free of the habit, and exit from the revolving door.

Exit stage This is the stage in which people are settled into a changed behaviour, such as stopping smoking permanently.

By identifying where clients are in the stages of change, health promoters can tailor their interventions to the particular stage. For example, behaviour change strategies are appropriate for someone in the 'action' or 'maintenance' stages; education and awareness-raising is appropriate for someone in the 'pre-contemplation' stage; working for client self-empowerment is appropriate for someone in the 'contemplation' stage; strategies to help people to make decisions are useful for those in the 'commitment' stage.

The model is particularly useful in primary health care settings, because a patient's needs can be assessed and appropriate advice or information given, within the constraints of a few minutes' consultation. Research into the effectiveness of this approach is currently taking place in England and elsewhere. For example, for the first time in the UK we now have a baseline assessment of smoking in pregnancy by stage of change.[7] The application of the model has been the subject of challenge and debate,[8] but it is now well-used in research and the everyday work of health promoters.[9]

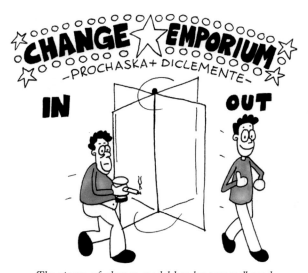

The stages of change model has become well used

See Chapter 5, Table 5.1: Aims and Methods in Health Promotion.

We now turn to the strategies and skills you require to help people to change. First, we look at motivation: an essential element in the application of the Stages of Change model. Then we outline strategies relating to two of the health promotion aims we discussed in Chapter 5: 'self-empowering' and 'changing attitudes and behaviour'.

Working with a Client's Motivation[10]

It is easy to think that motivation, or lack of it, is a personality trait. However, it is a state that changes throughout the course of a day depending on lots of different factors. If people are struggling to maintain their new behaviour, what gets them through this difficult time without relapsing? It is thought that both the *importance* of the new behaviour (in terms of the expectation of costs and benefits) and the *confidence* of the person being able to maintain the new behaviour are essential to prevent relapse. The following suggestions can help you explore the importance of the new behaviour with clients, and to build their confidence.

Ideas for Exploring Importance

- What are the good things about (the current behaviour)?
- What are some of the less good things about it?
- Summarise and ask 'And is there anything else?'
- Where does that leave you now?

Ideas for Building Confidence

- Get the client to identify as many solutions as possible which will help to prevent relapse.
- Ask 'What have you learned from previous attempts to change, about what works (or doesn't work) for you?'
- Ask 'Are there ways that you know have worked for other people?'
- Aim to help the client develop a clear plan but explain that it can be reviewed at any time.

It is essential to listen actively to the client when exploring readiness to change. Confidence can be divided into *self-efficacy* and *self-esteem*. Self-efficacy is concerned with a person's confidence in being able to make a specific change in behaviour; self-esteem is a more general sense of well-being that a person has about themselves. Self-efficacy can vary in different situations, and you can help your clients look at different approaches for improving self-efficacy in situations where they feel less confident.

Dangerous Assumptions About Motivation

Health promoters can become very focused on health issues, and may forget that there are other motives for change – and that health might not be one of them. The list below illustrates some of the other assumptions that are easy to make when counselling clients.

- This person ought to change.
- This person wants to change.
- It is the right time for this person to change.
- If this person decides not to change, this intervention has failed.
- A tough approach is always best.
- For this person, health is a prime motivator.
- I'm the expert. This person must follow my advice.

Working for Client Self-empowerment

Making health choices and carrying them out can bring benefits. These are not only the benefits that go with a healthier lifestyle (such as improved health and well-being), but also increased self-esteem from the feeling of taking active control over a part of life, such as being in control of the smoking habit rather than cigarettes being in control. In other words, making a positive choice about health can be a self-empowering process.

There are a number of different ways of working towards self-empowerment. Using the Stages of Change model is empowering, because people can follow their own progress. It encourages them to try to get to the next stage of the cycle, and not to see change as all-or-nothing. Also, the recognition that relapse is not the end of the world helps people to feel better about themselves.[11] Behaviour change messages can be tailor-made for individuals, for example through providing clients with access to specially designed computer programs.[12] Other methods include group work and experiential learning, individual counselling and therapy, and advocacy. We consider them all in the following sections, except therapy, which is beyond the scope of this book. (In any case, unless you are a mental health specialist, most people you work with probably do not need in-depth therapy but could benefit from counselling.)

The process of empowering people involves modifying the way they feel about themselves through improving their self-awareness and self-esteem. It involves helping them to think critically about their values and beliefs and build up their own values and beliefs system. This is in contrast to traditional teaching, which operates largely in the hope that the 'right' attitudes and values will be 'caught' by learners.

In the next section we outline some strategies you may find useful for helping clients to become more self-aware (having greater insight into, and understanding of, themselves, their attitudes, motivations, and feelings), and to help them clarify their values and attitudes.

Strategies for Increasing Self-awareness, Clarifying Values and Changing Attitudes

See Chapter 13 on working with groups.

Many of the strategies that are useful for increasing self-awareness, clarifying values, developing beliefs systems and changing attitudes (i.e. for the 'contemplation' stage of change) are designed for group work. However, some of them can be adapted for health promoters to use in one-to-one situations, to give clients to use by themselves.

See Chapter 12 on helping people to learn.

All these strategies use the principle of experiential learning, which emphasises the importance of personal experience as a source of learning.[13] It encourages 'active' learning through undertaking exercises and other activities designed, for example, to increase self-awareness or aid decision making. Some experiential learning methods are now described.

Deciding What Change to Focus On

Some clients could benefit from making several changes to improve their health, and it can be tempting to address all of them at the same time. But people are often at different stages of readiness to change over different issues. For example, a person considering making improvements to his diet might be ready to make one change (such as eating more fruit) but not ready to make others, such as changing to lower fat milk; an overweight person may be ready to take more exercise but not to change his eating habits. By writing down all the areas or issues that could be changed and asking 'Are there any of these you think you could discuss changing?' you can get agreement to discuss one particular topic.[14]

Ranking or Categorising

Ranking is a way of analysing an issue in order to distinguish the relative importance of different aspects. It is therefore useful for clarifying values. For example, in Exercise 1.1

See Chapter 1, section What Does Being Healthy Mean to You? (Chapter 1) readers are asked to rank aspects of 'being healthy'. Health is a value and that exercise is designed to help readers to clarify which aspects of health they value most.

Another approach to increasing self-awareness and values clarification is to generate a list of items, and then code them into different categories. Exercise 14.1 illustrates this approach; it is designed to raise awareness of the link between enjoyment and health.

Exercise 14.1   Enjoyment and Health

Quickly list as many things as you can think of that you enjoy doing. Write them down the left-hand side of a piece of paper. On the right-hand side, code each item according to the following categories.

£ – any items that involve spending money.
A – any items that you do alone.
P – any items you do with other people.
R – any items that involve some kind of risk.
F – any items that help to keep you fit.
C – any items that involve creativity.
D – any items that involve consumption of drugs (including alcohol and tobacco).
H+ – any items that positively affect your health.
H– – any items that negatively affect your health.

Items may be coded in more than one category. For example, if one of the things you enjoy is going out to the pub for a drink, this may be coded £, P and D, as well as H+ and/or H–.

What have you learned about enjoyment and health through doing this exercise?

Using Polarised Views

This is a way of getting people to clarify their views about a particular issue. Views about the issue are polarised – that is, phrased to reflect extremely different views. For example, if the issue was 'Is jogging good for you?' polarised views could be summed up as 'Jogging kills people and only very fit athletes should do it' or 'Jogging is very beneficial to health and all people would be fitter if they took it up'. Examples of polarised views can be described by the group leader or taken from writings that express opposite views.

The group leader may ask people to work in pairs, with each individual acting as if he fully adopted one of the points of view for the duration of the exercise, whatever his personal opinions. First, each person writes down all the arguments he can think of that support his position, without discussing it with his partner at this stage. After a few minutes, the partners are asked to start arguing the case, usually for about 15 minutes. The leader then lists the points in favour of each view by asking each pair in turn to contribute one point, until all the points have been collected. She then asks the group to comment on what they have learnt. In this way, members of the group can consider a whole range of arguments, which helps them to understand other people's

Another example of a values clarification exercise using the polarised arguments approach is Exercise 3.1 in Chapter 3.

points of view, tolerate differences of opinion, clarify their own views, and perhaps see the issue in a new light.

Using a Values Continuum

This is an extension of the polarised argument technique. It helps people to understand the spread of opinion on a particular issue and to clarify where they stand.

The leader describes two extremes of opinion and asks the group to imagine that these can be represented by two points, A and B, joined by a straight line. With a small group this line can be across a room; with a large group it could be drawn on the blackboard. The group members are then asked to mark or place themselves at a point along the line that best reflects their own view. For instance, in the jogging example discussed above, pro-joggers place themselves at one end, with the most extreme at the farthest point, people with moderate views stand around the middle, and the most ardent anti-joggers stand at the other end. The leader asks each person to state his views briefly as he takes up his position. Other people are asked not to interrupt or comment until everyone has taken up a position, or has passed if they choose not to participate.

The values continuum technique is used in the last task of Exercise 3.1 in Chapter 3.

This technique can encourage a more detailed discussion of the range of possible options than the polarised argument technique. On the other hand, if everyone seems moderate, a better discussion may be stimulated by the polarised argument technique.

Using Role Play

Role play generally means taking on the role of another person in a specified situation, and acting out what that other person might do and say in that situation. This helps people to understand what it feels like to be in another person's shoes. For example, adults role playing an unemployed young person may be helped to understand feelings of rejection and boredom. Health promoters role playing non-English-speaking patients visiting a clinic may be helped to understand how those patients feel, especially if the role play is given added authenticity by using a foreign language that the health promoters do not speak.

It is also possible to role play oneself in a new situation. This is a useful way of practising a new skill or rehearsing for a future event. For example, patients can role play a consultation with a doctor in order to practise the skills of presenting their health problems to doctors.

For an example of a role-play exercise, see Exercise 12.2 in Chapter 12.

Using Structured Activities

See Chapter 13, section on getting groups going, for icebreaker ideas.

Structured activities, usually for a group of people but sometimes for one or two people only, can be used to meet a variety of aims. One is to help people to get to know each other ('icebreakers'); other activities are devised to help people trust each other, communicate more openly or to increase self-awareness.[15]

For example, activities can be used to help people to identify 'irrational beliefs'. Irrational beliefs are misconceptions that hinder people from achieving their goals. They are usually expressed in terms of 'must', 'should', or 'ought'. There are three major irrational beliefs:[16]

■ 'I must win everybody's approval otherwise I am worthless'.

- 'Other people must treat me exactly how I want them to (and if they don't they must be blamed and punished)'.
- 'Life must give me everything I want and nothing I don't want'.

These beliefs lead to self-defeating thinking, which in turn can affect health. It can lead to health-related behaviour with destructive consequences, such as emotional disorders, heavy drinking and physical ailments. The quiz in Exercise 14.2 aims to help you to identify your own irrational beliefs.

Exercise 14.2   Beliefs Quiz

Look at the following statements and put a tick in the appropriate column:

	Agree	Disagree
1. I believe in the saying that 'A leopard cannot change his spots'.	☐	☐
2. I believe that 'wait and see' is a good philosophy for life.	☐	☐
3. I want everyone to like me.	☐	☐
4. I usually put off important decisions.	☐	☐

Now identify your rational beliefs and your irrational beliefs (misconceptions):

Q 1. If you agreed with this statement you may believe that the past has a lot to do with determining the present and that people are largely unchangeable. 'I'm made that way.' The idea that you are no good at playing sports, for example, can be used to avoid trying out new behaviour and learning the skills necessary to participate in a sport. The truth is that people who take risks, experiment and work on things, generally find that they can become reasonably competent at most of the things they attempt. (Not necessarily perfect, but good enough.)

Q 2. If you agreed with this statement you may believe that human happiness can be achieved by hoping for the best – and waiting to see what happens. This belief could result in you becoming merely a spectator in life – watching television every night and somnolent on a sunlounger for the whole of your holidays. Getting more actively involved could be more satisfying and actually provide you with more energy. If you feel too 'burnt out', now may be the time to take a close look at how you are managing your life and make some changes.

Q 3. If you agree with this statement you may believe you are only as good as other people think you are. Because of this you may feel worthless if, despite your efforts, people don't seem to like you. Having the approval of others is pleasant, but in order to run our own lives we shall almost certainly have to do some things some people do not like. Work on giving yourself the approval you deserve.

Q 4. If you agreed with this statement you may believe that life's problems will go away if you avoid them. Don't waste your time hoping that things will work out – make them.

Strategies for Decision Making

As a health promoter, it is likely that you will often be involved in counselling with the aim of helping people to make a choice, such as which treatment to have, whether an elderly person should stay put or move into residential accommodation, whether to have a blood test for HIV, or how to select healthy foods in particular circumstances. Research has shown that brief counselling sessions can be effective in bringing about health-related behaviour change.[17]

See Chapter 10 on Fundamentals of Communication.

Basic skills of counselling to help people to make decisions (the 'commitment' stage of change) are those we discussed in Chapter 10: understanding non-verbal communication, listening, helping people to talk, asking questions, and obtaining feedback.[18] We do not discuss counselling in depth here, but include suggestions for further study at the end of this chapter.[19]

There are at least five stages involved.[20] These stages may seem familiar to you because counselling involves a framework of planning and evaluating similar to the one we used in Chapter 5.

See Chapter 5, The Basic Planning and Evaluation Process.

Stage 1. Identify the Need and Create the Climate

Carl Rogers (a 'founding father' of counselling) has identified the qualities necessary for a counsellor to establish a climate in which a client can 'open up'.[21] These are warmth, openness, genuineness, empathy, and unconditional positive regard. Unconditional positive regard is the quality of totally respecting the worth and dignity of a person, irrespective of whether you like the person or agree with his views or behaviour.

The practical aspects of creating the climate include ensuring that you will not be interrupted and cannot be overheard, that you have sufficient time, and that you are comfortably seated in chairs of the same height, with the counsellor adopting an open posture and making direct eye contact when appropriate.

Stage 2. Explore the Needs and the Concerns

Through giving full attention and actively listening, by encouraging the client to talk and by asking questions, the counsellor begins to establish trust and to enable the client to move from superficial issues to deeper needs and concerns.

Stage 3. Help the Client to Set Goals and Identify Options

Having gained a new perspective on the issues and concerns, it becomes possible for the client to identify goals and ways these might be achieved. The counsellor could help the client to identify themes or to get a clearer vision of the future by asking key questions, such as:

'How would you feel if … ?'

'If things were exactly how you wanted them to be, how would they be different from now … ?'

'Have you ever felt like that on other occasions … ?'

The counsellor may also provide the client with information in order to establish options:

'If you do X what's likely to happen is ...'

'If you do Y the chances are that ...'

'You might find it helpful to consider that ...' and so on.

Stage 4. Help the Client to Decide Which Option to Choose

The important thing about this stage is that the choice must be the client's, not the counsellor's. Making decisions – that is, choosing between alternative options – is a highly complex process. It involves:

- weighing up the pros and cons of the alternative options
- considering the likely consequences of pursuing each alternative
- deciding which is the best alternative
- having the confidence to pursue the best alternative.

If the client is reluctant to commit to a decision, then both parties need to consider whether it is worth undertaking further work at stages two and three.

If the client chooses an alternative that the counsellor feels won't work, she should nevertheless back the client's choice and help him to develop an action plan (knowing that if it doesn't work, the door is still open for exploring other options).

Stage 5. Help the Client to Develop an Action Plan

See next section, Strategies for Changing Behaviour.

Having made a decision, the client now needs to think about turning that decision into action. He may need to identify coping strategies and sources of support. Once an action plan has been agreed, the final details are to set a review date and to clarify how progress will be monitored.

Strategies for Changing Behaviour

Having made a choice, people may need considerable help to carry their decision through into the 'action' stage of change. A number of techniques developed from behavioural psychology are useful, and the philosophy behind them (that people are responsible for their own behaviour and are capable of exercising control over it) is as important as the techniques themselves.[22] A variety of material has been developed to help people to change different aspects of their behaviour, such as stopping smoking, controlling drinking, changing eating habits, and taking up exercise.[23] Some useful techniques are as follows.

Self-monitoring

Self-monitoring involves keeping a detailed and precise account, often in the form of a diary, of behaviour that is to be changed. Its aim is to help people to analyse their pattern of behaviour and become fully aware of what they are doing, which is a starting point for gaining control. Secondly, the 'diary' provides a baseline against which progress can be checked.

Self-monitoring involves answering questions such as:

| Example 14.1 | **Counselling About a Health Choice** |

A health visitor has the task of helping a mother to decide what to do about having her baby vaccinated. The stages could be:

Stages 1 and 2. Identify and explore the need

For example, is the mother worried about having the child vaccinated at all, or is it just the whooping cough vaccination which is worrying? Is it *when* to have the child vaccinated, or *if*?

Stage 3. Help the client to set goals and establish options

For example, the parent may identify the goal of her child having the best possible chance of staying healthy.

The options might be: no vaccinations at all, some vaccinations, or all the vaccinations.

Stage 4. Help the client to decide which option to choose

- Weigh up the pros and cons – the health visitor provides unbiased information on the risks from catching each disease compared with the risks of having the vaccinations.
- Consider the likely consequences of pursuing each alternative: for the child in terms of health risk, for the parent, in terms of anxiety, guilt and responsibility, for other people in terms of spreading the diseases.

Stage 5. Help the client to develop an action plan

For example, the mother may decide to go ahead with the vaccination programme, but also to join a mother's group, in order to get support from other mothers facing the same anxieties and decisions. The health visitor suggests to the mother that she keeps a record of the vaccinations for future reference, and provides her with a record card for her child. They set a date for the first vaccination.

- How frequently does the problem occur?
- When the problem occurs, what else is happening, both externally (in the environment), and internally (in thoughts and feelings)?
- What event leads up to the problem?
- What happens afterwards: the consequences?

Example 14.2 is a smoker's diary.

Identifying Costs, Benefits and Rewards

The cost of changing behaviour can be considerable, involving deprivation of 'crutches', such as cigarettes, and pleasures, such as eating and drinking – or there may be a heavy price to pay in terms of time, effort, and perhaps money. So it is helpful to identify the benefits clearly, and set up a system of rewards to encourage perseverance.

Benefits may be long-term, such as better health or increased life expectancy. They may be abstract ('it will prove I've got will-power'), or in other people's interests ('for

Example 14.2	A Smoker's Diary

Day . . . (Complete one of these charts every day.)

Each time you smoke a cigarette, note down in the columns:

1. **The time.**
2. **How urgent your craving for a cigarette is, on a scale of 1–10 (1, very little craving; 10, extremely high craving).**
3. **Where you smoke the cigarette.**
4. **Whether you are alone or who you are with.**
5. **Do you smoke it with drinks (coffee, tea, alcohol)?**
6. **Do you smoke it after a meal?**
7. **What else are you doing at the time (e.g. chatting, reading the paper, working, talking on the phone)?**
8. **Why did you decide to smoke this cigarette?**
9. **What do you feel about it afterwards?**

Time	Craving	Where	Who with	With drinks	After meal	Doing what	Why	Afterwards

Total number of cigarettes smoked today = _____

the family's sake'). These benefits may be important but it is also necessary to find immediate, short-term rewards that people genuinely enjoy, such as small treats.

Setting Targets and Evaluating Progress

Targets should be realistic rather than idealistic. Losing an average of one pound in weight a week is realistic for most people; losing a stone in a month usually is not. People may have unrealistic hopes and expectations about what can be achieved, which lead to disappointment and a sense of failure when they don't meet the target.

In order to evaluate progress, it is necessary to keep a record of behaviour so that achievements can be seen clearly. Progress should be assessed once the 'new' behaviour has been given a fair trial, perhaps for two or three weeks, although short-term reviews ('How have I done today?') can also be useful.

If the target is not being achieved, possible reasons must be looked for and changes made. For example:

■ Is the target too difficult? Should it be lowered?
■ Are the rewards too distant? Is there a more immediate reward that could be more encouraging?
■ Is there an unforeseen crisis or illness? If so, encouragement to continue self-monitoring and to look on the setback as a learning experience may be needed.

- Are other people unhelpful? More strategies to cope with the negative influence of other people may be needed.
- Are there other problems which require help, such as learning to cope with anxiety or stress?

Devising Coping Strategies

Changing behaviour can mean coping with numerous difficulties, for at least a short period of time, until the new behaviour becomes a normal part of life. Someone who is stopping smoking has to cope with problems such as the craving he feels, the need to put something in his mouth, not knowing what to do with his hands, doing without his accustomed 'tension-reliever' in moments of stress, and resisting the offer of a cigarette.

People adopt a wide variety of coping strategies, and it is often useful to get a group to share their ideas about what helps them to cope. The list of strategies here is certainly not exhaustive.

- Finding a substitute, such as substituting chewing gum or eating low-calorie foods instead of high-calorie ones.
- Changing some routines and habits that are closely associated with the 'problem' behaviour. Examples are drinking tea or fruit juice instead of coffee, because coffee is closely associated with cigarettes.
- Making it difficult to carry on with the 'problem' behaviour by, for example, keeping cigarettes in an inconvenient place, sitting in the no-smoking area of a restaurant, and deciding to restrict eating to mealtimes, not between meals.

What all these strategies have in common is that they require only a small step to achieve a large degree of help for self-control. Other strategies may be:

- Getting support from other people in the same situation, who might be from a weight control group, a smoking cessation clinic, or a self-help group. Another helpful way of getting support is by linking with another person on the understanding that each may telephone or meet the other if they need help.
- Practising ways of responding to unhelpful social pressures, for example refusing the offer of a cigarette or a drink.
- Adopting a one-day-at-a-time approach. The prospect of the whole of the rest of life without a cigarette may be overwhelming, but the prospect of one day without one is far more tolerable. Even shorter time-spans may be helpful, such as putting off eating, drinking or smoking for just five minutes at a time.
- Learning relaxation techniques and other ways (such as exercise) of relieving stress. Simple relaxation routines that can be practised at any time and place can be helpful in coping with stressful moments when the 'old' reaction would have been to reach for a drink or a cigarette.

Using Strategies Effectively

We have discussed a number of different strategies that you can use when you are trying to help clients to increase their self-awareness, clarify their values and beliefs, change their attitudes and behaviour, and maintain behaviour change; in other words

Gemma is a single parent. She has a toddler who constantly wakes her at night. She has used various strategies, including trying to tire him out physically just before bedtime, keeping him up later, leaving toys for him to play with in the night, and playing with him herself in the night. She has started to buy vodka cocktails and cans of lager in the supermarket to drink in the evenings to help her relax and now finds that she needs another drink to help her get back to sleep after getting up in the night.

She phones her health visitor – Mary – for help. Mary goes to see her and asks her to describe a typical day (and night) in order to understand the situation better. She asks Gemma to describe the situations she struggled with, how she felt at the time and what she did. As Gemma's story unfolds Mary gains knowledge of Gemma's variation in mood states, existing coping strategies and support base.

Mary gets Gemma to reflect on her daily achievements and emphasises that it must be a struggle for her without much sleep. Gemma says she wants to do something to help her child sleep better. Mary explores how confident Gemma feels in being able to make some changes. Mary also asks Gemma if she knows of anything that seems to help her child to relax, and using her suggestions they devise a suitable bedtime routine for Gemma to try out. Mary recognises that Gemma is concerned about her drinking and asks her for suggestions of what she could do about it. Gemma says she feels that her drinking is related to her stressful situation and that once her child sleeps better she will feel more in control.

Finally, Mary suggests that she should come back to see Gemma in two weeks' time to discuss whether the new routines are helping her child to sleep. Gemma agrees. Mary makes a note to ask Gemma about her drinking on the next visit.

- **What strategies does Mary, the health visitor, use to help Gemma?**
- **What other strategies could Mary have used?**
- **What strategies might Mary want to use at the follow-up visit?**

to move them through the Stages of Change cycle. Research emphasises that, while it may be relatively easy to influence attitudes and behaviour short-term, it can be very difficult for people to sustain behaviour change over the longer term.[24] In order to use these strategies with maximum effect there are a number of principles to bear in mind.

Advocacy and Working in Partnership with Lay People

Some people may need extra help to make health choices. Advocacy is generally taken to mean representing the interests of people who cannot speak up for themselves because of illness, disability or other disadvantage. In the context of health promotion, it is better seen as a variety of ways of empowering those people who are disempowered in our society. It is concerned with using every possible means to assist people to become independent and self-advocating.

There can be deep conflicts of loyalty for health promoters who take on an advocacy role. There may be a need to challenge employers, or those in authority, about services that fail to meet people's needs.

For example, if a patient complains to a community mental health nurse that his drugs are making him feel drowsy and generally unwell, but the doctor insists he should continue to take them, where should the nurse's loyalties lie: to the patient, to the doctor, to the health service (which funds her) or to her profession (which controls her registration)? How can the nurse most effectively act as an advocate in this situation?

Because of such conflicts of loyalties, many advocacy schemes use non-professional workers who come from a similar background to those they are empowering. For example, 'Maternity Links' schemes provide workers as advocates and interpreters for Asian mothers who do not speak English. The workers are Asian themselves but able to speak English as well as their own mother tongue, and the organisation may be run with health service funding but managed independently.

In order to reach and influence disadvantaged groups of people successfully, many projects involve professionals working in partnership with lay volunteers. For example, a community mothers programme involved non-professional mothers as volunteers working with disadvantaged first-time mothers to improve their parenting skills.[25] A randomised controlled trial demonstrated that this approach was effective.

Making Healthier Choices Easy Choices

See Chapter 1, section What Affects Health? and Chapter 16, section Changing Policy and Practice.

People do not make health choices in a vacuum; they make them in the context of their own environment, subject to all the pressures and influences that surround them. If this environment is conducive to a healthier lifestyle, clients have greater freedom to choose the 'healthier' alternatives and change their behaviour. For example, the provision of cycleways makes it easier to take regular exercise by cycling to work; provision of litter bins, combined with frequent emptying, helps people to maintain a litter-free environment; a no-smoking policy in public places such as shopping malls and cinemas helps people not to smoke. National and local policies can create a climate where it is easier to adopt healthier behaviour.

Relating to Clients

See Chapter 10, section on exploring relationships with clients.

Research consistently shows that the degree of client change is related to helper empathy; in other words, clients are more likely to change if the health promoter understands the client, sees things from his point of view, and accepts him on his own terms. Achieving this relationship may be the most difficult part of helping people to change.

Sometimes it is difficult to start a discussion about changing behaviour, and establishing good rapport is essential for an honest discussion and openness for change. One way you can understand your client (and also assess readiness to change) is to ask the client to take you through a typical day with reference to a particular behaviour.

Furthermore, the attitude and behaviour of the health promoter herself is likely to influence the outcome. For example, it has long been known that doctors who themselves smoke are less likely to be effective in helping people to choose to stop smoking.[26] The experiences of health promoters in trying to change their own behaviour can be valuable in helping them to understand the difficulties that their clients experience. However, it is important to remember that everyone is different and that, although for some people making a particular change may be easy, for others a similar change is very difficult.

Dealing with Resistance

It is sometimes difficult for health promoters to stop providing advice when they know that a particular behaviour, such as stopping smoking, can have huge benefits for the patient. It is important to recognise when your clients are showing signs of resisting the suggestion to change. When you see this resistance, it is better to back off and express empathy, emphasising that it is the patient's personal choice and that he has control over his choices. Useful strategies for these clients at a later date are to reassess readiness to change, establish how important the behaviour change is to them, and how confident they feel about making the change.

Using Learning Methods Sensitively

People invest a great deal of emotion in their values and attitudes, which means that the exercises we have described here, especially those that are designed to encourage people to explore feelings (such as role play), need to be handled with care and sensitivity. Special training in the use of experiential teaching methods is recommended but, at the very least, group leaders should not attempt to use them unless they have experienced them first themselves. Some points to remember are as follows.

- Explain the activities carefully and thoroughly, and check to ensure that everybody understands what the exercise is for and what they are expected to do.
- Emphasise that participation is entirely voluntary.
- Allow plenty of time for discussion at the end. If people's opinions and cherished ideas have been challenged, they are likely to feel strongly about it. Increased self-awareness may be a very uncomfortable experience too. The group leader should ensure that people have time to express their feelings and get any support that they need before they leave the group.
- Ensure that there is an atmosphere of confidentiality and trust, so that people feel free to explore their views and feelings in safety. If they feel they may be laughed at or gossiped about, they will not participate fully, if at all.
- Save your own views to the end, after the group members have had a chance to think things through for themselves. Be open and honest about yourself and your values, and if you are also confused, say so!

PRACTICE POINTS

- For individuals to be ready to change a particular behaviour they need to feel confident in being able to adopt the new behaviour. The new behaviour also needs to be important to them and have clear benefits. You may need to help clients develop a number of competencies (often called 'life skills') to do with social interaction, assertiveness and time management, and possibly specific skills (for example, in order to participate in a physical exercise programme).

- In order to devise the appropriate strategy for each individual you need to start by exploring clients' health knowledge and beliefs related to the issue of concern, the stage they are at in the 'revolving door' of change, and what outcomes they desire. Asking the client to describe a typical day in relation to the behaviour is a useful approach.

PRACTICE POINTS

- You need to be aware that clients may be resistant to change. In these situations it is best to back off, emphasising that it is the client's personal choice and that he is in control. At a later date you could go back to explore again the individual's confidence about changing and how important the change is to him.

- You need to tailor an action plan to the specific needs of each client.

- You need to provide positive consequences for desired healthy behaviour (such as praise or rewards) in order to maintain behaviour change.

- You can improve success by combining a number of strategies. For example, a patient who is being rehabilitated after a heart attack could have an interview with a hospital doctor, backed up by a home visit from a nurse to encourage family members to support the patient, and small-group self-help sessions to help patients to manage their problems.

- Records are important for follow-up. They are most effective if they are kept and 'owned' by the individual concerned, for example in the form of a diary.

- Providing a supportive environment can be the key to success, so that people find it easier to make and maintain a healthier lifestyle.

Recommended Reading

On Health Behaviour

➤ Stroebe W, Stroebe M S 2000 Social psychology and health, 2nd edn. Buckingham: Open University Press
➤ Taylor S E 1998 Health psychology, 4th edn. Part 2. New York: McGraw-Hill International Editions

On Models of Behaviour Change

➤ Naidoo J, Wills J 2000 Health promotion: foundations for practice, 2nd edn. Chapter 11. London: Baillière Tindall
➤ Tones K, Tilford S 2001 Health education: effectiveness, efficiency and equity, 3rd edn. Chapter 2. Cheltenham: Nelson Thornes

On Helping People to Change Health-related Behaviour

➤ Hunt P, Hillsdon M 1996 Changing eating and exercise behaviour. Oxford: Blackwell
➤ Miller W R, Rollnick S 2002 Motivational interviewing – preparing people for change. New York: Guilford Press
➤ Rollnick S, Mason P, Butler C 1999 Health behaviour change – a guide for practitioners. London: Churchill Livingstone

➤ Squire A 2002 Health and well-being for older people: foundations for practice. London: Baillière Tindall in association with the Royal College of Nursing. (Chapter 14 is about helping older people towards healthier living.)

On Counselling

➤ Burnard P 1999 Counselling skills for health professionals. Cheltenham: Nelson Thornes
➤ Egan G 2001 The skilled helper: a problem-management and opportunity development approach to helping, 7th edn. New York: Thomson Learning
➤ Etherington K 2001 Counsellors in health settings. London: Jessica Kingsley
➤ Hough M 2002 A practical approach to counselling. Harlow, Essex: Pearson Education. (This provides an overview of different approaches to counselling, including a section on group counselling.)
➤ Katz J, Peberdy A, Douglas J (eds) 2000 Promoting health: knowledge and practice, 2nd edn. Chapter 9. Basingstoke: The Open University in association with Palgrave

On Working with Young People and Families

➤ Carr A (ed.) 2000 What works with children and adolescents? A critical review of psychological interventions with children, adolescents and their families. London: Routledge

A Model of Empowering Health for Those with Chronic Illnesses

➤ McGonical G 1998 Empowering health in chronic illness: a conceptual model. British Journal of Therapy and Rehabilitation 5 (11), 591–595

Notes and References

1   The Health Belief Model is the oldest and best known. See:

Becker M H (ed.) 1974 The health belief model and personal health behaviour. Thorofare, New Jersey: Slack.

In essence, this model suggests that when people are faced with pressure to change their behaviour they will weigh up the pros and cons, and what they decide to do will depend on their perceptions of factors such as how serious they think an illness or danger is. However, the Health Belief Model has been criticised because it assumes that people are rational (and we know that they often act irrationally!) and because it ignores powerful influences on behaviour such as family and friends.

The Theory of Reasoned Action is a model which emphasises the influence of 'significant others'. See:

Ajzen I, Fishbein M 1980 Understanding attitudes and predicting social behaviour. Englewood Cliffs: Prentice Hall

However, it too, sees human behaviour as essentially rational.

See Tones K, Tilford S 2001 Health education: effectiveness, efficiency and equity, 3rd edn. Chapter 2. Cheltenham: Nelson Thornes, for more on both of these models.

2   Tones B K 1987 Devising strategies for preventing drug misuse: the role of the Health Action Model. Health Education Research 2, 305–317.

Tones K, Tilford S 2001 Health education: effectiveness, efficiency and equity, 3rd edn. Chapter 2. Cheltenham: Nelson Thornes

3   Tones K 1995 Making a change for the better. Healthlines, November, p. 17. (Reproduced with permission from the Health Education Authority.)

4   Prochaska J O, DiClemente C 1982 Transtheoretical therapy: towards a more integrative model of change. Psychotherapy: Theory, Research and Practice 19 (3), 276–288

5   Batten E 1999 The transtheoretical model: profiling smoking in pregnancy. In: Perkins, E, Simnett I, Wright L (eds) Evidence based health promotion. Chichester: Wiley, pp. 76–88

6   The stages of change we use are adapted from:

Prochaska J, DiClemente C 1984 The transtheoretical approach: crossing traditional boundaries of therapy. Harnewood, Illinois: Dow-Jones

Neesham C 1993 A model for change. Healthlines, September, 15–17. Figure 14.2 reproduced by kind permission of the Health Development Agency.

7   Batten E 1999 The transtheoretical model: profiling smoking in pregnancy. In: Perkins, E, Simnett I, Wright L (eds) Evidence-based health promotion. Chichester: Wiley, pp. 76–88

8   A number of authors have challenged the application of the 'Stages of Change' model, including:

Ashworth P 1997 Breakthrough or bandwagon? Are interventions tailored to Stage of Change more effective than non-staged interventions? Health Education Journal 56, 166–174

Buxton K, Wyse J, Mercer T 1996 How applicable is the Stages of Change model to exercise behaviour? Health Education Journal 55, 239–257

Duncan P, Cribb A 1996 Helping people change – an ethical approach? Health Education Research 11 (3), 339–348

Whitehead M 1997 Editorial: how useful is the 'stages of change' model? Health Education Journal 56, 111–112

Whitelaw S, Baldwin S, Bunton R, Flynn D 2000 The status of evidence and outcomes in Stages of Change research. Health Education Research 15 (6), 707–718

9   Examples of using the Stages of Change approach:

Aveyard P et al 1999 Cluster randomized controlled trial of expert system based on transtheoretical ("stages of change") model for smoking prevention and cessation in schools. British Medical Journal 319, 948–953.

Aveyard P et al 2001 The change-in-stage and updated smoking status results from a cluster-randomized trial of smoking prevention and cessation using the transtheoretical model among British adolescents. Preventive Medicine 33, 313–324

Batten L et al 1999 Stage of change, low income and benefit status: a profile of women's smoking in early pregnancy. Health Education Journal 58, 378–388

Naylor P J, Simmonds G, Riddoch C, Velleman G, Turton P 1999 Comparison of stage-matched and unmatched interventions to promote exercise behaviour in the primary care setting. Health Education Research 14 (5), 653–666.

10   This section is based on: Rollnick S, Mason P, Butler C 1999 Health behaviour change – a guide for practitioners. London: Churchill Livingstone

11   Research shows that focusing on the prevention of relapse can be effective. See:

Marlett G, George W 1995 Relapse prevention: introduction and overview of the model. British Journal of Addiction 79, 261–273

12   Kreuter M, Stretcher V 1996 Do tailored behaviour change messages enhance the effectiveness of health risk appraisal? Results from a randomised trial. Health Education Research 11 (1), 97–105

13   Experiential learning has evolved from two sources. One is from the theories of the American philosopher John Dewey. Another is from humanistic psychology. Humanistic psychology sees people as free decision-makers actively controlling their own destinies. We discussed some limitations to this viewpoint in Chapter 3, but humanistic psychology has had a huge influence on health care, education and health promotion both in the UK and worldwide. The literature is vast. One classic text still worth reading (and available in print) is:

Rogers C R 1967 On becoming a person: a therapist's view of psychotherapy. London: Constable

14   From ideas in: Rollnick S, Mason P, Butler C 1999 Health behaviour change – a guide for practitioners. London: Churchill Livingstone

15   Brandes D 1998 Gamester's handbook three. Cheltenham: Nelson Thornes

16   Irrational beliefs can be identified and changed through 'rational emotive behaviour therapy'. For basic introductions to the principles and practice of this, see:

Dryden W 1996 Inquiries in rational emotive behaviour therapy. London: Sage

Dryden W 1995 Brief rational emotive behaviour therapy. Chichester: Wiley

See also:
Curwen B, Palmer S, Ruddell P 2000 Brief cognitive behaviour therapy. London: Sage

17   There are many occasions when a discussion between health promoter and client can only be brief. A technique has been developed which is essentially a brief and effective approach to empowering others, useful for clients who are at the 'commitment' (ready to change) stage of change. It focuses on building the confidence of the client that he has the capacity to change, through focusing on successes (what the client is already doing to reach the goals), rather than focusing on mistakes or failures. See:

De Jong P, Berg I K 1998 Interviewing for solutions. Pacific Grove CA: Brookes/Cole

18   For a useful introduction to counselling skills, see:

Burnard P 1999 Counselling skills for health professionals. London: Nelson Thornes

19   Counselling for those working with lesbian, gay or bisexual clients:

Davies D, Neal C (eds) 1996 Pink therapy: a guide for counsellors and therapists working with lesbian, gay and bisexual clients. Buckingham: Open University Press

Counselling in schools:

Sederholm G 2001 Counselling young people in school. London: Jessica Kingsley

Counselling older people:

O'Leary E 1996 Counselling older adults: perspectives, approaches and research. London: Chapman & Hall

Terry P 1997 Counselling the elderly and their carers. Basingstoke: Macmillan

Counselling in the workplace:

Carroll M 1996 Workplace counselling. London: Sage

Counselling people with alcohol problems:

Velleman R 2001 Counselling for alcohol problems. 2nd edn. London: Sage

Bryant-Jefferies R 2001 Counselling the person beyond the alcohol problem. London: Jessica Kingsley

Counselling in terminal care and bereavement:

Parkes C M, Pelf M, Couldrick A 1996 Counselling in terminal care and bereavement. Leicester: British Psychological Society

Counselling people under stress:

Ellis A, Gordon J, Neenan M, Palmer S 1997 Stress counselling: a rational emotive behaviour approach. London: Cassell

20   We have adapted our five stages from:

Burnard P 1985 Learning human skills: a guide for nurses. Oxford: Heinemann Nursing

Inskipp F 1993 Counselling: the trainer's handbook, Revised edition. Cambridge: National Extension College

21 Rogers C R 1983 Freedom to learn for the eighties. Columbus, Ohio: Charles E Merril

22 For a general introduction to health behaviour and behaviour change, see:

Stroebe W, Stroebe M S 2000 Social psychology and health, 2nd edn. Buckingham: Open University Press

23 For examples, see the NHS Health Promotion Department in your local area. Your local GP surgery or NHS walk-in centre may also have leaflets.

24 Pill R, Peters T J, Robling M R 1993 How important is health behaviour to the health of mothers of lower socio-economic status? Journal of Public Health Medicine 15 (1), 77

25 Settles B H, Davies J E, Grasse-Bachman C, Janvier K A, Rosas S R 2000 Developing community and peer support for young parents: process and outcome evaluation inputs in prevention programs. Family Science Review 13, 182–196

26 Pincherle G, Wright H B 1970 Smoking habits of business executives: doctor variations in reducing consumption. Practitioner 205, 209–212.

15 Working with Communities

SUMMARY

We introduce this chapter with an explanation of the term 'community-based work in health promotion' and the range of activities it may include. We discuss some key terms and principles before looking at three particular ways of working with communities: community participation, community development, and community health projects. Each of these includes an exercise, and there is also a case study of a community development project. We finish by looking at the competencies health promoters need to develop when working with communities.

See Defining Health Promotion in Chapter 2.

See Chapter 7, section Local Health Strategies and Initiatives, for information on government-funded initiatives focusing on disadvantaged communities.

As we have discussed in previous chapters, health promotion is the process of enabling people to increase control over, and improve, their health.[1] The challenge this presents is never more apparent than when considering people in the community who may be disadvantaged and discriminated against, and who feel powerless to do anything about their health. This chapter is about taking on that challenge, and working in the community with groups of people in a way that *does* enable them take more control over their health.

Community-based Work in Health Promotion

By *community-based work in health promotion* we mean work that directly involves the health promoter in working with groups of the public in a sustained way which will enable them to increase control over, and improve, their health. It may involve different kinds of activities, including:

- community development work
- setting up a group and working with members on health issues (such as a group with learning difficulties addressing issues of sexual health)
- working on projects or campaigns focusing on a particular health issue (such as sickle-cell disease or drug misuse)
- outreach work, which means workers going out to meet people where they are, rather than expecting people to come to them (such as community workers on sexual health, who might work with people in the sex industry on the streets or in clubs and massage parlours)
- providing health information services (such as well-women information centres)

- health-related work undertaken by organisations with wider remits (such as health courses for older people run by national older people's organisations)
- advocacy projects (such as organisations undertaking interpreting and/or advocacy for Asian women)
- self-help groups getting together for mutual support on health problems.[2]

This list begins to identify specific tasks health promoters may find themselves tackling, but first we need to clarify some of the key terms and principles involved in community-based work.

Key Terms

Community

A community may be thought of as a network of people. The link between them may be:

- where they live (such as a housing estate or neighbourhood)
- the work they do (such as 'the farming community')
- their ethnic background (such as 'the Jewish community')
- the way they live (such as 'new age' travellers or homeless people)
- or other factors they have in common.

The people in the network come together on the basis of a shared experience or concern, and identify for themselves which communities they feel they belong to. Networks may be formal or informal.

Community Work

This means working with community groups and organisations to overcome the community's problems and improve people's conditions of life. Community work aims to enhance the sense of solidarity and competence in the community. A **community worker** is usually a paid worker undertaking community work.

Community Health Work

This is community work with a focus on health concerns, but generally health is defined broadly to include social and economic aspects, so that community health work may encompass almost as broad a range of activities as community work without a specific health remit.

Community Action

This means activity carried out by people under their own control in order to improve their collective conditions. It may involve campaigning, negotiating with or challenging authorities and those with power.

Community Participation

This is about involving the community in health work that is led by someone outside the community; for example a worker employed by a statutory agency. The degree of participation may vary enormously.

Community Development

This means working to stimulate and encourage communities to express their needs and to support them in their collective action. It is not about dealing with people's problems on a one-to-one basis; it aims to develop the potential of a community as a whole. A **community development approach to health** involves working with groups of people to identify their own health concerns, and to take appropriate action. **Community development health workers** are essentially facilitators, locally based, whose role is to help people in the community to acquire the skills, knowledge and confidence to act on health issues. They are usually community workers by background, rather than health professionals.

Community Health Projects

This is a loose term applied to programmes of work that are organised by agencies for the improvement of health in a community, or to local organisations aiming to improve health by supporting some combination of community activity, self-help, community action, and/or community development.[3]

Finally, it is worth mentioning that in the health service the word 'community' is often used as an adjective to describe anything that is not based in hospital. Examples are **community care**, **community nurses** and **community services**.

Community participation, community development and community health projects will be explored in greater depth later in the chapter, but first we look at some principles of community health work.

Principles of Community-based Work

We identify four key principles, as follows.

1.   The Centrality of the Community

It is the community which defines its own needs, not the health workers. Community-based work is essentially a 'bottom-up' process, rather than a 'top-down' process where those with power and authority make the decisions. Community workers recognise and value the health experience and knowledge that exists in the community, and seek to use it for everyone's benefit.

2.   The Facilitator Role of the Community Health Worker

Community health workers do not perceive themselves as 'experts' in health, but as facilitators whose role is to validate, encourage and empower people to define their own health needs and to meet them. They start where the community is, recognising and valuing people's own abilities and experiences. They involve people in the community health work from the very beginning, encouraging and supporting them in working together. Knowledge and skills are shared and demystified. Community health workers aim to complement as well as challenge statutory services by making people's access to statutory agencies easier, and making the agencies more accountable to the people they serve.

3.   The Importance of Addressing Inequalities

See Chapter 1, section
Inequalities in Health.

A central concern in community-based health work is the need to challenge and change the many forms of disadvantage, oppression and discrimination that people face, and which adversely affect their health. There is acute awareness of the need to address inequalities in health and health services, and to focus on the social, environmental and economic determinants of health.

Work therefore focuses particularly on the needs of disadvantaged groups, which is why work with women and minority ethnic and black groups is prominent. Another example is people with learning difficulties, who need help to empower them to take more control over their own lives. A central way of working is to bring people in such groups together for support and information sharing, and to enable them to bring about change through collective action. There is no denying that the work is political, because it means working towards greater equality and social justice. It means working with people who experience powerlessness and inequality as part of their everyday lives, and working towards a redistribution of resources and power.

4.   A Broad Perspective on Health

Health is perceived broadly and holistically as positive well-being, including social, emotional, mental and societal aspects as well as physical ones. It is not seen merely as the absence of disease, and is not limited by medical or epidemiological views of what constitutes a health problem or issue. Health is seen to be affected by social, environmental, economic and political factors.

Community Participation

Participation is a word that is used widely to mean a range of activities, from those that are merely tokenistic to those which are firmly rooted in the concept of empowerment. Partnership, public participation and public decision making are all key issues in health services and local authorities. However, in reality many organisations make decisions without having any wish to engage with the public.

In this section we look at two aspects where you may be involved: first in planning new developments, and then in identifying practical ways of supporting the principle of community participation.

Community Participation in Planning

See also section
Public Views in Chapter 6.

The amount of community participation in planning health work organised by an agency (such as an NHS organisation or local authority) can vary along a spectrum of none to high, as shown in Table 15.1.[4] In the health service, such participation is usually called 'public involvement' or 'service user involvement'.

Ways of Developing Community Participation

Community participation can be encouraged and supported in many ways at different levels. We suggest some ways in which you may be able to develop community

Table 15.1	Community Participation (Public Involvement) in Planning Health Work
No participation	The community is told nothing, and is not involved in any way.
Very low participation	The community is informed. The agency makes a plan and announces it. The community is convened or notified in other ways in order to be informed; compliance is expected.
Low participation	The community is offered 'token' consultation. The agency tries to promote a plan and seeks support or at least sufficient sanction so that the plan can go ahead. It is unwilling to modify the plan unless absolutely necessary.
Moderate participation	The community advises through a consultation process. The agency presents a plan and invites questions, comments and recommendations. It is prepared to modify the plan.
High participation	The community plan jointly. Representatives of the agency and the community sit down together from the beginning to devise a plan.
Very high participation	The community has delegated authority. The agency identifies and presents an issue to the community, defines the limits and asks the community to make a series of decisions that can be embodied in a plan which it will accept.
Highest participation	The community has control. The agency asks the community to identify the issue and make all the key decisions about goals and plans. It is willing to help the community at each step to accomplish its goals, even to the extent of delegating administrative control of the work.

participation, particularly if you work for a public sector agency such as a local authority or the health service.[5]

Be open about policies and plans Publicise your policies, invite comments and recommendations on your plans, involve representatives on planning and management groups.

Plan for the community's expressed needs When planning services, help the community to express its own needs as it sees them, and take this into account when planning services.

Decentralise planning Set up planning and management of health and allied services on a neighbourhood basis, encouraging and enabling the public's involvement.

Develop joint forums Develop joint forums, such as patient participation groups in doctors' practices, where lay people and professionals can work together in partnerships. Mental health services often have joint forums to involve service users in service development.

Develop networks Encourage individuals or groups to come together, thus increasing their collective knowledge and power to change things. Value inter-agency links: gain the support of workers from different organisations because competition and lack of understanding of each other's roles and cultures can hinder progress.

Use electronic networking.[6] Electronic community networks can provide community information and a means of communication within and between communities. For example, rural communities with poor transport facilities can use electronic networks (e-mail and websites), which go some way towards addressing the problem of social exclusion caused by lack of information. Not only can groups and individuals find and supply information, they can participate in democratic processes. For example, local government can provide information and go one step further by creating 'virtual' councillors' surgeries.

Provide support, advice and training for community groups Provide opportunities for lay people to develop their knowledge, confidence and skills, such as in running groups, speaking in public, or finding their way around bureaucratic statutory organisations. This could be provided through informal discussions, perhaps on a 'drop-in' basis, structured training courses or via electronic networks.

Provide information Provide information about health issues, details of useful local and national organisations, leaflets, posters, books and websites.

Provide help with funding and resources Help local groups to obtain funding from statutory agencies, and provide other sorts of practical help such as a place to meet or facilities to photocopy materials. Short-term funding can hinder projects as it can result in frequent staff turnover.

Provide help with evaluation Being able to show real changes in resources, services and other visible achievements increases respect and confidence from communities, funders and agencies.

| Exercise 15.1 | **Developing Community Participation in Your Work** |

Consider the following list of ways in which you can encourage community participation in working for health.

- Be open about policies and plans
- Plan for the community's expressed needs
- De-centralise planning
- Develop joint forums
- Develop networks
- Provide support, advice and training for community groups
- Provide information
- Provide help with funding and resources
- Provide help with evaluation
- Support advocacy projects

(If you are not sure what is meant by these, look back at the explanations above.)

To what extent do you think these things are desirable?

To what extent do you do these things already?

From this list, can you identify ways in which you would like to increase community participation in your work?

Can you identify any other ways in which you would like to increase community participation in your work?

Given that there may be some obstacles to doing what you would ideally like to do, can you identify a practical way forward for acting on at least one of the things you would like to do?

Work individually, in pairs or small groups.

Support advocacy projects Support projects that enable people who are otherwise excluded to have a voice, such as interpreting/advocacy schemes for Asian patients.

Community Development

However much you might seek people's participation, it may be that they feel so alienated, dissatisfied or overwhelmed with problems that participation is the last thing they want to do. In this situation, it is necessary to develop a climate and culture where participation can happen. You need to encourage, enable and support people, and *community development* is a way of doing this. Evidence suggests that encouraging autonomy and strengthening social networks are prerequisites for good health.[7]

Community development is much more than community participation. It means working with people to identify their own health concerns, and to support and facilitate them in their collective action. It means adhering firmly to the principles of community-based work we outlined above, with the community development worker having the role of a facilitator.

Exercise 15.2 is designed to help you to consider what community development work means in practice.

See also Chapter 9, Case Study 9.1, about community development work with minority ethnic communities in Hillingdon, London.

Case Study 15.1 illustrates community development in practice, demonstrating how the community and the community's own expressed needs were central, the workers acted as facilitators, inequalities in health were addressed, and a broad perspective on health was taken. It also shows how local people were empowered to take action.

Some Implications of the Community Development Approach

If you choose to adopt a community development approach, it is important to appreciate the implications. The experience of community development projects around the country has shown that five areas of tension are likely to surface.[10] We identify these below, and some ways of trying to prevent them.

1.   Different Priorities

Priorities chosen by communities may not be the same as those of local statutory agencies or indeed the body who is funding the work. A common difference is that health problems as defined by health workers are likely to be about physical health problems, risk factors for major illnesses, and low uptake of health services, such as low-birthweight babies, heavy drinking and poor immunisation rates. Community priorities, on the other hand, are often about social conditions, such as housing, poor childcare provision, and lack of good public transport. This must be clearly understood and accepted at the outset of any community development work.

2.   A Threat to Local Health Workers

If local people gain confidence and become more articulate through the process of community development, they are likely to voice concern and criticism about local health services. Furthermore, the prospect of members of the community taking an active role in policy making and planning may be alien to many managers and field workers in statutory agencies. A thorough educational grounding in the rationale and

Exercise 15.2	Thinking About Community Development[8]

Working individually, or in pairs or small groups, work through the following questionnaire. If you are working with other people, discuss the reasons for the answers you give. You do not have to reach a consensus – after you have listened to each other's views, you can agree to disagree.

Tick whether you think each of the following statements is true or false:

Community development is about: True   False

1.   Fostering a sense of community among people

2.   Helping people to see the root causes of their ill health

3.   Enabling a statutory authority to show it 'cares'

4.   Getting involved in a political process

5.   Doing away with 'experts' and 'professionals'

6.   Confronting forms of discrimination such as racism and sexism

7.   Saving money on services by helping people to help themselves

8.   Promoting equal access to resources such as health services

9.   Enabling a community worker to become a leader/spokesperson for the community

10. Helping people to develop confidence and become more articulate about their needs

11. Campaigning for a better environment such as improved housing, transport and play facilities

12. Controlling social unrest, e.g. by providing activities for bored young people

13. Helping working-class people become more like middle-class people in terms of their attitudes and behaviour

14. Recognising and valuing the skills, knowledge and expertise of individuals and groups in the community

15. Beginning a process of redistributing wealth, power and resources

Now add any other points you think community development is, or is not, about.

principles of community-based work is required, although setting this up and getting people to listen may in itself be a daunting task.

3.   No Instant Results

Community development work is slow. It takes time to get to know a community and to build up trust with local people, and it may be years before there is any tangible out-

| Case study 15.1 | Community Development in Hull: Developing Our Communities[9] |

Developing Our Communities (DOC) started in January 1996 and is funded from a variety of sources including the New Opportunities Fund (in 2001, the National Lottery Charities Board changed this name to the Community Fund), NHS trusts, and the Single Regeneration Budget (government funding for economic and social development).

Hull DOC community workers started by getting to know people and the communities by listening to their hopes, aspirations and needs. Each community had different identities and cultures and many factors had an impact on the quality of life. The initial work built trust, confidence and a sense of value and self-worth within the communities. It included outreach to marginalised people so that confidence and learning increased, community networks were strengthened and people felt more able to have a collective voice in decision-making processes.

Examples of DOC's work included:

■ Carrying out a participatory appraisal – involving communities in looking at what was going on in the area and finding ways collectively to improve community life.

■ Community celebrations – bringing people together to facilitate a community event such as community plays, lunches or parties.

■ Community information – developing an interactive website with communities.

■ Meeting people in their locality – community workers have office space in the community and provide facilities and resources to the community. Community workers attend community group meetings.

■ Creating an informal local reference group so that residents can network, raise issues and prioritise work for Hull DOC. This includes nominating people to sit on the 'Community Chest' panel, which awards grants to community groups.

■ Food initiatives, such as food co-ops, developed by the food community worker to increase access to low-cost food.

■ Measuring success – both the process and outcomes.

come. A common problem is that projects with fixed-term funding for a year or two are often expected to achieve substantial outcomes in these short timescales, which is unrealistic. Secure funding for several years, with achievable objectives, is fundamental to success.

4.   A Token Gesture or an Easy Option

Well-meaning authorities who want to 'do something' (or to be seen to be doing something) about inequalities in health may set up a community health project as a way of addressing the issue. Clearly it cannot be 'the answer' to complex and deeply rooted causes of poor health; at best it can make a valuable contribution, but at worst it can divert attention from the real political solutions to the problems.

5.   Evaluation Conflicts

Outside agencies may expect to see results in terms of traditional 'outcomes' such as improved immunisation rates, a measurable change in community behaviour (less drunkenness, vandalism or crime, for example) or lower rates of hospital admission.

However, the objectives of a community development project are rarely couched in such terms, and are more likely to be concerned with far less easily measured results such as increased self-confidence, increased public participation in health planning, or better communication between the community and statutory agencies. Once again, education in the process, principles, aims and likely outcomes is essential for all concerned.

Community Health Projects

We now turn from thinking about community development to considering how you might be involved in a community health project. (We defined this earlier as a programme of work organised by an agency or a local organisation with the aim of improving health by some combination of community activity, self-help, community action and/or community development.) For example, you might want to set up a project to work with young parents on a housing estate with the aim of improving their confidence, skills and mutual support in parenting, or with older people in a particular area to encourage social activities with a health benefit, such as relaxation and exercise groups, tea dances, or lunch clubs.

See Chapter 5, The Basic Planning and Evaluation Process.

In order to think systematically about setting up and running a community health project, we suggest using the Planning and Evaluation Flowchart from Chapter 5. Additional help can be gained from reading the growing number of community health projects that have been written up so that the processes, successes and failures, and lessons learnt, can be shared.[11]

The experience of community health workers has highlighted specific issues that it is helpful to consider. These points are discussed below, set out within the planning and evaluation framework.[12] Figure 15.1 summarises the planning and evaluation flowchart, highlighting issues particularly relevant to community health project work. This is not a comprehensive guide to setting up and running community health projects; it is intended to be complementary to the information in Chapter 5.

Stage 1. Identifying Needs and Priorities

At this stage, two particular issues are: how do you get to know the community and who do you consult?

Getting to know the community and its needs Get all the relevant information you can about the health of the community. Search out data from local health services and the local authority.

Try contacting neighbourhood centres, community groups, voluntary organisations and tenants' associations. People who might be able to put you in touch with these include local workers in health and social services, local churches and schools, the local Council for Voluntary Service, and the local Council for Racial Equality. Talk to members of the public, perhaps at local markets and festivals. It might be useful to hold public meetings or conduct a small survey.

Talk to local professionals, but bear in mind that professional perceptions will often stem from a problem-centred view of a locality; for example, police may talk about crime, social workers about the numbers of children on the 'at-risk' register.

Fig 15.1   Flowchart for Planning and Evaluating Health Promotion, with Special Reference to Community Health Work

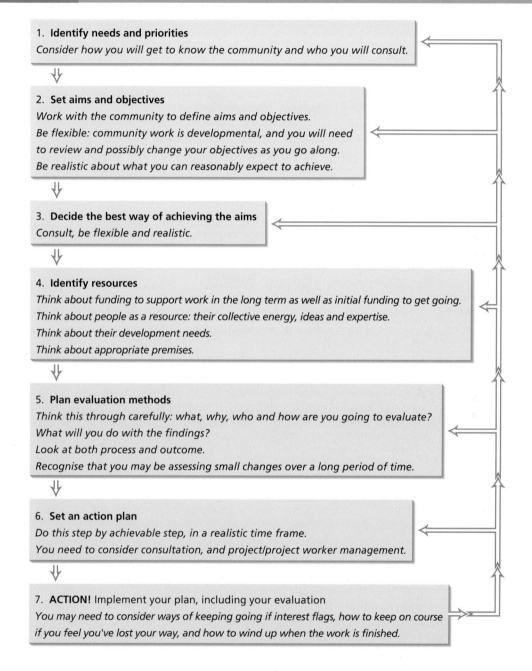

1. Identify needs and priorities
Consider how you will get to know the community and who you will consult.

2. Set aims and objectives
Work with the community to define aims and objectives.
Be flexible: community work is developmental, and you will need
to review and possibly change your objectives as you go along.
Be realistic about what you can reasonably expect to achieve.

3. Decide the best way of achieving the aims
Consult, be flexible and realistic.

4. Identify resources
Think about funding to support work in the long term as well as initial funding to get going.
Think about people as a resource: their collective energy, ideas and expertise.
Think about their development needs.
Think about appropriate premises.

5. Plan evaluation methods
Think this through carefully: what, why, who and how are you going to evaluate?
What will you do with the findings?
Look at both process and outcome.
Recognise that you may be assessing small changes over a long period of time.

6. Set an action plan
Do this step by achievable step, in a realistic time frame.
You need to consider consultation, and project/project worker management.

7. ACTION! Implement your plan, including your evaluation
You may need to consider ways of keeping going if interest flags, how to keep on course
if you feel you've lost your way, and how to wind up when the work is finished.

Local newspapers may be a useful source of information about the needs, interests and activities of a locality, and may even have a library service to select material on a particular issue for you. Another approach is to walk – not drive – around the neighbourhood. Groups of young people on street corners, smells from fast-food shops, and the range and price of goods in shop windows can reveal a lot about local lifestyle and socioeconomic conditions.

Consulting before setting up Consult with local health and social service workers at a very early stage. Consult with the community only if you are sure the project is going to happen: consultation before funding is secure, for example, could raise people's expectations falsely, waste their time and diminish their trust.

Stages 2 and 3. Setting Aims and Objectives, and Deciding the Best Way of Achieving Them

Key issues here are about being flexible and realistic. It is helpful to consult the people you have already made contact with, and the management group/steering group of the project (if there is one). These people may help you to set realistic, achievable aims and objectives, and to work out the best means of achieving them.

Flexibility is vital because community work is essentially a developmental process, so you need to review and modify your objectives regularly. Objectives may change, and indeed should change, if new opportunities arise and/or previous objectives no longer seem achievable or compatible with changing needs.

Be realistic: this applies to identifying what you plan to achieve, and when. For example, if you are planning a community development approach, ensure that you have a realistic time scale; three years is suggested as a reasonable minimum.

Stage 4. Identifying Resources

Funding Many projects are funded by statutory organisations, such as the local authorities or the health service, sometimes in partnership. Other projects may be funded from the voluntary sector through funding from government grants and independent funds. Short-term, marginal projects are rarely cost effective and can lead to disillusionment in communities as well as workers. Uncertain funding arrangements can increase difficulties in planning and evaluating work and can divert efforts from project work to fundraising. It is also important to think about long-term funding, otherwise there is a danger of work being dropped when funding runs out after perhaps only one or two years.

People By bringing people with a common interest or experience together, you may find that the collective energy of the group generates ideas for future action and you can begin to share the work. This means that your role may also begin to change, from being an initiator to being a supporter.

It is also important to think about the training and development needs of the people who are the key resource of the project. Not only project workers but also the project management committee (if there is one) and local health professionals may need help in understanding what this type of work is all about. What training is needed, who will do it and how will it be funded?

Premises You need to consider what premises you need: rooms for meeting in (large and small meetings), a room for a crèche, a place to keep and use equipment such as video equipment and photocopiers, a library/place where people can look up information and use computers with access to the Internet and e-mail. Is there access for wheelchairs, pushchairs and prams? Running water and toilets? Facilities for making refreshments or meals? Good access by public transport? Well-lit premises so that people feel safe going there after dark?

You also need to consider the 'image' of possible premises: if you are offered space in a clinic, for example, this may mean that people perceive the project to be part of the statutory health services.

Stage 5. Planning Evaluation Methods

It is vital that evaluation is planned before any work starts, as this will avoid misunderstandings and false expectations. All parties (funders, managers, workers, participants) need to agree on key issues:[13]

- Why are you undertaking an evaluation? Who and what is it for?
- What will you be evaluating?
- How will you do it? What methods will you use?
- Who will do it? Will you evaluate yourselves or will you use someone who is not involved in the work as an external evaluator?
- Who will be involved in the evaluation process? Will it involve the community, the workers, the funders, the steering group?
- What will you do with your evaluation findings? Will you publish a report? Who will be responsible for publication? Who will the evaluation report be distributed to? Who will own it? Will findings be widely disseminated, e.g. in journal articles?

Bear in mind the possibility of evaluation conflicts, which we discussed in the previous section, and make sure that your evaluation looks at process, impact and outcome, and identifies realistic ways of assessing what may be very small changes over long periods of time. It will probably not be possible to evaluate every element of a project so it may be necessary to prioritise which elements will be assessed.

It may be helpful to think in terms of charting changes as they occur, using a framework to record these systematically. An example of this approach is the 'Outcome Measures Checklist' used in a community health project described in Case Study 15.2.

Stage 6. Setting an Action Plan

There are many things to consider here, but the main one is to identify what you plan to do, step by achievable step.

You may need to build the following activities into your action plan:

Reviewing aims and priorities It is necessary to review continuously the aims and priorities originally set down for the project, and compare them with those of the people who are now involved. You may need to modify your original aims, and constantly check out whose agenda you are working to – your own or the community's?

Consulting and being accountable to the community We recommended consultation before you set up, but this needs to continue all through. Once your project is established, you have a continuing responsibility to tell the community about its role and what work is going on. This could be through meetings, newsletters, electronic networks and open days, for example.

Arranging a management committee or steering group A management committee or steering group should provide a secure foundation for the project, taking responsibility for its continued development, its policies, and management tasks such as fundraising and recruiting. It should also provide support for the workers. Usually

Case study 15.2	A Checklist for Charting Changes in a Community[14]

A 3-year project ran on a housing estate where residents were identified as being at high risk for heart disease. Using a community development approach, a community health worker worked with local residents on issues which residents identified as important. Over the life of the project, changes were noted, many of which became embedded as permanent features in the community. These changes were charted by the project worker in a systematic way, using the following **outcome measures checklist.**

Type of change	Information recorded	Examples
Participation of target population in health-related action	Numbers and characteristics (age range, sex, etc.) of people who attend groups and community activities	Number and age range of young parents attending a new parent and toddler group
Perceived changes in knowledge, attitude and behaviour of target population	Changes in attitude towards participation in group and community activity; change in beliefs about ability to have control over one's own life and the power of group action; changes in the subjective experience of belonging to a community; changes in the capacity of local groups to identify problems and collaborate to solve these	Action group set up by local people to get better play facilities on the estate. Led to establishment of local play group run by local women. Many members stopped smoking
Changes in demand for health-related services	Changes in demand or requests for services or facilities	Groups requested talks from health visitors on health issues. Request for more accessible primary health care facilities on the estate
Changes in the availability of support, facilities and resources for people wanting to change lifestyle	Changes in group and community activities, informal social and support networks within the community	New groups to support young single parents. 'Get Cooking' group to help people learn to cook healthier food for their family. Exercise group for older people
Other physical changes to the environment	Any changes to the built or natural environment	Playground built. Traffic calming schemes introduced
Changes in knowledge, attitudes, skills and practices of local health and allied workers	Changes in attitudes towards local residents to exercise choice and control over the services they receive, or changes in ways of working	Local health visitors use experienced local mothers to support young new parents
Changes in policy and procedures by local statutory and voluntary organisations	Changes that enable local people to have more say in decisions about local services	Consultation with local residents about location and design of new GP surgery on the estate
Dissemination of good practice	What information was sent out and why, talks, presentations, papers published and any evidence that good practice elsewhere has been affected	Article in community health journal. Community health projects featured in health authority public health report
Any other outcomes	Any other outcomes, expected or unexpected, which fall into the above categories	

the workers are members of the group; they should not be expected to run the management committee themselves, but sometimes this is the case. This is not desirable because it leads to confusion about who is managing whom, and puts an unreasonable burden on the workers.

A management group could consist of both local workers, such as health visitors and social workers, and local people, perhaps representing groups the project is in contact with.

It may be helpful to get the members of a management committee/steering committee together for a day, to talk through the issues, clarify aims and foster a sense of teamwork.

Writing job descriptions Paid project workers need clear job descriptions, specifying what is included. For example, does the job include fundraising, doing your own typing, servicing or even running the management committee meetings, keeping the accounts, evaluating, writing progress reports?

Ensuring support for the project workers Recognise the value of networking as a means of informal training and support. By 'networking' we mean making time and resources available to meet other people doing similar work and to link with other community health projects in different parts of the country. This enables information and ideas to be shared, problems discussed and encouragement given, fostering a vital sense of not 'going it alone'. Access to e-mail and the Internet can help. The need to ensure that project workers are not isolated in what may be very slow and at times discouraging work cannot be over-stressed.

Networking also means that more people will know about your project and you may get more support. Consider developing a website to promote your project. Other people, too, may benefit if they have also been experiencing isolation.

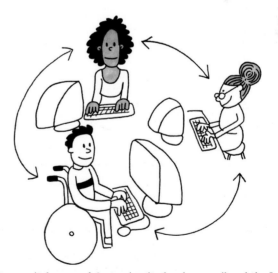

Networking fosters a vital sense of 'not going it alone' – e-mail and the Internet can help

Formalising your project group It may be helpful at some stage to look at the costs and benefits of formalising a project group that started off as a loose collection of interested people. The advantages of having a formal organisation are that it can apply for financial help and for recognition as a legitimate body; the disadvantages might be that control could be exercised from outside, or that members are attracted who turn out to be more of a hindrance than a help. The local Council for Voluntary Service can be extremely useful because it provides a helpful service for newly formed groups, and affiliation to the Council brings credibility in itself.

Dealing with friends and enemies The issues your project is concerned with will probably have a local history, and be likely to have both lost and won support in the past. You need to identify other interest groups, and decide how to tackle them. Study the tactics and arguments of any 'opposition' and plan your strategy.

Stage 7. Implementing Your Plan

As you implement your plan, you may run into difficulties because of flagging interest, a feeling of losing your way, and, finally, that the project has to come to an end. Some suggestions about these three issues are as follows.

Keeping going With the passage of time, people may lose their enthusiasm. You may be able to provide additional impetus by having the advantage of being involved as a whole or part of your paid work. You need to be sensitive to the many ways by which a project can lose its way, and in such circumstances you may be able to help by:

- discovering what similar activities are taking place elsewhere and circulating details
- drawing the issue to the attention of relevant statutory agencies, and conveying the response to the group
- helping the group to produce its own health promotion materials such as posters, leaflets, website or video, and distributing them
- looking at other health promotion material on topics of interest
- encouraging members of the project to talk about their work to other people, such as groups of interested professionals and students
- sending memos or e-mails to everyone to remind them of meetings
- providing practical support such as photocopying or access to a computer
- introducing new members.

Working out what to do next If you feel that you have lost your way, it can help to write down what information you have found, what contacts you have made, what needs and aims you have identified and what you have done so far. Then seek the views of your management/steering group (if there is one) or the impartial views of someone who has not been involved. Exercise 15.3 may help to provide a focus for working out what to do next.

Leavings and endings There comes a point when your involvement has to stop, maybe because you change your job or the priorities of your work, or because the project work has been taken on by local people. Occasionally, you will need to recognise that you have done all you could do, and that there is no potential in the project any more. Ending your involvement provides the opportunity for a final evaluation of what has been achieved and what your own contribution has been, and for making recommendations for future action.

| Exercise 15.3 | **Planning Community Health Work** |

The following exercise may be useful when you are starting community health work or taking stock part way through a piece of work.

Complete the following statements as far as you can:

The key issue is . . .
The people I need to talk to are . . .
The documents I need to read are . . .
I can get to know more about the community by . . .
The information that is likely to be available is . . .
I intend to look for this information by . . .
Work done on this issue elsewhere is . . .
The people who are likely to be supportive are . . .
The people I should avoid offending are . . .
The period of time I can spend on this issue is . . .
The amount of time I can give it during this period is . . .
The person/people I will talk to in order to work out what to do next is . . .

Developing Competence in Community Work

To be a successful community health worker, you need to develop a range of knowledge and skills, and have certain crucial values and attitudes.[15]

In terms of values and attitudes, you will need to be committed to the principles and ideals of community-based work which we outlined earlier in this chapter: the centrality of the community, your own role as a facilitator rather than an 'expert', the importance of addressing inequalities, and a broad perspective on health.

See Chapter 1, section Inequalities in Health and Chapter 3.

In order to hold these values and attitudes with depth and conviction, you will need knowledge of key issues, such as the extent and cause of inequalities in health, the effects of racism, sexism and other forms of oppression on health, and awareness of the structures, policies and powers which influence the lives and health of communities. You will also need to be clear about your own particular political ideologies.

See the section above on getting to know the community and its needs, Chapter 4, section Agents and Agencies of Health Promotion and Exercise 4.1, and Chapter 6, section Finding and Using Information.

Other areas of knowledge include knowledge of local health resources: who and where to go to for information, advice and materials on health issues. Knowledge of local health services and social services is vital; so is understanding how local statutory and voluntary agencies work, and how to use 'the system' effectively. An understanding of the community itself is of course vital too.

A range of skills is required. It is important to have skills of raising awareness of inequalities and discrimination, and being able to counter these by taking positive action when appropriate and working in an anti-discriminatory way.

See Chapters 5, 7, 8 for planning and managing; 10 for communication; 11 for using communication tools; 13 for working with groups.

Other skills are to do with working with people: being able to communicate well, facilitate groups and have effective meetings, for example. You also need skills of planning and management, using and producing health promotion materials, and working for political change.

A list of useful agencies is given at the end of this chapter.[16]

PRACTICE POINTS

■ Community-based work means working with communities (rather than individuals) over a period of time to enable them to increase control over, and improve, their health. It may involve you in community development work, specific community health projects and group work.

■ A key principle is that community work is 'bottom-up', not 'top-down'. This means that you respond to issues that the community identifies, rather than working on issues identified by people outside the community, such as health workers from statutory agencies.

■ Community health workers are facilitators rather than health experts, whose role is to develop the community's ability to identify health needs and meet them.

■ Work is often focused on addressing inequalities and working with people who are disadvantaged.

■ Health is interpreted widely to encompass social, emotional and societal well-being.

■ It is important for you to encourage community participation as much as possible in health planning and health promotion activity, and to consider all the ways of doing this.

■ You need particular skills and processes for successful community development work and community health projects. You need to be aware of the potential conflicts and difficulties inherent in this kind of work.

Recommended Reading

On Community Work

➤ Twelvetrees A 1998 Community work, 3rd edn. Basingstoke: Palgrave. (A practical guide for community workers.)

On Community Participation

➤ Heller T, Muston R, Sidell M, Lloyd C 2001 Working for health. London: The Open University in association with Sage Publications. Chapter 20, User Involvement and Participation in the NHS: A Personal Perspective.

➤ Labyrinth Consultancy 2000 Community participation for health: a review of good practice in community participation health projects and initiatives. London: Health Education Authority. (This report describes factors that help and hinder community participation as well as providing guidelines for good practice.)

On Community Health Work

➤ *Community Health Action* is the journal of Community Health UK. Each issue contains reports and articles on community health work, with a focus on a specific themes in each issue. (For address see Note 16 below.)

➤ Jones L, Sidell M (eds) 1997 The challenge of promoting health – exploration and action. Basingstoke: Macmillan/Open University. (Part 1, Promoting health at the local level – the collective approach, has chapters dealing with working with primary health care teams, local communities, community action, participation, evaluation of community action.)

➤ Naidoo J, Wills J 2000 Health promotion: foundations for practice, 2nd edn. London: Baillière Tindall. (Chapter 10 covers working with communities and community development.)

➤ North Cumbria Health Development Unit 2001 Building healthy communities: a resource pack for multi-agency health improvement. Available from

North Cumbria Health Development Unit, Workington Infirmary, Infirmary Road, Workington, Cumbria, CA14 2UN.

➤ Standing Conference for Community Development 2001 Strategic Framework for Community Development Sheffield: SCCD. (The framework describes what community development is and the values that underpin it. The process of community development is described as well as the resources required for effective community development. The roles of evaluation, quality and networking are considered.)

➤ Tones K, Tilford S 2001 Health education: effectiveness, efficiency and equity, 3rd edn. Cheltenham: Nelson Thornes. (Chapter 9 discusses the meaning of community, community development, participation, networks and community health projects.)

On Community Health Work with Ethnic Minority Groups

➤ Paton A, Higgins J 2000 Health promotion and ethnic minority groups. In: Kerr J (ed.) Community health promotion: challenges for practice, Chapter 11. London: Baillière Tindall

International Examples of Community Involvement in Health Development

➤ Kahssay M H, Oakley P (eds) 1999 Community involvement in health development: a review of the concept and practice. Geneva: World Health Organization. (Provides a methodology for community involvement and focuses on three case studies in Bolivia, Nepal and Senegal.)

On Tackling Poverty

➤ Ideas, analysis, information and examples of action to tackle poverty, including community health action are available from the UKPHA, 7th Floor, Fleming House, Renfrew Street, Glasgow, G3 6ST Tel: 0870 0101931 Website: www.ukpha.org.uk/poverty.htm

➤ Naidoo J, Wills J 1998 Practising health promotion: dilemmas and challenges. London: Baillière Tindall.

(Chapter 4, Promoting equity in health promotion: health and poverty, discusses looking at strategies for promoting health in poverty, including community development approaches.)

On Evaluation of Community Health Work

➤ Charities Evaluation Service Evaluating ourselves series: titles include Monitoring ourselves, Managing evaluation, and Developing aims and objectives. (For address see Note 16 below.)

➤ Community Health Action is the journal of Community Health UK. Issue 41, Vol. 4, 1996 contains useful articles on the theme of evaluation. (For address see Note 16 below.)

➤ Luck M, Jesson J 1996 Evaluation of community health development. Community Health UK. (An overview of community health development and evaluation, with particular reference to a project in Corby. For address see Note 16 below.)

➤ Roberts E 2000 Evaluating your health project: a guide for community health development workers and local people. Bristol: Health Promotion Service Avon. (Available from the Health Promotion Manager, Bristol North Primary Care Trust, King Square House, King Square, Bristol BS2 8EE.)

➤ The Scottish Community Development Centre 2000 Learning, evaluation and planning handbook. Glasgow: The Scottish Community Development Centre. Available from the Scottish Community Development Centre, 329 Baltic Chambers, 50 Wellington Street, Glasgow, G2 6HJ. Tel: 0141 248 1964. Also on website (www.scdc.org.uk)

On Working with Voluntary Organisations

➤ Hanvey C, Philpot T (eds) 1996 Sweet charity – the role and workings of voluntary organisations. London: Routledge. (Covers a range of aspects of voluntary organisation work, including campaigning, fund-raising, marketing and management.)

Notes and References

1   Definition in:

World Health Organization 1984 Health promotion: a WHO discussion document on the concepts and principles. Reprinted in: Journal of the Institute of Health Education 23(1), 1985. (For discussion of this definition, see Chapter 2.)

2   Adapted from: London Community Health Resource & National Council for Voluntary Organisations 1987 Guide to community health projects. London: National Community Health Resource

3   These definitions draw on the work of:

Channon G 1990 in Adams L, Smithies J (eds) Community participation and health promotion. London: Health Education Authority

The definition of community development also draws on:

Association of Metropolitan Authorities 1989 Community development, the local authority role. London: Association of Metropolitan Authorities

4   This framework is adapted from:

Brager C, Sprecht H 1973 Community organising. Columbia: Columbia University Press

5   These suggestions are adapted from:

Adams L, Smithies J 1990 Community participation and health promotion. London: Health Education Authority

Labyrinth Consultancy 2000 Community participation for health: a review of good practice in community participation health projects and initiatives. London: Health Education Authority

6   For more information for getting communities on line and building electronic communities visit the website www.partnerships.org.uk

7   Cooper H, Arber S, Fee L, Ginn J 1999 The influence of social support and social capital on health: a review and analysis of British data. London: Health Education Authority

8   Adapted from a questionnaire by Lee Adams and David Hawkins and reproduced by kind permission.

9   Hull Developing Our Communities 2001 Annual report. Hull: Hull DOC

For more information contact: Hull DOC, 86 Twelfth Avenue, Hull HU6 9LE. Tel: 01482 854550. Website: www.ourcoms.org.uk

10 Whitehead M 1989 Swimming upstream: trends and prospects in education for health. London: King's Fund Institute, p. 34

11 Examples of community health projects:

Bruce N et al (eds) 1996 Research and change in urban community health. Aldershot: Avebury. (An edited collection of conference contributions, including many chapters describing specific community health projects.)

Dwelly T 2001 Creative regeneration: lessons from ten community arts projects. Birmingham: Joseph Rowntree Foundation

Mitchell J 2000 Health promotion and community care: the neighbourhood health strategy. In: Kerr J (ed) Community Health Promotion: Challenges for Practice. Chapter 14. London: Baillière Tindall. (Describes a community development project in Stockport.)

The Health Education Journal (vol. 58, No 4, December 1999) contains several papers on the theme of community development, especially focusing on evaluation.

12 This section draws on material in:

Guidelines for setting up projects. In: Community Health Initiatives Resource Unit & London Community Health Resource 1987 Guide to community health projects, Chapter 4.

Henderson P, Thomas D N 1980 Skills in neighbourhood work. National Institute of Social Services Library, no. 39. London: George Allen & Unwin

Standing Conference for Community Development 2001 Strategic framework for community development. Sheffield: SCCD

Kings Fund 2001 Strategic action programme for healthy communities. London: Kings Fund. A set of key point documents are available free of charge from: The Administrator, Public Health Programme, Kings Fund, 11–13 Cavendish Square, London WIC 0AN. Tel: 020 7307 2672. Website: www.kingsfund.org.uk/ePublicHealth

13 Based on ideas in:

De Groot R 1996 Much is written, but little is read. Community Health Action, 1(41), 3.

14 Based on the 'Outcome Measures Checklist' developed for the Health Education Authority/Look After Your Heart-Avon Localities Project, which included a three-year community development project in an estate of high health need in Weston-Super-Mare, North Somerset. More about the project, and the checklist, can be found in:

Bruce N et al (eds) 1996 Research and change in urban community health. Aldershot: Avebury. (Chapter 18 is on the HEA/LAYH-Avon Localities project on the Bournville Estate, Weston-Super-Mare.)

Ewles L, Miles U, Velleman G 1995 Promoting heart health on an urban housing estate. Community Health Action, 35, 12–14.

Ewles L, Miles U, Velleman G 1996 Lessons learnt from a community heart disease prevention project. Journal of the Institute of Health Education 34(1), 15–19

15 This section is derived from:

Smithies J 1987 Training needs of community health workers. National Community Health Resource. Unpublished report on community health workers training project.

See also: North Cumbria Health Development Unit 2001 Building healthy communities: a resource pack for multi-agency health improvement. Available from North Cumbria Health Development Unit, Workington Infirmary, Infirmary Road, Workington, Cumbria, CA14 2UN

16   Useful agencies are:

Community Health UK, 3 The Yard, PO Box 2977, Freshford, Bath BA2 7YR. Tel 01225 723779. Fax 01225 722024. Website: www.chuk.org. E-mail: mail@chuk.org. This organisation exists to promote and support community health development in the UK. It acts as a source of information and advice; supports projects and provides forums for community health groups; enables community health workers to share experiences through publications, conferences and other events; creates links and fosters partnerships between the voluntary sector and statutory services; promotes collaborative work by linking groups and individuals sharing common interests and concerns. It has a membership subscription scheme.

SCCD Standing Conference for Community Development (supporting people who support communities), Floor 4, Furnival House, 48 Furnival Gate, Sheffield S1 4QP. Tel 0114 270 1718. Fax: 0114 276 7496. Website: www.comm-dev.co.uk. E-mail: admin@sccd.solis.co.uk. This organisation provides support to local networks through the provision of information and networking events. SCCD believes that new policies relating to community development should be based on tried and tested practice, reflecting the skills and experience that exist in the field. It is a membership subscription scheme, with members receiving regular copies of SCCD News and being entitled to attend their conferences.

Two agencies that can help with evaluation of community health work are:

Charities Evaluation Service, 4 Coldbath Square, London EC1R 5HL. Tel: 0207 713 5722. Provides training, external evaluation, consultancy, advice, information and publications.

The Association for Research in the Voluntary and Community Sector (ARVAC), 2D Aberdeen Studios, 22–24 Highbury Grove, London N5 2EA. Tel: 0207 704 2315. Website: www.arvac.org. ARVAC is a research network with members from academic, voluntary, community and statutory organisations. It provides training, publications and information.

Community Matters, Charlton House, 36 Hunslet Road, Leeds, LS10 1JN. Tel: 0113 245 6634 Website: www.comm-dev.co.uk. Community Matters produces publications and provides training to enable its members and other community organisations to share good practice.

16 Changing Policy and Practice

SUMMARY

We consider how health policy at local and national level is made, how it can be influenced, and discuss how health promoters can challenge health-damaging policies. We look at the characteristics of power and influence and the politics of influence, illustrated with a case study. We follow with sections on developing and implementing policies, a case study exercise on policy implementation, and end with a section on campaigning.

See Chapter 7, section Linking Your Work into Broader Health Promotion Plans and Strategies, for information on national and local public health strategies and plans.

Health promoters are engaged in influencing policies and practices that affect health. By a 'policy' we mean a broad statement of the principles of how to proceed in relation to a specific issue, such as a national policy on transport, a local authority policy on housing, or a policy on how to deal with alcohol issues in a workplace. Policies can be at any level, from national to the day-to-day work of a health promoter.

In order to influence policy and practice, you need to understand how power is distributed and exercised between people at any level, from a group of colleagues to those in positions of great authority or influence. You need to be able to use that knowledge to affect decisions. (This process of understanding the distribution of power and how it is used, and using that knowledge to further your work, is what we mean by 'being political'.)

Changing policy and practice includes working with statutory, voluntary and commercial organisations to influence them to develop health-promoting policies for their staff and to produce health-enhancing products and services. It also includes working for healthy public policies and economic and regulatory changes requiring campaigning, lobbying and taking political action.

We discuss another relevant and important aspect – implementing change – in Chapter 8, section on managing change.

In this chapter we look first at local and national health policy and the contribution of health promoters to making and influencing policies. We then focus on three practical aspects of changing policy and practice that we see as especially relevant in health promotion: understanding the politics of influence, developing and implementing health promotion policies, and campaigning.

Making and Influencing Local and National Health Policy

First we consider who makes health policy at the local and national levels, the mechanism for implementation, and opportunities for influence.

The importance of making policy changes as an integral part of health promotion is increasingly being recognised. We are concerned here with both local and national policies, because health promoters working at a local level can press for the introduction of policies at both levels and have an influence on how they are implemented. Furthermore, the development of local policies cannot be divorced from government policies: central government's policy and allocation of funds shape the nature of, and the resources for, health service, local authority and voluntary organisation work at local level. The evolution of national policy is in turn influenced by representations from health services and local authorities, voluntary agencies and other bodies.

National health promotion agencies and public health organisations are also active in the field of policy development.[1]

Local Health Policy

At a local level, during the last decade healthy public policies and priorities have increasingly been jointly agreed by health, local authority and voluntary agencies, which has improved their effectiveness.[2] With the introduction in the late 1990s of Health Improvement Programmes (subsequently Health Improvement and Modernisation Plans, HIMPs), Neighbourhood Renewal Strategies and Community Strategies, health and partner agencies are required to deliver joint plans for health and well-being.[3] This means that policies can be agreed by local authorities, primary care trusts (accountable to strategic health authorities), and other relevant community organisations such as the Commission for Racial Equality, trade unions, housing associations and voluntary organisations. The Local Strategic Partnerships (LSPs) are one vehicle by which this policy-making process is put into action.[4]

The structure of the NHS, including PCTs and Strategic Health Authorities, is outlined in Chapter 4. We say more about LSPs later in this chapter.

Some health organisations and local authorities undertake *health impact assessments* or *environmental impact assessments* of their services.[5] This involves examining the impact on health and/or the environment of all current and planned policies and activities. The purpose is to develop practical ways in which current health and environmental impact of services could be improved and to inform the development of a corporate approach to new health and environmental policies.

See Chapter 7, section Health Impact Assessment.

Health Policy in the NHS

The task of commissioning health services and programmes was undertaken by health authorities until 2002, when it passed to primary care trusts (PCTs). (*Commissioning* health services means deciding what health services and programmes are needed to improve the health status of the local population and ensuring that they are provided.) Performance agreements are now made between PCTs and their new strategic health authority, to which they are accountable.

See Figure 4.2 in Chapter 4 for the structure of the NHS in England.

PCTs provide opportunities for the public to comment on health service plans. There are representatives of the public on PCT management boards (usually called lay representatives) and PCTs generally consult the public on any significant proposals for change. Individuals, groups, professional associations and others are able to express their views on, for example, the balance of money spent on treatment and care compared with health promotion and disease prevention. Some PCT board members have responsibility for ensuring that the PCT properly addresses specific areas of work such as inequalities in health or involving the public in health service planning.

Implementing National Health Policies at Local Level

National strategies for health are outlined in detail *in* Chapter 7, and referred to in Chapters 1 and 4.

Formal national strategies for health have been in place since the early 1990s. Here we discuss how national health policy, and national strategies for health, are implemented in the NHS.

National strategies for health set national targets for health, which are ways of expressing specific health outcomes. PCTs and partner agencies from the public, private and voluntary sectors translate these national targets into local ones, and may add other local targets. These targets, and the priorities and objectives they are derived from, are an important influence on decisions about providing health promotion programmes and activities.

For example, the *National Service Framework for Coronary Heart Disease*[6] – a national document which sets out the standards for services about prevention and treatment of heart disease and strokes – sets national targets for reduced death rates from heart disease and stroke, and targets that focus on changes in risk behaviour, such as smoking. These targets are translated into local targets in local HIMPs. HIMPs therefore include health promotion programmes on smoking prevention, such as providing smoking cessation help as part of maternity services, or ensuring that hospitals are smoke-free zones. In this way, national strategies become part of local health service provision.

See also Chapter 7, section Local Health Strategies and Initiatives, for more about HIMPs and other local plans and strategies.

Local Strategic Partnerships and Community Strategies

The local authority contribution to health gain is made at a strategic level through LSPs, and the development of Community Strategies.[7] LSPs bring together people from the public, private and voluntary sectors. They aim to avoid duplication and to rationalise separate partnerships and plans to make it easier to deliver action around health improvement, education and crime, for example. HIMPS (for which the health services are predominantly responsible) come under this broader umbrella as part of a local Community Plan. The Neighbourhood Renewal Strategy is the driving force behind these partnerships and plans and has a direct impact on health gain.[8]

See also Chapter 7, section Local Health Strategies and Initiatives, for more about local plans and strategies.

Local Agenda 21

Another important way in which health services and local authorities can work together at local level is through cooperating in implementing Local Agenda 21 strategies. These are agreements forged by governments at the Earth Summit in Rio de Janeiro in 1992, sometimes referred to as 'green plans', which focus on ways of achieving *sustainable development*.[9] Sustainable development means development that meets the needs of the present without damaging the health or environment of future generations. It is about the life we experience as individuals and communities in our local environment, but also about the far-reaching effects of our lifestyles on other parts of the world.

Local authorities often work with each other and consult their communities about future developments. Health services form part of such alliances – cooperating, for example, on cycleways and the use of public land for people to pursue healthy activities in a safe environment. Public participation in Local Agenda 21 is an important part of the process. Health promoters, in both their working role and their role as private citizens, can play their part.

The Voice of the Consumer in the NHS

In *The NHS Plan* (2000)[10] the government made a clear commitment to the NHS of the 21st century, being responsive to the needs of all individuals and groups within society. Citizens and patients should to have their voice heard about health-related public policies, planning and provision of services.

How is this voice heard? Ultimately, it is through the democratic process and the right to vote for the elected government. In the 1990s the government took a number of steps to enable consumers to express their views on health services more directly. One of the most obvious examples was *The Patient's Charter*, which set out patients' rights and the standards of service that patients could expect from the NHS.[11]

The *NHS Charter* replaced the *Patient's Charter* in 2001, clarifying how people can access NHS services, what commitment people can expect from the NHS and what their rights and responsibilities are as patients.[12] A new Patient Advice and Liaison Service (PALS) was set up in every NHS trust for patients to get their concerns addressed. Other measures announced in *The NHS Plan* to ensure that citizens and patients have more influence at all levels of the NHS include:

- independent local advisory forums (made up of local residents) to act as sounding boards for policies and priorities such as those set out in the local HIMP
- increased lay representation on regulatory bodies (such as the General Medical Council), boards (such as the national NHS Modernisation Board) and commissions (such as the Commission for Health Improvement – a national body responsible for ensuring good quality services in the NHS)
- a new Citizens' Council, to advise the National Institute for Clinical Excellence (a national body which oversees standards of clinical practice).

All these forums are relevant to health promotion policies and programmes.

Challenging Health-damaging Policy[13]

A question health promoters often pose is: what can you do when you are faced with policies that you perceive as health damaging?

This question often induces feelings of helplessness and frustration because such policies come from 'high places' such as national government or (closer to home) your own employer or even your own direct manager. To protest may seem a futile waste of energy and can cause a conflict of loyalty between wanting to press for what you see as right and what is decreed to be right by your employing authority. To protest or take action may be seen as 'trouble-making' or 'too political'.

There is no easy answer to this issue, but there are some positive steps worth considering.

- **Use your vote**. At the next general or local election, look at the health implications in the policy manifestos. Raise questions about health policy with doorstep canvassers, at public meetings and by writing to candidates. All this can be done in your capacity as a private citizen rather than a health worker.
- **Use your professional association or trade union**. These groups can raise issues at a national and local level, and can be a powerful voice. You can play your part by joining and supporting their activities, and raising the issues you feel strongly about.

- **Use your representative**. There are many people whose job is to represent your interests. At European Union or national level, it is your Member of the European Parliament (MEP) or your MP. So if you want to raise an issue at these levels, lobby your MEP or MP: send letters, telephone, attend 'surgeries'. At local level, do the same with your local councillor.[14] You could also contact your professional association or union local branch representative.

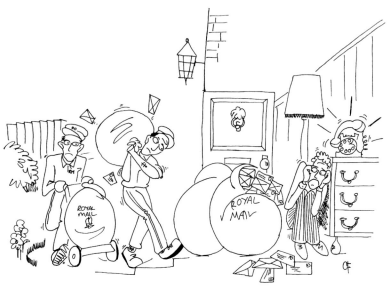

Lobby your MP

- **Use your collective power**. If you are concerned about an issue at your place of work, it may help to find out if colleagues feel the same. If they do, join together so that you raise the issue collectively, which is likely to give it more impact and take the heat off any one individual. Or at a national level, join with others who share your concern to improve health and challenge health-damaging policies. For example, the UK Public Health Association (UKPHA) aims to widen the focus of health policy in the UK towards creating a healthy environment, reducing inequalities and improving quality of life.[15]

However, many areas of policy development are not controversial, and indeed can be a positive and rewarding part of the day-to-day work of health promoters. The main thrust is likely to be in developing, changing and implementing local policies. To do this you need to understand the characteristics of power and influence and to be competent at exerting influence when necessary. We look at this in the next sections.

Characteristics of Power and Influence

Power is the ability to influence others. There are four generally recognised types of power that are relevant to health promotion work:

- **Position power** is the power vested in someone because of their position in an organisation. For example, the chief executive of a local authority has position power.

■ **Resource power** is the power to allocate, or limit, resources, including money and staff. It often goes hand-in-hand with position power. For example, a senior manager in the health service has both position power and the power to regulate the use of resources. You have a real source of power if you have the authority to control the allocation of any resources that people want. Every health promoter will have some power because people want the skills or services on offer.

■ **Expert power** is power related to special expertise. Consultants in the health service will have the expert power associated with their clinical speciality.

■ **Personal power** is the power that comes from the personal attributes of a person – including strong personality, charisma and ability to inspire. It is closely related to leadership qualities, such as above-average intelligence, initiative, self-confidence and the ability to rise above a situation and see it in perspective (the 'helicopter' trait). However, effective leaders are not always charismatic, and what makes a leader effective in one situation may cause them to be less effective in changed circumstances. The classic example of this is Sir Winston Churchill: the attributes that made him effective in wartime were not so appropriate in peacetime.

You may sometimes be in the position of wishing to exert influence on people who have a stronger power base. For example, a health visitor may wish to influence a general practitioner to adopt a policy of supporting the running of antenatal clinics in the local ethnic minority group's community centre, or a community worker may want to lobby local councillors about the need for more recreational facilities for young people on a housing estate. To do this requires skills in influencing.

See Chapter 5, The Basic Planning and Evaluation Process.

Before attempting to influence someone who is more powerful, first consider (as always) the basic questions in the planning process, such as: What are your aims? What resources do you need? Is the investment going to be worth it? Could the aim be achieved more easily another way?

The Politics of Influence[16]

The elements of any strategy aiming to change policy and practice could include:

■ key aspects of planning
■ making allies
■ networking
■ making deals and negotiating.

We now consider each of these in turn.

Planning

Three particular aspects of planning are useful to consider: undertaking a force field analysis, identifying stakeholders, and considering your timing.

Undertake a force field analysis A force field analysis identifies the helping and hindering forces in your situation and helps to pinpoint how you can influence the process to make progress towards change. You identify how you can increase the power of the helping forces and decrease the power of the hindering forces.

There is an example of a force field analysis at the end of Chapter 4, Exercise 4.2.

Identify the stakeholders The stakeholders are those people with a vested interest in the issue, who wish to influence what is done and how it is done. They are obviously powerful forces in the situation. It could be difficult to identify all the stakeholders, because some of them may not wish to be visible and try to work covertly through others.

Time your action It is also important to consider when to introduce a proposal or when to delay. If people are already preoccupied with other major issues, it might not be the right time to make a new proposal. On the other hand, if a proposal will help other people to attain their own objectives, now may be a good time.

Making Allies

Identify which of the stakeholders could be allies, and gain their trust and confidence in order to establish and maintain an alliance. It helps to pay attention to their concerns, values, beliefs and behaviour patterns, and to see what you need to do in order to form an effective working alliance.

For example, if you are concerned about the way in which people with disabilities are treated in an organisation, you might identify the person in charge of human resources as a key stakeholder. So find out: is she concerned about it? Does she think it is important for her organisation? What kind of way does she work: is she likely to respond best to a lively discussion on the subject or to a well-argued paper on the need for policy, backed up with facts and figures? Does she like time to make decisions? Will she be happy to leave you to take the lead, or will she want to feel that the initiative lies with her?

Networking

Many people working in organisations belong to one or more interest groups who meet to discuss, debate and exchange information on issues that concern the members. These interest groups are networks. By playing an active role in networks, people can extend their influence. Networks provide access to information that can help with making a case, to people with experience of successful influencing, and to other resources. There are different types of networks:

Professional networks Members are from the same profession. Professional networks may attempt to influence employers and organisations to reconsider their policies or to develop new policies for the future. Professional networks institute criteria for professional practice and are active in the professional development of their members.

Elitist networks Members of an elitist group can join by invitation only. The network operates by personal contact and personal introduction, such as 'old boy' links. Members of such networks may have considerable power and influence, often through their position in organisations.

Pressure groups Members wish to pursue certain objectives, which may be environmental, social or political. In order to enter a particular network it may be necessary to identify the 'gatekeepers' who control entry, and other people who are influential in the network and could act as a sponsor for someone seeking to join. Having entered a network it is important to support the values and established ways of working. Later, having been accepted, it may be possible to challenge accepted practices.

Making Deals and Negotiating

Making deals is common practice in most organisations. Individuals or groups agree to support a proposal in return for agreement on something that benefits them. In order to make deals successfully, it pays to know the person with whom you are dealing, paying careful attention to the values and intentions of the other party and what you could realistically expect from them.

For detailed descriptions of these steps and how best to approach negotiations, see the suggestions for further reading at the end of this chapter.

Negotiation is the art of creating agreement on a specific issue between two or more parties with different views. Successful negotiation takes place when there is a desire to solve problems and the parties genuinely commit to going through a number of steps.

Case study 16.1   **The Politics of Influence – Health and Safety at Work**

Bob is an environmental health officer working for Midshire City Council. His aim is to improve the implementation of the health and safety at work policy of the council. He makes a list of the *helping* forces and the *hindering* forces:

Helping:

- the existing safety officers
- existing codes of practice, for example, sight checks for VDU operators
- a councillor who is a health lecturer at the university
- a human resources officer interested in improving the working environment for staff
- an existing commitment to appoint an occupational health nurse.

Hindering:

- the cost of any improvements (the council has severe financial constraints)
- staff time to attend health and safety training
- problems with recruiting an occupational health nurse
- deficiencies in the structure of council buildings (poor ventilation, open-plan offices, lack of showers for those staff wishing to take physical exercise during the day)
- lack of councillors' commitment to improve health and safety conditions for staff
- lack of access to council buildings for disabled people.

He identifies the stakeholders as:

- the staff themselves
- the trade unions
- departmental managers, senior and chief officers
- the councillors
- the public health specialist and the health promotion specialist from the local PCT.

He further identifies key stakeholders as:

- officers in the department of engineering because they enforce building regulations
- council members on the health committee
- the director of personnel.

He then identifies ways of increasing the helping forces and decreasing the hindering forces. Through making an ally of the interested human resources officer he is able to increase the commitment of the director of human resources, who is also a chief officer. One short-term outcome is that an occupational health nurse is recruited. Another outcome is a plan agreed by the human resources department and the trade unions for training staff in health and safety.

By joining a local network of people interested in health promotion he is able to find out what is going on elsewhere, and this gives him some useful ideas, including sources of help in stress management training which he incorporates into the training plan.

He makes a deal with the engineering depart-ment by agreeing to assist with monitoring con-struction sites of new buildings in order to prevent accidents on the site. In return, they agree to assist with a plan for improving sound-proofing and modifications to open-plan offices. Their commitment grows after a report shows that accidents on construction sites are reduced. He discusses with them the issue of raising with council members the plan for modifying coun-cil buildings.

Finally, he makes an ally of the councillor at the university by offering to provide an input to some of the courses. This councillor is on the health committee and provides him with useful advice on how to approach the com-mittee and how to prepare documents for its consideration.

On Being 'Political' . . .

A final point is about 'political' behaviour, by which we mean finding out about who holds power, and working to use this information to change a situation. When is it acceptable and when is it unethical?

Being 'political' can smack of being devious and manipulative. Many people view political behaviour with suspicion and will therefore not be easily influenced by it. Most people mistrust those who seek to manipulate covertly, or who coerce, lie, or deliber-ately withhold information that affects others. We do not support any of these tactics.

But to ignore the politics within organisations is unwise, because it results in fail-ure to make a realistic appraisal of situations, and failure to make the best of the oppor-tunities for positive health promotion. Furthermore, we contend that it is possible to be 'political' without losing professional integrity. For example, we suggest that deals are best made as the outcome of open negotiations, and that relationships should be based on genuineness, trust, goodwill and mutual respect.

Developing and Implementing Policies

In this section, we look first at the range of health promotion policies, and then at prac-tical guidelines on how to develop and implement polices.

First, what kind of health promotion policies are there? Many are about health issues that relate to workplaces or other settings. Common examples of settings are workplaces, schools, communities and hospitals. Other policies can be about health issues in a range of contexts, such as a national policy on HIV prevention, which would cover action across many different population groups and settings. For some health issues, such as smoking at work, it is common practice to have a policy. Other exam-ples of health issues where there are often policies are mental health, food and healthy eating, alcohol and exercise.

We now look in more detail at policies in specific settings.

Policies on Promoting Health in Workplaces

The benefits of health promotion at work are well established and reviews of the liter-ature identify the major benefits as a decrease in absenteeism and staff turnover, and an increase in productivity and morale.[17] For general workplace policies, the World Health

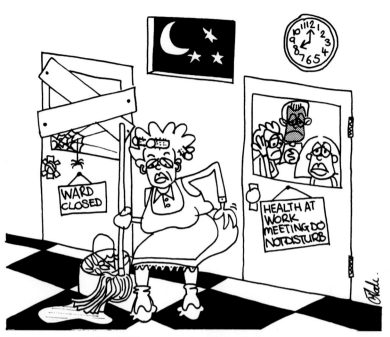

The NHS promotes healthy workplaces

Organization (WHO) provided policy guidance in 1988, which is still of relevance today.[18] In 1996 the European Commission set up the European Network for Workplace Health Promotion.[19] Leading employers and trade unions have begun to take on a wider concept of health at work, including giving priority to issues such as smoking, alcohol, and stress.

'Health at Work in the NHS' is an initiative originally launched in 1992 by the Secretary of State as part of the national strategy for health.[20] It aims to:

- introduce a systematic healthy workplace programme throughout the NHS
- engage all NHS staff in health-promoting activities.

The idea is that the NHS becomes an exemplary employer, demonstrating to others that a healthy workforce benefits both individual staff members and the organisation as a whole. This will help the NHS to provide better services, because healthy staff are more able to care for others.[21]

Finally, the Health and Safety Executive is a source of information on all regulations governing health and safety in the workplace.[22]

Policies on Promoting Health in Hospitals

'Health Promoting Hospitals' is a WHO initiative, originally designed to improve health and environmental conditions for both staff and patients by reviewing and implementing a range of health-promoting policies and activities.[23] The first phase of a WHO Europe pilot hospital project, which in England was based at Preston Hospitals Acute NHS Trust, finished at the end of 1996.[24]

Many hospitals have taken up the idea of being a health-promoting hospital, but it can be difficult in practice to inform and involve everyone in an institution as large and complex as a hospital.

Promoting Health in Urban Settings: 'Healthy Cities'

See Chapter 15 for principles of 'bottom-up' working.

A number of other settings have also been the focus of WHO initiatives. In 1987 the WHO's regional office for Europe initiated a 'Healthy Cities' project, aiming to work from the bottom up, not from the top down, and to involve collaborative work between local government, health authorities, local businesses, community organisations and, of course, individual citizens.

The Health for All (UK) Network is the coordinating body for action on Healthy Cities within the UK.[25] The Healthy Cities work in Liverpool is a good example of what can be achieved.[26] Liverpool was the first city in the UK to produce a City Health Plan (April 1996), which aims to get everyone moving in the same direction to take action on the underlying causes of ill health. Priority areas include the environment, the economy, housing, crime, education, and transport.

Policies on Promoting Health in Schools

See Local Authorities in Chapter 4 for more about health promotion in educational institutions.

Schools have long been regarded as an important setting for health promotion. The European Network of Health Promoting Schools (ENHPS), involving 37 countries, set out to show that schools can be powerful agents for change through the adoption of 'whole school' approaches.[27] This means that the school promotes health not only by a programme of social, personal and health education for the pupils but also by looking at the way the school is run (does it, for example, promote a sense of positive self-esteem and care for others in all it does?), and the health and well-being of teachers and other staff, parents and the wider community who have contact with the school. An evaluation of schools in England found that, with the right support and planning, tangible learning and health gains could be achieved.[28]

See Chapter 4, section on national health promotion agencies, for more about the Health Development Agency.

The government's commitment to the whole school approach to health and learning was confirmed in 1998, with the introduction of the National Healthy School Standard (NHSS) as a joint venture between the Department for Education and Skills and the Department of Health.[29] The Young People's Team, based at the Health Development Agency, supports the development of health and education partnerships at the local level, to help schools implement changes that will improve the environment and ethos of the school, thereby promoting better health and learning.

Health promotion programmes can also cover higher education settings; the WHO leads an initiative on 'Healthy Universities'.[30]

Policies on Promoting Health in Prisons

All prisons are required to develop health promotion programmes and some are developing prison HIMPs. The WHO Regional Office for Europe launched the Health in Prisons Project (HIPP) in 1995 to promote health in prisons, and is working to develop an award scheme for health-promoting prisons.[31]

Guidelines on Developing and Implementing a Policy

Many health promoters have a role in developing and implementing polices in specific settings such as a workplace or a hospital. An example is an alcohol policy in a workplace, as we outline in Exercise 16.1. The process of developing and implementing a health promotion policy involves four aspects: preparation, implementation, education and training, and evaluation.[32] We consider each of these in turn.

Exercise 16.1   A Workplace Alcohol Policy

Westshire NHS hospital trust is encouraged by a national 'sensible drinking' initiative to develop a policy on alcohol for its workforce.

A Senior Health Promotion Specialist working with Westshire trust convenes a working group to develop a policy, which includes representatives of human resources officers, general management, consultant psychiatrists, trade unions and the local voluntary organisation on alcohol.

The working group meets four times, and produces a draft policy. The policy specifies that the trust sees sensible drinking as everyone's responsibility and that all employees will receive basic information about sensible drinking. It also covers the trust's responsibility to develop an environment conducive to self-referral by anyone with an alcohol problem, early identification of alcohol-related problems and the provision of expert confidential help. It looks at the provision of alcohol on trust premises, and specifies that non-alcoholic drinks should be provided as an alternative at all social functions where alcohol is served, and that alcohol consumption should be discouraged at non-social functions.

This draft policy goes to the trust board. It receives a lukewarm reception, and there is much concern that it will interfere with personnel policies on dealing with people who drink on duty. There is also discussion and disagreement about what constitutes 'social' and 'non-social' functions, and resistance to the idea of curtailing 'social' drinking (i.e. selling alcohol at the doctors' bar) and serving it at working lunches, publicity events such as the opening of new clinics, and leaving parties.

Nevertheless, it is passed for consultation, and comes back to the board for final approval. The board members are still unenthusiastic, and one major change they make alters the working group's recommendations on implementation. These were that many different staff groups had a key role, including human resources, health promotion, general management and the training department. This is changed so that responsibility for implementation rests entirely with the trust Director of Human Resources. The alcohol policy is finally approved formally by the trust board.

In the meantime, the trust has been engaged in a major strategic review that has affected many of its services, and there follows a long period of substantial organisational change. Two years after the alcohol policy was approved, it had still not been implemented. There had been no education of the workforce about 'sensible drinking' and no change in the way alcohol was served and sold on trust premises.

Looking at the stages for developing and implementing a workplace policy in the section above, and the section on 'The politics of influence', consider these questions:

- What steps were taken that helped the policy development?
- What else could have been done?
- Why did the policy receive such a lukewarm reception by the trust board? Could anything have been done to prevent this?
- Why was the policy never implemented? Could anything have been done to ensure that the implementation stage actually happened?
- Are there any other significant points to note about the lessons learnt from this case study?

1.   Preparation of the Policy

The formulation of a policy by any organisation is a corporate matter, so the usual starting point is to convene a working group. This group:

- clarifies its terms of reference and elects a Chair
- identifies the need for a policy
- identifies the committee, department or senior person who has overall responsibility for taking the policy forward
- identifies key personnel to consult with and convince of the need for a policy
- establishes a timescale for policy development
- prepares a draft policy and consults widely
- prepares the final draft policy for approval.

In the case of a workplace policy, it is important to involve trade unions. This can be achieved either by including trade union representatives on the working group or by setting up an effective framework for consultation and negotiation. This may be crucial in persuading the workforce to look positively on the new policy.

It is also important that an identified senior member of staff or manager, with political 'clout', acts as a 'champion' for the policy. This person will be crucial in getting the commitment of other managers to the policy.

2.   Implementation of the Policy

This starts with planning, which will include:

- setting aims and objectives
- setting up a system for monitoring and evaluation
- identifying resources and defining key implementation tasks
- defining the role of key personnel
- developing an action plan.

Key personnel should be encouraged to participate actively in identifying their roles and in discussing boundaries and overlap in roles, so that the potential for conflict and confusion is reduced. For example, managers have the primary responsibility for ensuring that their staff are fully conversant with workplace policies and understand what is expected of them. Nevertheless, the trade unions also have a role in informing the workforce of the policy. These sources of information hopefully will be complementary and spell out the same, not contradictory, messages. The open discussion of these issues will help to increase commitment to making the policy work.

Any policy that is not the subject of regular review risks becoming obsolete. So the working group must reconvene at intervals to consider issues such as:

- Does the workforce know about and understand the policy?
- Have attitudes to the health issue covered by the policy changed? If so, how? How do staff feel about the policy?
- Has the behaviour of individual staff changed? Does this include changes in working practices and/or individual lifestyles?
- Are staff getting any help they need?
- Are managers and trade unions supporting the policy?

- Are indicators showing that the policy is making progress towards the attainment of its aims and objectives? For example, in the case of a workplace policy, have absenteeism and sickness reduced? Or have accident rates decreased? Has work performance improved? Is morale better?
- How can we improve the effectiveness of the policy?

3.   Education and Training

This is a continuous process, not a one-off event. Wherever possible it should be integrated into existing provision for professional and managerial staff development. The purposes of education and training include:

- securing the commitment of management (e.g. of elected members, chief officers and senior management in the case of a local authority)
- obtaining the commitment of the whole workforce or group at which the policy is aimed (e.g. the prison population or the staff of a business)
- providing those responsible for implementing the policy with the necessary skills
- overcoming prejudices, discrimination and stereotyping where relevant (for example, in policies on alcohol and HIV/AIDS)
- encouraging and assisting the workforce, or the particular groups of people the policy is concerned with, to make choices and individual lifestyle changes.

4.   Evaluation

See the section Plan Evaluation Methods in Chapter 5 for further suggestions.

This should include evaluation of both process and outcomes. It will require the collection of information, both baseline and on-going.

Campaigning

You, or clients with whom you work, may feel strongly about changing policy or practice about a health issue, and decide that the way forward is to mount a campaign. Or you may wish to run a local campaign to back up a national one, such as local events and publicity to support a national promotion of breastfeeding.

Campaigns can range from short-lived local ones with the objective of making a single change ('save our local cottage hospital') to long-term national ones such as annual 'drinking and driving' campaigns. Pressure groups are made up of the people who are running the campaign, such as the 'Save our Cottage Hospital Campaign Group'. Examples of national pressure groups are Shelter[33] (on homelessness) and Friends of the Earth[34] (on environmental issues). Some pressure groups (such as Shelter) may provide direct services as well as acting as a pressure group.

Principles of Campaigning

Some important principles to keep in mind if you are setting up a campaign:[35]

- **Be persistent:** success requires persistent effort, so you must be committed and prepared to put in a lot of time and energy over as long a period as necessary – which may be a very long time.

- **Be professional:** give care and attention to details (such as well-written letters, preferably not hand written, with the name of the campaign clearly evident), and ensure that activities such as keeping records are undertaken properly.
- **Keep a sense of perspective:** your campaign may be vitally important to you, but being perceived as a fanatical crank (or even being a fanatical crank!) will do your cause no good.
- **Reflect your ideals in your behaviour:** it is no good, for example, campaigning to clean up your neighbourhood if your own front garden looks like a tip. Neither is it helpful to campaign for equal opportunities if the place where your own organisation meets does not have good access for people with disabilities.
- **Be positive:** for example, call yourselves the 'Save the Cottage Hospital Campaign Group' rather than 'Group Against Closing the Cottage Hospital'. Shelter is called the 'National Campaign for the Homeless', not the 'Campaign against Bad Housing'.
- **Join with others:** rival pressure groups campaigning on similar (or even identical) issues waste a lot of time and effort. If someone is already campaigning on 'your' issue, join them rather than setting up a rival organisation. Or if there is more than one organisation working on similar issues, form a coalition. For example, the Save the Cottage Hospital Campaign Group could link with the local Patient Advice and Liaison Service if its members are also concerned about the issue.
- **Where you can, do something as you go along:** for example, if you are campaigning to clean up your neighbourhood, you could organise a one-off 'litter collection day' as well as lobbying your local council for better refuse collection and more litter bins.
- **Involve as many people as possible:** this is not only to harness their support but also to let people see for themselves what is wrong and what needs to change.

Planning a Campaign

See also Chapter 5 for help with planning that applies to planning a campaign.

When you plan a campaign, it helps to go through the same planning process as you would with any other kind of health promotion activity:

- identify your aims clearly
- decide the best way of achieving them (public meetings? press coverage? lobbying MPs and local councillors? getting up a petition?)
- identify your resources (do you need to fundraise?)
- clarify how you will know if your aim is achieved (e.g. when the NHS trust promises to reconsider the closure of the hospital or has formally agreed to keep it open for a specified length of time?)
- set an action plan of who is going to do what and when.

PRACTICE POINTS

- Recognise that you and all health promoters are in the business of influencing policy and practice at many levels, from national to local and day to day.

- If you want to influence policy and practice, you require careful and long-term planning and timing. You need to know how national and local health promotion policy is created, developed and changed, and how you can have a voice by commenting on proposals and plans.

- Know the rights and standards you can expect from NHS services, and comment on those which you and your clients receive.

- Challenge health-damaging policy by working with others, using your vote and by collective action.

- Identify how you could be more effective in influencing policy through reviewing your skills in planning, networking, negotiating, and joint working.

- Start policy change by identifying key stakeholders and looking at issues from each of their viewpoints; use techniques such as force field analysis to establish how to move forward.

- When campaigning on health issues, pay attention to careful planning and be persistent, professional and positive; involve as many other people as possible.

- Keep the ethical aspects of activities in mind when campaigning, lobbying and working towards changing health policy and practice; work with other people to build up trust and mutual respect.

Recommended Reading

On Public Policy and the Politics of Health

➤ Baggott R 2000 Public health: policy and politics. London: Macmillan Press

➤ Heller T, Muston R, Sidell M, Lloyd C 2001 Working for health. Chapter 20, User involvement and participation in the NHS: a personal perspective. London: The Open University in association with Sage Publications

➤ Jones L, Sidell M (eds) 1997 The challenge of promoting health – exploration and action. Basingstoke: Macmillan/Open University. (Part 2, Promoting health through public policy, includes chapters on making and changing public policy; and politics of health.)

➤ Naidoo J, Wills J 2000 Health promotion: foundations for practice, 2nd edn. Chapter 7, The politics of health promotion. London: Baillière Tindall

On Power and Influence

➤ Davis A 1997 An 'insider' looking out: the politics of physical activity in England. In: Sidell M, Jones L,

Katz J, Peberdy A (eds) Debates and dilemmas in promoting health, Chapter 30. Basingstoke: Macmillan/Open University Press. (A case study on the politics and policy issues in relation to sport, physical activity, transport and health policy.)

➤ Gavel M, Glantz S (May 1999) in tobacco control archives: www.library.ucsf.edu/tobacco/fl/ (A case study hat analyses tobacco industry political power and influence in Florida from 1979 to 1999.)

➤ Lee B, Covey SR 1998 The power principle: influence with honor. New York: Simon and Schuster

On Negotiating Agreements

➤ Harvard Business Review 2000 Negotiation and conflict resolution. Harvard: Harvard Business School Press

➤ Kraus S 2001 Strategic negotiation in multiagent environments. Cambridge, Massachusetts: Massachusetts Institute of Technology Press

➤ Shell G R 2000 Bargaining for advantage: negotiation strategies for reasonable people. Harmondsworth: Penguin Books

On the Links Between Health Promotion and Sustainable Development

➤ Russell S B, de Viggiani N 1997 Promoting sustainable health: integrating health promotion and sustainable development. Journal of Contemporary Health 6, 48–52

On Promoting Health in Different Settings

➤ Naidoo J, Wills J 2000 Health promotion: foundations for practice, 2nd edn. London: Baillière Tindall.

(Part 3 covers health promotion in the workplace, schools, neighbourhoods, primary health care and hospitals.)

➤ Tones K, Tilford S 2001 Health education: effectiveness, efficiency and equity, 3rd edn. Cheltenham: Nelson Thornes. (Part 2 includes health promotion in schools, health care settings and workplaces.)

On Campaigning

➤ Gilchrist K 2002 Promoting your cause: a guide for fundraisers and campaigners. London: Directory of Social Change

➤ Lattimer M 2000 The campaigning handbook, 2nd edn. London: Directory of Social Change

Notes and References

1 Examples of policy development and guidance by national agencies on health promotion issues and/or in health promotion settings are:

Department of Health 2001 The strategy for sexual health and HIV (www.doh.gov.uk/jointunit/jip.htm)

Access to Health Development Agency policy documents on HIV/AIDS is through the NHPIS website: www.hda-online.org.uk/nhpis/resources.html

Alcohol Concern has called for a national strategy to tackle alcohol dependence, as twice as many people are dependent on alcohol as on all other drugs:

Alcohol Concern 1999 Proposals for a National Alcohol Strategy for England. Available from: Alcohol Concern, 32–36 Loman Street, London SE1 0EE. Also available through the website: www.alcoholconcern.org.uk

For a national survey to assess School Health Policies and Programmes (SHPPS), see:

Journal of School Health 71 (7), September 2001, and the SHPPS website: www.cdc.gov/nccdphp/dash/shpps/

The Health Education Board for Scotland (HEBS) has defined its policy in a series of strategic statements on oral health promotion, promotion of physical activity, mental health promotion, and accident prevention and safety promotion. Other HEBS policy documents include a smoking cessation policy for Scotland. To access these documents, see HEBSWEB 2001: www.hebs.scot.nhs.uk/strategy/index.cfm

Health Promotion Wales (now the Health Promotion Division of the National Assembly for Wales) has produced a series of booklets (Healthy Schools for Wales) aimed at helping to develop health policy, including:

Alcohol, Smoking, Implementing food policies in schools, and Sex education.

2 An example of a policy developed by partnerships including the local council, health authority and other bodies is:

Sheffield – see Healthy Sheffield Information Pack April 1997. For current information on Healthy Sheffield contact the Healthy City Office, Room 223, Old Town Hall, Pinstone Street, Sheffield S1 2HH. Tel: 0114 273 5868.

3 For further information on HIMPs, community strategies and neighbourhood renewal see:

www.doh.uk/hrforhimps/

www.local-regions.dtlr.gov.uk/index.htm

www.regeneration.dtlr.gov.uk/neighbourhood/index.htm

www.cabinet-office.gov.uk/seu/2001/Action_Plan/default.htm

4 For further information on LSPs see: www.local-regions.dtlr.gov.uk/index.htm

5 For a useful introduction to health impact assessment see: A short guide to health impact assessment – informing healthy decisions. Commissioned in 2000 by the NHS Executive, London. Available at: www.londonshealth.gov.uk, including fuller details and some practical tools for use in different situations.

See also:

Scott-Samuel A 2001 Health impact assessment. In: Heller T, Muston R, Sidell M, Lloyd C 2001 Working for health, Chapter 14. London: The Open University in association with Sage Publications

6 Department of Health 1999 National service framework for coronary heart disease. London: The Stationery Office

7 For further information on LSPs and community strategies and the power to promote community well-being see: www.local-regions.dtlr.gov.uk/index.htm

8 For further information see: www.cabinet-office.gov.uk/seu/2001.Action_Plan/default.htm

9 For information on Local Agenda 21 contact:

Improvement and Development Agency, Sustainable Development Unit, Layden House, 76–78 Turnmill Street, London E1M 5QU

Forum for the Future, 149 Morley Hill, Enfield, Middlesex EN2 0BQ

Going for Green website: www.gfg.icinet.co.uk

10 Department of Health 2000 The NHS plan. A plan for investment. A plan for reform. London: The Stationery Office

In preparing for the NHS Plan the government conducted a major consultation with the public (and NHS staff) to elicit their views on the NHS and how it could be improved. This included written responses, opinion research and the Office for Public Management talking to groups of people and patient organisations. Concerns voiced included the need for more prevention services and information on healthy living. For further information see: www.doh.gov.uk/nhsplan

11 Department of Health 1992 The patient's charter. London: HMSO

This was updated in 1995: The patient's charter and you. London: Department of Health

12 For more information on the NHS charter see: www.doh.gov.uk/nhs/nhscharter

13 For critical analysis of today's health policy and public health issues, see recent copies of the *Health Matters* magazine. The journal *Critical Public Health*, published by Carfax Publishing, also provides a forum for debate.

14 You can find out who your MP and local councillor are, and details of their 'surgeries', from local libraries and Citizens Advice Bureaux.

15 UK Public Health Association, 7th Floor, Holborn Gate, 330 High Holborn, London, WC1V 7BA. Tel: 0870 0101930. Email: info@ukpha.org.uk Website: www.ukpha.org.uk

16 This section is partly based on:

Kakabadse A P 1982 The politics of interpersonal influence. Leadership and organisation development 3 (3). Bradford: MCB University Press

17 For further details and references on workplace health see:

Orme J 2001 Overview of health promotion in the workplace. In Scriven A, Orme J (eds) Health promotion: professional perspectives, 2nd edn. Basingstoke: Palgrave/Open University

18 World Health Organization 1988 Health promotion for working populations. Report of a WHO Expert Committee, Technical Report Series No. 765. WHO: Geneva

The WHO has also published the results of a survey of health promotion in European organisations:

Malzon R A, Lindsay G B 1992 Health promotion at the worksite: a survey of large organisations in Europe. European Occupational Health Series No. 4. Copenhagen: WHO

19 See: www.bkk.de

The European Information Centre of the European Network for Workplace Health Promotion produces a newsletter and good practice guides, which is available from: Bkk Bundesverband, European Information Centre, Krmprinzenstr. 6, 45128 Essen, Germany.

20 Health Education Authority/NHS Management Executive (1992) Health at work in the NHS: action pack. London: HEA

21 For further information about the success and issues related to the Health at Work in the NHS (HAWNHS) programme see:

Health Education Authority 1999 Developing and sustaining workplace health in the NHS. London: HEA

See also the HAWNHS Website: www.hawnhs.hda-online.org.uk

22 Health and Safety Executive, Health Directorate, working to reduce illness caused or made worse by work: Securing health together, Health and Safety Executive, 7NW Rose Court, 2 Southwark Bridge, London SE1 9HS. Tel: 020 7717 6978. Website: www.hse.gov.uk/action/index.htm

23 See:

Health Education Authority 1993 Health promoting hospitals: principles and practice. London: HEA

NHS Executive 1994 The health of the nation: health promoting hospitals. London: Department of Health

24 For information on the English National Network of Health Promoting Hospitals and Trusts contact:

North West Lancashire Health Promotion Unit, Progress Business Park, Orders Lane, Kirkham, Lancashire PR4 2TZ. Tel: 01772 686 031

The 9th International Conference on Health Promoting Hospitals was held in Copenhagen, Denmark 16–18 May

2001. For information on this, contact Johannes Moeller, The School of Public Health, WHO Collaborating Center, University of Bielefeld, Germany.

25 For further information contact the Health for All (UK) Network website: www.independent.livjm.ac.uk/healthforall/whatis.htm

The World Health Organization's website also provides links to the Healthy Cities project: www.who.dk

Each Healthy City has its own website. For example, Glasgow Healthy City Partnership's website: www.glasgow.gov.uk/healthycities

Belfast Healthy Cities website: www.belfasthealthycities.com

26 Castings C, Springett J 1997 Joint working and the production of a City Health Plan: the Liverpool experience. Health Promotion International 12(1), 9–19.

27 The European Network of Health Promoting Schools is a tri-partite project launched by the WHO Regional Office for Europe, the European Commission and the Council of Europe. See: www.who.dk/enhps/page/int.html

28 This evaluation was carried out by the National Foundation of Educational Research (NFER):

Health Education Authority 1997 The health promoting school: an evaluation of the ENHPS project in England. London: Health Education Authority

29 The National Healthy School Standard (NHSS) initiative supports the development of healthy schools in England through local education and health partnerships. See: www.wiredforhealth.gov.uk

30 Abercrombie N 1998 Universities and health in the twenty first century. In: Tsouros A, Dowding G, Thompson J, Dooris M (eds) Health promoting universities: concept, experience and framework for action. Copenhagen: World Health Organization

31 For further information contact the WHO Collaborating Centre on health in prisons:

The Directorate of Health Care, HM Prison Service, Cleland House, Page Street, London SW1P 4LN.

See also the HIPP website: www.hipp-europe.org/

32 This was originally based on:

Simnett I, Chiles M 1989 A practical guide to developing and implementing alcohol policies. Bristol: Frenchay Health Authority, and:

Health and Consumer Services, Sheffield City Council 1989 Guidelines for local authorities on the development, implementation and evaluation of an alcohol policy for their staff. London: Health Education Authority

33 Shelter, 88 Old Street, London EC1V 9HU.

34 Friends of the Earth, 26–28 Underwood Street, London N1 7JQ.

35 This section was originally adapted from some material in Chapter 2 of:

Wilson D 1984 Pressure: the A to Z of campaigning in Britain. London: Heinemann. Although this text is nearly 20 years old, the principles still apply today.

Jargon Explained

This glossary contains explanations of jargon and abbreviations used in this book, and in health promotion and public health generally. (Refer to the Index to find where terms are used in the text.)

Words in *italics* appear in this list as separate entries.

Advocacy Representing the interests of people who cannot speak up for themselves because of illness, disability, or other disadvantage.

Agenda 21 A world-wide movement to address environmental concerns for the 21st century, focusing on *sustainable development*. All local authorities are required to develop a Local Agenda 21 Strategy.

Aim Broad statement of what you are trying to achieve (e.g. in a health programme or activity).

Audit Systematic examination of a service in order to check and improve its quality.

Care trust NHS organisation that provides *health and social care* services, formed by the merger of local authority social care services with NHS primary and community health services. Care trusts started to be set up in 2002.

Commission for Health Improvement (CHI) A national body responsible for ensuring good-quality services in the NHS.

Commissioning In the context of commissioning health services, this means deciding what health services and programmes are needed to improve the health status of the local population and ensuring that they are provided.

Communicable disease Diseases that can be transmitted from one person to another; often called infectious or contagious diseases.

Community action Activity carried out by people under their own control in order to improve their collective conditions. It may involve campaigning, negotiating with, or challenging authorities and those with power.

Community development Working with people to identify their concerns, and support them in collective action for the good of the community as whole.

Community Health Council (CHC) An independent body that advised the local NHS until it was replaced in 2002 by *Patient Advice and Liaison Services* (*PALS*). Sometimes known as 'the patients' watchdog'.

Community health project A programme of work organised by an agency or a local organisation with the aim of improving health by some combination of community activity, self-help, *community action* and/or *community development*.

Community health services/community services Health services provided in people's homes or from premises in the community such as GP surgeries, health centres, clinics and small community hospitals (as distinct from services provided in major hospitals).

Community health work This is *community work* with a focus on health concerns, but generally health is defined broadly to include social and economic aspects, so that community health work may encompass almost as broad a range of activities as community work that does not have a specific health remit.

Community strategy Local plan led by local authorities with the aim of improving economic, social and environmental well-being.

Community work Working with community groups and organisations to overcome the community's problems and improve people's conditions of life. Community work aims to enhance the sense of solidarity and competence in the community.

Comparative need Comparison between similar groups of people, some in receipt of something such as a service and some not. Those who are not are then defined as being in comparative need. (See also *Expressed need, Felt need* and *Normative need.*)

Competencies The combination of knowledge, attitudes and skills needed to do a particular job.

Connexions Government-funded local partnership designed to provide help, support and guidance for all teenagers.

Coronary heart disease (CHD) Heart disease caused by poor circulation of blood to the heart muscle because the blood vessels have become blocked. This may show up as a heart attack or chest pain (angina).

Cost–benefit analysis The process of comparing the benefits with the costs (e.g. of a health programme or activity).

Cost-effectiveness analysis Comparing the costs and outcomes of alternative activities to achieve the same goal (e.g. comparing the cost of a telephone helpline with nicotine replacement therapy to achieve the goal of successfully helping people to stop smoking).

Cross-sectoral Working across the boundaries of different *sectors*, e.g. health services working together with businesses and voluntary organisations. Sometimes also called intersectoral.

Demography The study of the statistics about a population, such as birth, death and age profile.

Educational objectives What an educator would like clients to know, feel and do as a result of the education.

Effectiveness The extent to which a programme, activity, service or treatment achieves the result it aimed for (e.g. the effectiveness of a public health programme would mean the extent to which it had achieved objectives such a specified positive change in the population's health).

Efficiency A term applied to a programme or activity to denote how good the *process* (as distinct from the *outcome*) is in terms of, for example, value for money or use of time; it is about how results are achieved compared with other ways of achieving them.

Epidemiology The study of the distribution, determinants and control of disease in populations.

Ethnicity Racial origin or cultural background.

Ethnic minority Group differentiated from the main population of a community by racial origin or cultural background.

Evaluation The process of assessing what has been achieved (the *outcome*) and how it has been achieved (the *process*).

Evidence-based Based on reliable evidence that something works. For example, 'evidence-based health promotion' means health promotion projects or programmes based on sound research that shows they are likely to be successful in achieving their aims.

Expressed need What people say they need; expressed requests or demands. (See also *Comparative need, Felt need* and *Normative need*.)

Facilitation/facilitator The process of making/a person who makes something more easily achieved. For example, a group facilitator will help a group of people to get to know each other and discuss things together, but will not be the dominant leader.

Felt need Need that people feel; what they want. This is not necessarily what they say they need. (See also *Comparative need, Expressed need* and *Normative need*.)

Green Paper A government policy document issued for consultation. Becomes a *White Paper* when it is finalised and formally agreed as government policy.

Health 21 A policy framework published by the *World Health Organization* in 1999, which set out 21 targets for the European region in the 21st century.

Health Action Zone Area of high health need selected by government for special funding and health programmes.

Health alliance Partnership of two or more organisations working together to promote health. Often also called health 'partnership'.

Health and social care services A wide range of services to meet people's health and social needs. Health care tends to mean services provided by the NHS, and social care usually refers to services provided by local authorities, especially social services departments. In many instances services are provided by both. They may also be provided by the *voluntary sector*.

Health at Work in the NHS A government initiative started in 1992, which aimed to introduce a systematic healthy workplace programme throughout the NHS and engage all NHS staff in health-promoting activities.

Health authority The statutory NHS organisation responsible for health services for a defined population until abolished in 2002, when its responsibilities were largely taken on (in England) by *primary care trusts* and *care trusts*.

Health Development Agency National public body established in 2000, which is a resource for public health work in England. Its remit includes maintaining a data base of research evidence about what works to improve health and providing information about the effectiveness of health improvement programmes. There are comparable bodies in Scotland (the Health Education Board for Scotland), Wales (the Health Promotion Division of the National Assembly for Wales), and Northern Ireland (the Health Promotion Agency for Northern Ireland).

Health education Planned opportunities for people to learn about health, and to undertake voluntary changes in their behaviour.

Health For All A movement started in the 1980s by the *World Health Organization*. It included *health targets* for year 2000 and stressed basic principles of promoting positive health through health promotion and disease prevention; reducing *inequalities in health*; community participation; cooperation between health authorities, local authorities and others with an impact on health; and a focus on *primary care* as the main basis of the health care system.

Health gain A measurable improvement in health status, in an individual or a population, attributable to earlier intervention.

Health gap The difference between the overall health of the more wealthy and more deprived communities in a population.

Health impact assessment (HIA) Systematic process of estimating the effects of a specified action – a programme, policy or project – on the health of a defined population. For example, what difference a new transport policy would have on the health of the population affected by it.

Health Improvement and Modernisation Plan (HIMP) A three-year local rolling plan of action to improve health and services for health and social care, led by local NHS organisations such as *primary care trusts*. (Formerly known as Health Improvement Programme.)

Health in Prisons Project (HIPP) *WHO* initiative launched in 1995 to promote health in prisons.

Health Promoting Hospitals A *WHO* initiative that aims to improve health and environmental conditions for both staff and patients in hospitals.

Health promotion The process of enabling people to increase control over, and to improve, their health.

Health-related behaviour Things people habitually do in their daily life that affect their health. Usually refers to issues such as whether they smoke, whether they take exercise, what they eat, their sexual behaviour, how much alcohol they drink, drug use. Sometimes simply called 'health behaviour'.

Health target A quantified, measurable improvement in health status, by a given date, which achieves a health objective. It provides a yardstick against which progress can be monitored.

Healthy Cities A *WHO* initiative started in 1987 to improve health in urban areas. Involves collaborative work between local government, health services, local businesses, community organisations, and citizens. The *Health for All* (UK) Network is the coordinating body for action on Healthy Cities within the UK.

Healthy Living Centres Centres or networks of activity that aim to promote good health, developed by partnerships with local participation. Funded from the National Lottery.

Healthy Universities *WHO* initiative to promote health in university settings.

High-risk approach Public health approach that prioritises people particularly at risk of ill health. (Compare with *whole-population approach*.)

Holistic In the health context (as in 'holistic approach to health') this means taking into account all aspects of a person – physical, mental, emotional, social – as well as their social, economic, and physical environment. (As distinct from an approach which focuses only on, for example, the physical functioning of the body.)

Impact A term sometimes used to describe short-term *outcomes*. For example, the impact of a programme to encourage women to attend for a breast cancer screening test (mammogram) might be assessed in terms of how many women attended; the long-term outcome could be a change in the rate of women who died of breast cancer.

Incidence The number of new episodes of illness arising in a population over a specified period of time.

Inequalities in health The gap between the health of different population groups, such as better-off and more deprived communities, or people with different ethnic backgrounds.

Input The resources that go into a programme or activity, including money, time, staff and materials.

Lifestyle The particular way of life of a person or group, often referring to *health-related behaviour* such as smoking, drinking, diet and exercise.

Local Strategic Partnership (LSP) Local NHS, local authority and other agencies working together to develop and implement local strategy for *neighbourhood renewal*.

Low birthweight The weight of a baby at birth of less than 2500 grams. High rates of low birthweight babies in a population indicate poor health overall.

Marketing When applied to health issues, this means identifying opportunities for satisfying the requirements of consumers or clients, and by doing so maximising the protection and/or improvement of their health.

Monitoring The process of regularly reviewing achievements and progress towards goals.

Morbidity/morbidity rate Illness/incidence of illness in a population in a given period.

Mortality/mortality rate Death/incidence of death in a population in a given period.

Multi-disciplinary Involving people from different professions (disciplines) and backgrounds.

National Healthy Schools Standard (NHSS) Government standard introduced in 1998 as a joint venture between the Department for Education and Skills and the Department of Health. Aims to develop health-promoting schools through programmes of social, personal and health education for the pupils, the way the school is run; and the health and well-being of staff, parents and the wider community who have contact with the school.

National Institute for Clinical Excellence (NICE) National body that provides patients, health professionals and the public with authoritative, robust and reliable guidance on 'best practice' in relation to drugs, treatments and services across the NHS.

National Occupational Standards Nationally agreed statements of best practice about what people are expected to do in their jobs.

National Service Framework (NSF) National document that sets out the pattern and level of service (standards) which should be provided for a major care area or disease group, such as mental health or heart disease.

National strategies for health Government strategies to improve the health of national populations. Strategies current in 2002:

Northern Ireland: *Health and Wellbeing: into the Next Millennium*

England: *Saving Lives: Our Healthier Nation*

Scotland: *Towards a Healthier Scotland*

Wales: *Improving Health in Wales: a summary plan for the NHS with its partners* and an action plan *Promoting Health and Wellbeing: Implementing the National Health Promotion Strategy.*

Neighbourhood Renewal Strategy Strategy developed by local agencies with a coordinated approach to tackle the social and economic conditions in the most deprived local authority areas.

Network A group of people who exchange information, contacts and experience for mutual benefit.

New Deal for Communities Government funding for deprived communities to support plans that bring together local people, community and voluntary organisations, public agencies and local business in an attempt to make improvements in health, employment, education, and the physical environment.

New public health An approach to public health that emerged in the 1980s. It shifted emphasis from a *lifestyle* approach focused on people's individual health behaviour to a new focus on political and social action to address underlying issues that affect health (such as poverty, employment, discrimination and the environment people live in).

NHS Direct A national NHS telephone help line (0845 4647) staffed by specially trained nurses.

NHS Plan Government plan for the NHS published in July 2000.

NHS trust An independent body within the NHS that provides health services in hospitals. Some NHS trusts provide specialised services, such as ambulance services or mental health services.

Non-governmental organisation (NGO) Organisation that is independent of government control.

Normative need Need defined by an expert or professional according to that person's or profession's standards. (See also *Comparative need, Felt need* and *Expressed need*.)

Objective Applied to a health programme or activity, this means the desired end state (or result, or *outcome*) to be achieved within a specified time period. Objectives are usually more specific and detailed than *aims*.

Opportunity costs Potential benefits, which will not be realised if one thing is done instead of another. For example, if there is only enough time and money for one health programme (A or B), and it is spent on A, the opportunity costs are the potential benefits of spending on B that will be forgone.

Ottawa Charter A document launched in 1986 at an international *World Health Organization* conference in Ottawa, Canada, which identified key themes for health promotion practice.

Outcome The end-product of a health programme or activity, expressed in whatever terms are appropriate (e.g. changes in people's attitudes or knowledge, changes in health policy, changes in the uptake of services, or changes in the rate of illness).

Patient Advice and Liaison Services (PALS) Established from April 2002 within NHS trusts to help patients, families and carers to resolve problems or air concerns. Replaced *Community Health Councils*.

Performance management Systematic management practices and monitoring systems, which support people so that they can achieve their work objectives.

Policy A broad statement of the principles of how to proceed in relation to a specific issue, such as a national policy on transport, a local authority policy on housing, or a policy on how to deal with alcohol issues in a workplace.

Premature death Death under 65 years of age. High rates of premature death in a population indicate poor health overall.

Prevalence Measure of how much illness there is in a population at a particular point in time or over a specified period.

Primary care Services that are people's first point of contact with the NHS, such as services provided by GPs, practice nurses, district nurses, and health visitors. (As distinct from *secondary care*, provided in hospitals.)

Primary care groups (PCGs) NHS bodies, first set up around 1999, formed from groups of GP practices in a locality. In the early 2000s PCGs became *primary care trusts* and were given more responsibilities.

Primary care trust (PCT) An NHS body whose main tasks are to assess local health needs, develop and implement *Health Improvement and Modernisation Plans*, provide *primary care* services and commission *secondary care* services from hospitals and specialised services run by *NHS trusts*. PCTs are run by a board whose members include GPs, nurses, representatives from local authority social services, and the lay public.

Primary health care team Health workers, usually based at a GP surgery or health centre, who provide *community health services*. They include GPs, district nurses, practice nurses, and health visitors.

Primary health education. *Health education* directed at healthy people, aiming to prevent ill health arising in the first place.

Primary prevention Stopping ill health arising in the first place. For example, eating a healthy diet, not smoking and taking enough exercise are factors in the primary prevention of heart disease.

Private sector A collective term for business and commercial organisations. (See also *Sector*.)

Process All the implementation stages of a health programme or activity that happen between *input* and *outcome*.

Project A one-off, time-limited programme of work with clearly identified start and finish times, aims and objectives.

Public health Preventing disease, prolonging life and promoting health through work focused on the population as a whole.

Public sector A collective term for organisations that are controlled by the state and publicly funded, such as the NHS, local authorities, police, fire, probation and prison services. Often also called statutory sector/services because they are governed by laws (statutes). (See also *Sector*.)

Qualitative Concerned with quality – how good or bad something is according to specified criteria, usually expressed as a description in words rather than numbers. For example, qualitative data about the outcome of a breast screening programme could include users' descriptions of how they felt about it: whether they found it painful, embarrassing, well-organised etc. (Compare with *quantitative*.)

Quality How 'good' something (such as health service) is when judged against a number of criteria.

Quality Protects Services for children in need, including vulnerable children in local authority care.

Quality standard An agreed level of performance negotiated within available resources.

Quantitative Concerned with measurable quantity, usually expressed in numbers. For example, quantitative data about the outcome of a breast screening programme could include the percentage of the women invited who actually attended, the percentage called back for further assessment, and (ultimately) the decrease in rates of illness and death from breast cancer. (Compare with *qualitative*.)

Resources A term often used in health education and health promotion to mean educational and/or publicity materials such as leaflets, posters, displays and videos.

Risk factor An attribute, such as a habit (e.g. smoking) or exposure to an environmental hazard, that increases the likelihood of developing an illness.

Saving Lives: Our Healthier Nation *National strategy for health* in England, published in 1999, which sets out priority areas (cancer, heart disease and stroke, accidents, mental health) and sets national targets.

Screening The application of a special test for everyone at risk of a particular disease to detect whether the disease is present at an early stage. It is used for diseases where early detection makes treatment more successful.

Secondary care Specialised health care services provided by hospital inpatient and outpatient services.

Secondary health education *Health education* directed at people who are already ill, to prevent ill health moving to a chronic or irreversible stage, and to restore people to their former state of health. Often involves educating patients about their condition and what to do about it.

Secondary prevention Intervention during the early stages of a disease to prevent further damage.

Sector Organisations are often categorised into three types: *public sector* (such as the NHS and local authorities), *private sector* (business and commerce) and *voluntary sector* (charities, not-for-profit and *voluntary organisations*).

Self-empowerment Ability to have control over your own life.

Self-esteem How good you feel about yourself; your opinion of yourself.

Single Regeneration Budget (SRB) Government funding for economic and social development.

Social capital Investment in the social fabric of society, so that communities have characteristics such as high levels of trust and supportive networks for the exchange of information, ideas, and practical help.

Social inclusion/exclusion A sense of belonging to/feeling alienated from the community in which a person lives.

Stages of Change A cycle of stages a person usually goes through when changing a health-related behaviour, such as stopping smoking. Stages are: (1) not yet thinking about it, (2) thinking about changing, (3) being ready to change, (4) action – making changes, (5) maintaining change; then either maintaining the changed behaviour permanently or (6) relapsing – often then repeating the cycle by thinking about changing again (2).

Statutory organisations/agencies *Public sector* organisations or agencies such as local authorities and NHS organisations.

Statutory sector Another term for the *public sector*.

Strategy A broad plan of action that specifies what is to be achieved, how and by when; it provides a framework for more detailed planning.

Sure Start Government schemes in areas of high health need, which aim to support parents and children under four.

Sustainable development Development that meets the needs of the present without damaging the health or environment of future generations.

Target group The people who are intended to benefit from a public health or health promotion activity.

Targets Quantified and measurable achievements to aim for, by specified dates, which provide yardsticks against which progress can be monitored. (See also *Health target*.)

Tertiary health education *Health education* directed at people whose ill health has not been, or could not be, prevented and who cannot be completely cured. Concerned with educating about how to make the most of the remaining potential for healthy living, and how to avoid unnecessary hardships, restrictions, and complications (e.g. in rehabilitation programmes following a stroke).

Victim-blaming Blaming people for their own ill health when it is rooted in their social and/or economic circumstances. For example blaming people for contracting lung cancer ('it's their own fault') because they smoke, but ignoring the reasons for smoking – which could include lack of education, no help available to stop smoking, or smoking used as a way of coping with stresses such as poverty, poor housing, single parenthood, or unemployment.

Voluntary organisations Not-for-profit organisations, ranging from large national ones to small groups of local people, run by volunteers but possibly employing paid staff. Small local voluntary organisations are often called community groups.

Voluntary sector A collective term for *voluntary organisations*, community groups and charities. (See also *Sector*.)

Walk-in Centre NHS service offering advice, information and treatment for health problems from specially trained nurses, with no appointment necessary.

White Paper Government policy, often accompanied by legislation. Usually follows a *Green Paper*.

Whole-population approach Public health approach that focuses on a whole community rather than on individuals who are identified as being in particular need. (Compare with *High-risk approach*.)

World Health Organization (WHO) An intergovernmental organisation within the United Nations system whose purpose is to help all people attain the highest possible level of health through public health programmes. Its headquarters are in Geneva, Switzerland.

Index

Note – A letter 'f' following a page number indicates a reference to a figure.